AVOIDING COMMON PREHOSPITAL ERRORS

AVOIDING COMMON PREHOSPITAL ERRORS

EDITORS

BENJAMIN J. LAWNER, DO, EMT-P, FAAEM
Assistant Professor
Department of Emergency Medicine
University of Maryland School of Medicine
Deputy Medical Director, Baltimore City
Fire Department
Baltimore, Maryland

COREY M. SLOVIS, MD, FACP, FACEP, FAAEM
Professor of Emergency Medicine
and Medicine
Chairman, Department of
Emergency Medicine
Vanderbilt University Medical Center
Medical Director, Metro Nashville Fire
Department and International Airport
Nashville, Tennessee

RAYMOND L. FOWLER, MD, FACEP
Professor of Emergency Medicine, Surgery,
Health Professions, and Emergency
Medical Education
University of Texas Southwestern
Medical Center
Attending Emergency Medicine Faculty
Parkland Memorial Hospital
Dallas, Texas

PAUL E. PEPE, MD, MPH, MACP, FCCM, FACEP
Chairman of the Division of Emergency
Medicine, Surgery, Medicine, Pediatrics,
and Public Health
Riggs Family Chair in Emergency Medicine
University of Texas Southwestern
Medical Center
Parkland Memorial Hospital
Dallas, Texas

AMAL MATTU, MD, FACEP, FAAEM
Professor and Vice Chair
Department of Emergency Medicine
University of Maryland School of Medicine
Baltimore, Maryland

SERIES EDITOR

LISA MARCUCCI, MD
Attending Physician
Department of Surgery and Critical
Care Medicine
Veterans Administration Hospital
Pittsburgh, Pennsylvania

Wolters Kluwer | Lippincott Williams & Wilkins
Health
Philadelphia · Baltimore · New York · London
Buenos Aires · Hong Kong · Sydney · Tokyo

Acquisitions Editor: Rebecca Gaertner
Product Manager: Tom Gibbons
Vendor Manager: Marian Bellus
Senior Manufacturing Manager: Benjamin Rivera
Marketing Manager: Kimberly Schonberger
Design Coordinator: Holly McLaughlin
Production Service: Aptara, Inc.

© 2013 by **LIPPINCOTT WILLIAMS & WILKINS, a WOLTERS KLUWER business**
Two Commerce Square
2001 Market Street
Philadelphia, PA 19103 USA
LWW.com

Printed in China

Library of Congress Cataloging-in-Publication Data
Avoiding common prehospital errors / Benjamin Lawner . . . [et al.].
    p. ; cm.
  Includes bibliographical references and index.
  ISBN 978-1-4511-3159-8 (alk. paper)
  I. Lawner, Benjamin.
  [DNLM: 1. Emergencies. 2. Disaster Planning. 3. Emergency Medical
Services. 4. Emergency Treatment. WB 105]

362.18—dc23   2012017022

To purchase additional copies of this book, call our customer service department at (800) 638-3030 or fax orders to (301) 223-2320. International customers should call (301) 223-2300.

Visit Lippincott Williams & Wilkins on the Internet: at LWW.com. Lippincott Williams & Wilkins customer service representatives are available from 8:30 am to 6 pm, EST.

10 9 8 7 6 5 4 3 2 1

CCS0812

ACKNOWLEDGMENTS

This book would not have been possible without the support of family and friends. I greatly appreciate their patience and inspiration. My resident and faculty colleagues at the University of Maryland are a continued source of encouragement, and I am privileged to be part of such a motivated group. A special thank you to prehospital providers for their diligence and commitment to excellence in patient care: your contributions do not go unnoticed!

Benjamin Lawner, DO

My deepest thanks to my family for their support and patience. Thanks also to the faculty and residents in emergency medicine at the University of Maryland for their inspiration. Finally, I wish to extend kudos to the prehospital providers around the world for their dedication and unending hard work, always in the interest of patient care.

Amal Mattu, MD

Thank you to all of the EMTs, Paramedics and EMS Physicians who have taught me so much and who made this book possible. I am deeply indebted to the Section Editors who devoted so much time and effort to make our text practical and understandable.

Corey Slovis, MD

My life in emergency medical services has taught me who the real heroes are in our field: the critical care technicians in the field who provide the life-saving assessments and treatments. I am grateful to have been along for this wonderful ride. My thanks go to the authors in our section who worked so hard to share their knowledge and expertise.

Ray Fowler, MD

One of my perennial mantras has been, "The earlier the intervention, the better the results!" However, that could be a two-edged sword if early interventions are not used appropriately — or if the wrong intervention, well-intended or not, has been provided. This outstanding text is a true labor of love that is fueled by a grass-roots approach to quality in public service and public safety. It provides us with another terrific tool to ensure that every patient will get the best care possible (and I emphasize "care": not "treatment" or "management," but the best possible care). Thanks to all of you who are entrusted to respond each day to deliver that most admirable of duties to those we serve.

Paul E. Pepe, MD, MPH

CONTRIBUTORS

STEPHEN C. ANDREWS, BA, MSN, ACNP
Hospitalist Nurse Practitioner, Maryland Inpatient Care Specialists, Glen Burnie, Maryland; Captain, EMS Operations, Kent Island Volunteer Fire Department, Chester, Maryland

ANDERS APGAR, MD, FACOG
OB/GYN Physician, Capital Women's Care, Rockville, Maryland

CHRISTOPHER S. AYRES, JD, NREMT-B
Ayres Law Office, P.C., Addison, Texas

R. JACK AYRES JR., JD, LEMT-P
Ayres Law Office, P.C., Addison, Texas

STEVEN BARMACH, MD
Chief Resident, Division of Emergency Medicine, Duke University Medical Center, Durham, North Carolina

BRIAN S. BASSHAM, MD
Clinical Fellow, Department of Pediatric Emergency Medicine, Vanderbilt University Medical Center, Nashville, Tennessee

DALE E. BECKER, NREMT-P
Captain, Howard County Department of Fire and Rescue, Columbia, Maryland

JEFF BEESON, DO, FACEP, EMT-P
Medical Director, MedStar EMS, Fort Worth, Texas

LEE BLAIR, RN/EMT-P
EMS Coordinator, Comprehensive Regional Pediatric Center Outreach Program, Department of Pediatric Emergency Services, Monroe Carell Jr. Children's Hospital at Vanderbilt, Nashville, Tennessee

STEPHEN BOCK, LP
EMS Division Chief, Farmers Branch Fire Department, Farmers Branch, Texas

PATRICK BRADY
PHI Air Medical, Richardson, Texas

SABINA A. BRAITHWAITE, MD, MPH
Medical Director, Wichita-Sedgwick County EMS System; Clinical Associate Professor of Emergency Medicine, University of Kansas, Kansas City; Clinical Associate Professor of Preventive Medicine and Public Health, University of Kansas, Wichita, Kansas

TIMOTHY E. BRENKERT, MD
Assistant Professor of Clinical Pediatrics, Division of Emergency Medicine, Cincinnati Children's Hospital Medical Center, Cincinnati, Ohio

JEREMY J. BRYWCZYNSKI, MD, FAAEM
Assistant Professor of Emergency Medicine, Medical Director Vanderbilt LifeFlight, Vanderbilt University Medical Center; Assistant Medical Director, Metro Nashville Fire Department, Nashville, Tennessee

BRENDAN J. CARMODY, MD
Attending Physician, Department of
Emergency Medicine, Suburban Hospital,
Johns Hopkins Medicine, Bethesda,
Maryland

THOMAS G. CHICCONE, MD, FACEP
Clinical Assistant Professsor, Department
of Emergency Medicine, University of
Maryland School of Medicine, Baltimore,
Maryland

ERIC CLAUSS, RN/CCEMT-P
Assistant Manager, CRPC Outreach
Program, Department of Pediatric
Emergency Services, Monroe Carell Jr.
Children's Hospital at Vanderbilt,
Nashville, Tennessee

CHRISTOPHER B. COLWELL, MD
Director of Service, Department of
Emergency Medicine Denver Health;
Professor and Vice Chair, Department
of Emergency Medicine, University of
Colorado School of Medicine, Denver,
Colorado

SEAN S. COVANT, DO
Assistant Professor of Emergency
Medicine, University of Texas
Southwestern Medical Center, Dallas,
Texas

ROBERT DICE, MS, RN, NREMT-P
Trauma/Burn Program Manager, Johns
Hopkins Bayview Medical Center,
Baltimore, Maryland

PATRICK C. DRAYNA, MD
Division of Pediatric Emergency Medicine,
Department of Pediatrics, Monroe Carell
Jr. Children's Hospital at Vanderbilt,
Nashville, Tennessee

JAMES V. DUNFORD, MD
City of San Diego Medical Director
(EMS); Professor Emeritus (Emergency
Medicine), UCSD School of Medicine,
San Diego, California

MARC ECKSTEIN, MD, MPH, FACEP
Medical Director, Los Angeles Fire
Department; Professor of Emergency
Medicine, Keck School of Medicine of the
University of Southern California, Los
Angeles, California

CRISTINA M. ESTRADA, MD
Assistant Professor, Pediatric Emergency
Medicine, Department of Pediatrics,
Vanderbilt Children's Hospital, Nashville,
Tennessee

PRESTON J. FEDOR, MD
Clinical Assistant Professor of Emergency
Medicine, Department of Surgery,
University of Texas Southwestern Medical
Center, Dallas, Texas

P. MARC FISCHER, MBA, NREMT-P
Firefighter/Paramedic/Instructor, Howard
County Fire and Rescue, Columbia,
Maryland

RAYMOND L. FOWLER, MD, FACEP
Professor of Emergency Medicine,
Surgery, Health Professions, and
Emergency Medical Education, University
of Texas Southwestern Medical Center,
Dallas, Texas

JOHN P. FREESE, MD
Chief Medical Director, Office of Medical
Affairs, Fire Department of New York
(FDNY), Brooklyn, New York

JON E. FRIESEN, MSOD
Paramedic, Instructor/Coordinator Major-Education Manager, Office of the Medical Director, Wichita/Sedgwick County EMS System, Wichita, Kansas

BRIAN FROELKE, MD, FACEP

THERESA M. GALLO, BS, NREMT-P
Master Firefighter/Paramedic, Howard County Fire and Rescue, Howard County, Maryland

MARIANNE GAUSCHE-HILL, MD, FACEP, FAAP
Professor of Clinical Medicine, David Geffen School of Medicine at UCLA; Vice Chair and Chief of the Division of Pediatric Emergency Medicine; Director, Pediatric Emergency Medicine and EMS Fellowships, Harbor–UCLA Medical Center, Department of Emergency Medicine, Torrance, California

CASSANDRA MARIA CHIRAS GODAR, BS, NREMT-P
EMS Data Analyst, Howard County Department of Fire and Rescue, Columbia, Maryland; Firefighter/EMT-P, Elkridge Volunteer Fire Department, Elkridge, Maryland

JEFFREY M. GOODLOE, MD, NREMT-P, FACEP
Medical Director, Medical Control Board, Emergency Medical Services System for Metropolitan Oklahoma City and Tulsa; Professor and EMS Division Director, Department of Emergency Medicine, University of Oklahoma School of Community Medicine, Tulsa, Oklahoma

KEVIN HIGH, RN, MPH, EMT
Trauma Program Manager, Associate in Emergency Medicine, Department of Emergency Medicine and Emergency Services; Clinical Associate, Vanderbilt LifeFlight, Vanderbilt Medical Center, Nashville, Tennessee

JOEL M. HIGUCHI, AAS, FIREFIGHTER, EMT-P, EMS I/C
Roseville Fire Department, Roseville, Michigan

JOSEPH E. HOLLEY JR., MD, FACEP
EMS Medical Director, State of Tennessee, Memphis Fire Department, Shelby County Fire Department and surrounding municipalities, Memphis, Tennessee

BENJAMIN KAUFMAN, RN, BS, NREMT-P
Montgomery County Fire Rescue Services, Montgomery County, Maryland

JACOB B. KEEPERMAN, MD
Assistant Professor of Emergency Medicine and Anesthesiology, Washington University School of Medicine; Attending Physician, Emergency Medicine and Critical Care Medicine, Barnes Jewish Hospital, St. Louis, Missouri

A.J. KIRK

BENJAMIN J. LAWNER, DO, EMT-P, FAAEM
Assistant Professor of Emergency Medicine, University of Maryland School of Medicine; Deputy Medical Director, Baltimore City Fire Department, Baltimore, Maryland

LAURIE M. LAWRENCE, MD
Assistant Professor of Emergency Medicine and Pediatrics, Vanderbilt University Medical Center, Nashville, Tennessee

DAVID LEHRFELD, MD
Assistant Professor of Emergency Medicine, Department of Surgery, University of Texas Southwestern Medical Center, Dallas, Texas

RICHARD LEONARD, AS, NREMT-P
EMS Training Officer, Bureau of Education and Training, Howard County Department of Fire and Rescue Services, Howard County, Maryland

MARK D. LEVINE, MD
Associate Professor of Emergency Medicine, Washington University School of Medicine; Medical Director, St. Louis Fire Department, St. Louis, Missouri

ELIZABETH M. LiCALZI, MD
Resident in Psychiatry, Department of Psychiatry, Vanderbilt University Medical Center, Nashville, Tennessee

MATTHEW R. LOCKLAIR, MD
Assistant Professor of Pediatrics and Emergency Medicine, Division of Pediatric Emergency Medicine, Monroe Carrel Jr. Children's Hospital at Vanderbilt, Nashville, Tennessee

MICHAEL T. LOHMEIER, MD, EMT-T

BRAD LONDON, LP, BS
Dallas Fire-Rescue Department Frisco, Texas

JESSICA L. MANKA
Firefighter/Medic, Shelby Township, Michigan; Paramedic IC, Fire Instructor, Macomb Community College, Warren, Michigan

SAMUEL A. MATTA, RN, BSN, CFRN, NREMT-P
Flight Nurse, PHI Air Medical Express Care 1, Baltimore, Maryland

JARED J. McKINNEY, MD
Assistant Professor of Emergency Medicine, Medical Director, Vanderbilt LifeFlight Event Medicine, Vanderbilt University Medical Center; Assistant Medical Director, Metro Nashville Fire Department; Chairman, Vanderbilt University Resuscitation Committee, Nashville, Tennessee

C. CRAWFORD MECHEM, MD, MS, FACEP
EMS Medical Director, Philadelphia Fire Department, Philadelphia, Pennsylvania

AZHER MERCHANT, MD
Attending Physician, Department of Emergency Medicine, Franklin Square Hospital Center, Baltimore, Maryland

MATTHEW T. MESSINGER, RN, EMT-P
Flight Nurse Paramedic, St. Mary's of Michigan-FlightCare, Saginaw, Michigan

JARROD M. MOSIER, MD
Assistant Professor of Emergency Medicine, Director of Emergency Medicine Critical Care, University of Arizona; Deputy Medical Director, Tucson Fire Department, Tucson, Arizona

HAWNWAN PHILIP MOY, MD
Washington University; Department of Emergency Medicine, Barnes Jewish Hospital, St. Louis, Missouri

ELIZABETH MOYE, BA, NREMT-P
Paramedic, Sussex County Paramedics, Delaware

J. BRENT MYERS, MD, MPH
Director/Medical Director, Wake County Department of Emergency Medical Services, Raleigh, North Carolina

MAXWELL PATTERSON
Paramedic, Parkwood Volunteer Fire Department, Durham, North Carolina

ALEXANDER J. PERRICONE, BS, EMT-P
Deputy Chief-EMS, Baltimore City Fire Department, Baltimore, Maryland

DAVID E. PERSSE, MD, FACEP
Professor of Surgery, Baylor College of Medicine; Physician Director, EMS Public Health Authority, Houston, Texas

JULIE PHILLIPS, MD
Clinical Fellow, Department of Pediatrics, Vanderbilt University, Nashville, Tennessee

CAPTAIN MARIO L. RAMIREZ, MD, MPP
Emergency Medicine Physician, United States Air Force

NEAL J. RICHMOND, MD, FACEP
Chief Executive Officer and Medical Director, Louisville Metro Emergency Medical Services, Louisville, Kentucky

WENDY RUGGERI, MD
Division of Emergency Medicine, University of Texas Southwestern Medical Center, Dallas, Texas

GILBERTO SALAZAR, MD
Assistant Professor of Emergency Medicine, EMS Physician, University of Texas Southwestern Medical Center, Dallas, Texas

JULIETTE M. SAUSSY, MD, FACEP
Assistant Clinical Professor, Section of Emergency Medicine, Louisiana State University School of Medicine, New Orleans, Louisiana

KATHLEEN S. SCHRANK, MD, FACEP, FACP
Professor of Medicine and Chief, Division of Emergency Medicine, University of Miami Miller School of Medicine; EMS Medical Director, City of Miami Fire Rescue, Miami, Florida

ELIZABETH L. SEAMAN, NREMT
AB in Psychology, Georgetown University, Washington, D.C.

KEVIN G. SEAMAN, MD, FACEP
Medical Director, Howard County Department of Fire and Rescue Services, Columbia, Maryland

CYNTHIA S. SHEN, DO, FACOEP, FACEP
Clinical Assistant Professor, Department of Emergency Medicine, University of Maryland School of Medicine, Baltimore, Maryland

COREY M. SLOVIS, MD, FACP, FACEP, FAAEM
Professor of Emergency Medicine and Medicine, Chairman, Department of Emergency Medicine, Vanderbilt University Medical Center; Medical Director, Metro Nashville Fire Department and International Airport, Nashville, Tennessee

FREDERICK W. SMITH, RN, EMT-PARAMEDIC
Nashville Metro Fire Department, Nashville, Tennessee

JILL D. SMITH, BSN, RN, CEN

SPENCER C. SMITH, MD
Clinical Instructor, University of Utah Health Care, Salt Lake City, Utah

CERISA SPEIGHT, FIREFIGHTER, NREMT-P
Howard County Department of Fire and Rescue Services, Howard County, Maryland

ROGER M. STONE, MD, MS, FACEP, FAAEM
Clinical Assistant Professor of Emergency Medicine, University of Maryland School of Medicine, Baltimore, Maryland; Medical Director, Montgomery County Fire Rescue, Rockville, Maryland; Associate Medical Director, Carroll County EMS Programs, Westminster, Maryland

GREGG TAGGARD, EMT-PARAMEDIC

CHRISTOPHER TOUZEAU, MS, RN, NREMT-P
Firefighter/Paramedic, Montgomery County Fire Rescue, Rockville, Maryland

JENNIFER TRIACA, RN, NREMT-P
Baltimore City Fire Department, Baltimore, Maryland

GREGORY R. VALCOURT, AAS, NREMT-P, CCP-C
Paramedic Instructor, Howard County Department of Fire and Rescue Services, Bureau of Education and Training, Marriottsville, Maryland

TERENCE VALENZUELA, MD, MPH
Medical Director, Tucson Fire Department; Professor of Emergency Medicine, College of Medicine, University of Arizona, Tucson, Arizona

BRUCE G. VANHOY, FP-C, NREMT-P
Flight Paramedic, PHI Air Medical Express Care 1, Baltimore, Maryland

MORGAN M. WALKER, RN, BA, BSN
Emergency Department, Mercy Medical Center, Baltimore, Maryland

KAREN WANGER, MDCM, FRCPC, FACEP
Clinical Associate Professor of Emergency Medicine, University of British Columbia, Vancouver, British Columbia; Emergency Physician, Providence Health Care; Medical Director, Whistler Fire Rescue Service, Whistler, British Columbia, Canada

BENJAMIN W. WEBSTER, MD
Attending Physician, Akron General
Medical Center, Akron, Ohio; Medical
Director, Copley Fire Department,
Copley, Ohio

JONATHAN C. WENDELL, MD
Assistant Professor, Division of Emergency
Medicine, Department of Surgery, Duke
University Health System, Durham, North
Carolina

JONATHAN WENK, MD
Chairman of Medical Education, Shady
Grove Adventist Hospital, Rockville,
Maryland

**VALERIE N. WHATLEY, MD,
FAAP**
Assistant Professor of Pediatrics and
Emergency Medicine, Department of
Pediatrics, Monroe Carell Jr. Children's
Hospital at Vanderbilt, Nashville,
Tennessee

**ELIZABETH WHEATLEY, BA,
NREMT-P**
Paramedic, Sussex County EMS,
Georgetown, Delaware

**SCOTT H. WHEATLEY, BS,
NREMT-P**
Sergeant, Special Operations, Queen
Anne's County Department of Emergency
Services, Centreville, Maryland

ABBY M. WILLIAMS, MD
Clinical Fellow, Division of Pediatric
Emergency Medicine, Department of
Pediatrics, Vanderbilt University Medical
Center, Nashville, Tennessee

AMANDA G. WILSON, MD
Assistant Professor, Psychiatry and
Emergency Medicine, Vanderbilt
University Medical Center, Nashville,
Tennessee

**JESSE YARBROUGH,
NREMT-P**
Operations Officer, Louisville Metro EMS,
Louisville, Kentucky

The practice of prehospital medicine can be extremely challenging. On a daily basis, providers may make life and death decisions on the basis of information that is often quickly gathered and is occasionally incomplete. Fortunately, the evidence base for emergency medical services is growing at a rapid pace. Prehospital care is now a recognized subspecialty for those EMS physicians who have developed the unique competencies involved in this most remarkable discipline in the house of medicine. More than ever before, EMS systems are in an excellent position to rapidly treat complex and critically ill patients.

While, traditionally, EMS was once considered an extension of hospital care into the "field" setting, prehospital care systems are now often driving improvements in in-hospital management through innovation, research, and associated quality processes for deciding transport destination policies. More and more providers are charged with complex medical decision-making, procedurally, logistically and clinically, in often volatile or time-sensitive conditions. Accordingly, to aid in those on-scene responsibilities, the authors of this textbook have attempted to compile evidence-based practice, coupled with well-earned experience and best practices opinion. It is hoped that the pearls contained within these pages function as a valuable resource for both novice and veteran providers alike. While the text focuses on core "high impact" areas of prehospital medicine such as airway management, cardiac arrest, trauma and respiratory emergencies, it also further enhances our overall goals and root philosophies of providing safety for each and every one of our patients. We believe that a better understanding of common patient presentations will ideally result in best practices and, hopefully, an avoidance of "common errors" as well.

CONTENTS

RESPIRATORY EMERGENCIES

CARDIAC EMERGENCIES AND ECG

MANAGEMENT OF CARDIAC ARREST

TRAUMA EMERGENCIES

Pediatric Emergencies

AEROMEDICAL/CRITICAL CARE CONSIDERATIONS

INCIDENT COMMAND/DISASTER

CUSTOMER SERVICE/MEDICOLEGAL

BEHAVIORAL/PSYCHIATRIC

OB/GYN EMERGENCIES

NEUROLOGIC EMERGENCIES

AVOIDING COMMON PREHOSPITAL ERRORS

AIRWAY MANAGEMENT

RESPIRATORY EMERGENCIES

CARDIAC EMERGENCIES AND ECG

MANAGEMENT OF CARDIAC ARREST

TRAUMA EMERGENCIES

PEDIATRIC EMERGENCIES

AEROMEDICAL/CRITICAL CARE
CONSIDERATIONS

INCIDENT COMMAND/DISASTER

CUSTOMER SERVICE/MEDICOLEGAL

BEHAVIORAL/PSYCHIATRIC

OB/GYN EMERGENCIES

NEUROLOGIC EMERGENCIES

DON'T HAVE A FAILED AIRWAY BECAUSE YOU FAILED TO PREPARE

BRENDAN J. CARMODY, MD
MARIANNE GAUSCHE-HILL, MD, FACEP, FAAP

INTRODUCTION

Airway management is the most important skill for prehospital providers to master. This chapter outlines the steps taken to prepare for intubation.

ASSESSMENT

Historically, the decision to insert an airway adjunct was based on the absence of a gag reflex. However, checking for a gag reflex should not be done as it contributes next to nothing to the management of the patient and may be counterproductive. Approximately 25% to 33% of the normal awake population lacks a gag reflex. For those with an intact gag reflex, stimulating it while supine may induce vomiting and aspiration, which are exactly what you are trying to prevent. Instead look in the mouth for food, foreign body, or the pooling of secretions. If the patient has a depressed level of consciousness and anything is found in the pharynx, take it out and put an airway in! How about taking time to check a formal Glasgow Coma Scale? Quick! What gets you 3 for motor and a 2 for verbal? Neither you nor your patient has time to look it up. Check the level of consciousness with your voice. If your patient's eyes open in response to your voice, put the laryngoscope down; they don't need to be intubated. If they don't respond to a truly painful stimulus, they probably require some sort of airway intervention. Is there something better than the sternal rub? Grab the clavicle with the thumb and forefinger and squeeze. No response to this maneuver strongly suggests the need for intervention. If you don't believe me, try this maneuver on your partner before your next run: you'll agree, it's the best.

POSITIONING

Extremes of head and neck positioning can lead to airway obstruction. The ideal "sniffing position" can be obtained by placing a small towel beneath the patient's head, then tilting the head backward. This is considered the best starting position, but other factors such as obesity or trauma make this maneuver less helpful or inappropriate. The jaw thrust is used in conjunction with head positioning to help open the airway.

BAG-MASK VENTILATION (BMV)

Assure adequate oxygenation after the patient is appropriately positioned. BMV should be avoided in the spontaneously breathing patient as it can cause gastric distention and increase risk of aspiration. Instead, the spontaneously breathing patient should receive high-flow oxygen via non–rebreather face mask. Pre-oxygenation prevents rapid desaturation during intubation attempts. Another neat trick is to place a nasal cannula on the patient during intubation attempts to further minimize desaturation. Anesthesiologists use this technique in the operating room! It is important to remove the nasal cannula when using the BMV as it prevents the user from achieving a tight mask seal. Almost all patients requiring ventilation can be managed with proper BMV. An oral or nasal airway should be deployed whenever BMV ventilation is utilized. Also, most providers ventilate too quickly. Planning proper ventilation rates by using the verbalization of "squeeze-release-release" helps to avoid this. The provider should squeeze the bag until the chest just begins to rise and then allow enough time for full exhalation.

EXTERNAL MANIPULATION

There's little question that complications increase with each attempt at laryngoscopy. Improve your chances at optimum glottis visualization with some simple tricks and tips…. A number of techniques can be used, but we have found a blending and modification of BURP and bimanual laryngoscopy most helpful in visualizing the cords.

Simultaneous with the insertion of the blade, the airway operator places his right hand on top of the assistant's right hand to manipulate the anterior laryngeal structures. The operator guides the assistant's hand through the manipulation (Backward, Upward, Rightward Pressure [BURP]) and leaves the assistant's hand in place when an optimal view is achieved. These manipulations require gentle pressure, which should be released if airway structures can't be visualized.

The operator is then free to place the endotracheal (ET) tube. The assistant's left hand can pull open the right side of the patient's mouth to maximize the area through which the ET tube can be passed. The beauty of this "modified bimanual laryngoscopy" is that the second person needs no prior airway experience and can be walked through the process, if need be, on the spot.

RESCUE AIRWAY DEVICES

Providers have a number of rescue devices to choose from, which rescue device you use depends on operator experience, available equipment, and patient condition. Providers must be familiar with all the devices on the rig and practice how and when to use them before the airway emergency arises.

SUMMARY

Proper planning and preparation will maximize success.

THINGS NOT TO DO

- Induce aspiration (by gagging the patient)
- Bag the spontaneously breathing patient
- Bag too fast—remember: "squeeze-release-release"
- Cricoid pressure, if too vigorous may obstruct the airway
- Rely on Glasgow Coma Scale as your sole measure of need for airway management
- ET intubation when BMV or other airway devices may be more appropriate
- Fail to familiarize yourself with all of the airway devices at your disposal

SELECTED READINGS

Davies AE, Kidd D, Stone SP, et al. Pharyngeal sensation and gag reflex in healthy subjects. *Lancet.* 1995;345:487–488.

Levitan RM, Kinkle WC, Levin WJ, et al. Laryngeal view during laryngoscopy: a randomized trial comparing cricoid pressure, backward-upward-rightward pressure, and bi-manual laryngoscopy. *Ann Emerg Med.* 2006;47:548–555.

Walls RM. Rapid sequence intubation. In: Walls RM, Murphy MF, eds. *Manual of Emergency Airway Management.* 3rd ed. Philadelphia, PA: Lippincott Williams & Wilkins; 2008: 24–25.

2

DON'T FORGET TO PROPERLY POSITION THE PATIENT PRIOR TO ATTEMPTING INTUBATION!

CHRISTOPHER TOUZEAU, MS, RN, NREMT-P
BENJAMIN KAUFMAN, RN, BS, NREMT-P

The success rates of paramedic field intubation fall below hospital success rates, and some scholars question whether prehospital intubation should even be attempted. One of the most important considerations for improving the success rate of orotracheal intubation is proper patient positioning. EMS providers have a tendency to intubate patients in the position in which they are found—on a bathroom floor, in a poorly lit area, and without sufficient space. While we may pride ourselves on performing skills in challenging environments, it is best to take a few moments to position our patient correctly. Optimizing the patient's position is critical to ensure first-pass success of intubation attempts, especially in the morbidly obese or pregnant patient.

The optimal position for orotracheal intubation requires flexion of the lower cervical spine and extension of the upper cervical spine *(Fig. 2.1)*. A simple and effective method of ensuring proper alignment is to look at the patient from the side and determine if the external ear canal aligns with the anterior clavicle and sternal notch. Several techniques can be utilized to properly place the patient in the optimal position. The simplest technique involves placing a firm pillow or blanket under the patient's head. This maneuver causes flexion of the lower cervical spine. Then, simply extend the head so that the patient's chin becomes the highest part of the body. This maneuver extends the upper cervical spine, and the patient is in the proper position for laryngoscopy. When performing laryngoscopy with the patient supine, along with ear-to-sternal notch positioning, the face plane of the patient should be parallel to the ceiling. A common error is to overextend or tilt the head backward. Atlanto-occipital extension pushes the base of tongue and epiglottis against the posterior hypo-pharyngeal wall. Not only does this make recognition of the epiglottis more difficult upon blade insertion, but this also narrows the space available to pass the laryngoscope and restricts laryngeal exposure. Extension creates an opposing tension on the anterior neck muscles as a simultaneous effort is made to distract the jaw open. This technique also requires very few supplies and no additional personnel to perform.

Another technique used to achieve the optimal position is called ramping. This technique is especially useful in the morbidly obese and pregnant

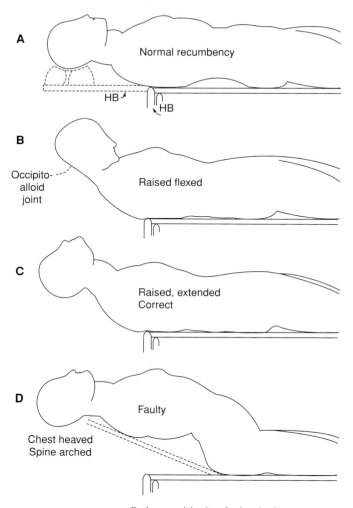

FIGURE 2.1. Patient positioning for intubation.

patient. Padding or blankets are placed under the patient in progressively thicker levels from the low thoracic region to the head. Though commercially available devices exist to "ramp" patients, they are often costly, require maintenance and storage space on the unit, and are not very EMS friendly as a result.

Providers can also achieve the desired ramping effect by raising the head of the stretcher to 20 or 30 degrees, placing padding behind the shoulders and head, and extending the patient's head into the optimal position. This technique requires the provider to be familiar with the process and comfortable performing direct laryngoscopy from a position above the patient, looking down. This technique takes advantage of gravity to help move the mandible anteriorly and inferiorly.

There are a number of things that can prevent providers from achieving the optimal position and hinder attempts at orotracheal intubation. Cervical spine immobility is a frequently encountered condition, especially in the elderly. Also, patients with cervical spine immobilization devices require special attention and an alternative approach to laryngoscopy. In these cases, a second provider will be required to maintain cervical spine stabilization during attempts at orotracheal intubation. Flexion and extension of the neck must be avoided, and laryngoscopy should be reserved for the most experienced and trained provider. Furthermore, all noninvasive airway management techniques should be attempted prior to attempting intubation of the patient with suspected cervical spine injury. Video laryngoscopes may provide additional exposure of airway structures while minimizing movement of the cervical spine.

Kyphosis and scoliosis are conditions that interfere with proper patient positioning. Changes in the shape of the spine and thoracic cage may cause excessive, and fixed, flexion of the cervical spine. Care must be taken to properly pad behind the back, shoulders, neck, and head in these patients, prior to attempting laryngoscopy.

Providers should exhaust all available noninvasive airway management tools and techniques prior to attempting orotracheal intubation. Use of bag-valve-mask resuscitators in conjunction with simple airway adjuncts such as nasal and oropharyngeal should be employed before making any attempts at intubation. Extraglottic devices such as the laryngeal mask airway (LMA), dual lumen devices such as the EasyTube, and obturator devices such as the KingLT are all great alternatives to direct laryngoscopy and orotracheal intubation. In addition, all of these devices can be inserted with the head in neutral alignment, and in the pregnant and morbidly obese without any special skills.

Remember to position your patient properly prior to intubation attempts. Positioning aligns the external auditory meatus with the sternal notch. This simple step brings the individual airway axes into the intubator's line of sight. Excessive head extension can actually interfere with a view of the glottic opening: don't crank the patient's head back during laryngoscopy! Finally, less invasive airway adjuncts and supraglottic airways are valuable additions to your toolbox. These devices can rapidly mitigate a difficult airway encounter and require less manipulation of the patient's head and cervical spine.

SELECTED READINGS

Bale E, Berrecloth R. The obese patient. Anaesthetic issues: airway and positioning. *J Perioper Pract.* 2010;20(8):294–299.

Deakin CD, King P, Thompson F. Prehospital advanced airway management by ambulance technicians and paramedics: is clinical practice sufficient to maintain skills? *Emerg Med J.* 2009;26(12):888–891.

Holmberg TJ, Bowman SM, Warner KJ, et al. The association between obesity and difficult prehospital tracheal intubation. *Anesth Analg.* 2011;112(5):1132–1138.

Jensen JL, Cheung KW, Tallon JM, et al. Comparison of tracheal intubation and alternative airway techniques performed in the prehospital setting by paramedics: a systematic review. *Can J Emerg Med.* 2010;12(2):135–140.

Rao SL, Kunselman AR, Schuler HG, et al. Laryngoscopy and tracheal intubation in the head-elevated position in obese patients: a randomized, controlled, equivalence trial. *Anesth Analg.* 2008;107(6):1912–1918.

3

WHICH PATIENTS SHOULD UNDERGO RSI?
ITS NOT JUST ABOUT THE CLENCHED JAW!

BENJAMIN KAUFMAN, RN, BS, NREMT-P
CHRISTOPHER TOUZEAU, MS, RN, NREMT-P

BACKGROUND

Rapid sequence intubation (RSI) is the induction of both unconsciousness and motor paralysis for the purpose of tracheal intubation. RSI is the most common method of emergency department intubation and the method of choice for the majority of emergency pediatric intubations. The technique is used to facilitate intubation and maximize chances for successful tube placement on the first attempt.

Studies indicate less than optimum success rates for endotracheal intubation. Researchers attribute the poor success rates to a lack of training opportunities, absent or inadequate ongoing education, and infrequency of clinical experience. Though prehospital RSI has been associated with poor patient outcomes, it has been shown to increase the success rate for endotracheal intubation. A study by Wang et al. in 2001 linked failed prehospital intubations to inadequate patient relaxation. So why are so many EMS medical directors and agencies reluctant to adopt RSI protocols? One major challenge to implementing an RSI program is determining which patients actually benefit from RSI.

EVIDENCE

In the emergency department setting, any conscious patient requiring intubation is a candidate for RSI. Generally speaking, the patient must be unable to tolerate direct laryngoscopy because of an intact gag reflex and meet at least one of the following conditions for intubation:

1) Failure to ventilate or oxygenate spontaneously
2) Failure to maintain airway patency
3) Rapid deterioration of clinical presentation
4) Anticipated clinical course (the patient will require deep sedation or transport away from the emergency department)

Virtually, all trained providers should be able to quickly recognize patients who are failing to ventilate and oxygenate. These patients often present with signs such as profound hypoxemia, air hunger, skin color and vital sign changes, and altered mentation. Paramedics are also adept in assessing airway patency. A patent airway is free from physical obstruction and should not impede the respiratory cycle. Seasoned clinicians may rely on instinct to anticipate a rapid deterioration of clinical presentation, and they can often anticipate a patient's clinical course simply from prior experiences. However, predicting clinical course can be quite challenging, and even veteran providers may find it difficult to articulate the justification for performing RSI. The following is a list of clinical presentations that many jurisdictions have incorporated into their RSI protocols to provide guidance on patient selection.

1) Rapid deterioration of mental status
2) Combativeness
3) Uncontrolled seizure activity
4) Significant facial trauma or swelling of the upper airway
5) Airway burns with inevitable airway loss
6) Waning level of consciousness
7) Respiratory exhaustion in medical cases
8) Periods of apnea
9) Clenched jaw
10) Severe intoxication with altered mental status
11) Angioedema from anaphylaxis/medication (i.e., ace inhibitors)

Traumatic brain injury (TBI) is not included in the list above because of the controversy behind prehospital intubation in the TBI patient. Although a recent study published in the Annals of Surgery (2010) suggests that severe TBI patients who undergo prehospital RSI show a slight improvement in neurologic outcomes, virtually all other TBI studies support withholding prehospital intubation in patients with a Glasgow Coma Scale (GCS) less than 8.

The paramedic should use these patient selection criteria in combination with the mechanism of injury in the case of trauma, or the nature of the medical presentation, to anticipate the clinical course and act quickly to preserve or restore the airway.

Patient selection is just one component of a successful RSI program. There are several challenges associated with establishing a prehospital RSI protocol. Success is directly linked to provider training, crew composition, meticulous quality assurance and quality improvement, and high skill frequency. Flight programs boast the highest success rates due to rigorous program requirements such as maintaining a mandatory minimum number of successful intubations for each provider.

BEST PRACTICE
RSI can be safely and effectively performed by EMS with few complications and without delaying transport. Medical directors should ensure that

providers who are authorized to perform RSI receive the proper initial and continuing education, are afforded sufficient live patient training opportunities, and undergo regularly scheduled skill assessments. Furthermore, RSI programs should adopt a comprehensive approach to airway management that incorporates techniques for rescuing the failed airway, rigorous quality assurance, and ongoing quality improvement objectives. It is critical for the RSI practitioner to master patient selection criteria. RSI is a complicated treatment strategy that requires appropriately selected patients and expertly trained providers. Performing RSI in patients with severe TBI remains controversial. Providers should assess the risks and benefits of the procedure and consider exhausting all other airway management techniques prior to performing RSI in the out-of-hospital setting.

SELECTED READINGS

Bernard SA. Prehospital rapid sequence intubation improves functional outcome for patients with severe traumatic brain injury: a randomized controlled trial. *Ann Surg.* 2010;252(6):959–965.

NAEMSP. Drug assisted intubation in the prehospital setting: Position statement of the National Association of Emergency Physicians. *Prehosp Emerg Care.* 2006;10(2):260.

Rapid Sequence Intubation (n.d.). Retrieved from http://www.scottishintensivecare.org.uk/education/RSI%20brochure.pdf.

Wang HE, Mann NC, Mears G, et al. Out-of-hospital airway management in the United States. *Resuscitation.* 2011;82(4):378–385.

Wang HE, O'Connor RE, Rubenstein H. Failed prehospital intubations: an analysis of emergency department course and outcomes. *Prehosp Emerg Care.* 2001;5(2):134–141.

4

IF A NONREBREATHER IS NOT CUTTING IT, SLAP ON THE PAP! USE NONINVASIVE POSITIVE PRESSURE VENTILATION IN PATIENTS WITH MODERATE TO SEVERE RESPIRATORY DISTRESS

STEVEN BARMACH, MD

The utilization of noninvasive negative pressure ventilation has been reported as far back as the 1700s, but did not achieve widespread use until the first half of the twentieth century, with the invention of the iron lung to combat the polio epidemic. Over the past few decades, negative pressure ventilation has become impractical and less popular. Intensive care units (ICUs), operating rooms (ORs), and emergency departments (EDs) now commonly treat patients in respiratory distress with noninvasive positive pressure ventilation (NIPPV), specifically with bilevel positive airway pressure (BiPAP) and with continuous positive airway pressure (CPAP). Because respiratory distress ranks as one of the most common prehospital encounters, the use of NIPPV has become an essential prehospital provider skill.

Several studies have examined the use of NIPPV in patients presenting with either a chronic obstructive pulmonary disease (COPD) exacerbation or an acute cardiogenic pulmonary edema. In a COPD flare, the patient has hyperinflated lungs, decreased diaphragmatic excursion, increased respiratory rate, increased intrinsic positive end-expiratory pressure, and consequently ineffectual tidal volumes. Noninvasive ventilator strategies decrease the work for the respiratory muscles and increase the tidal volume. This can aid in decreasing the respiratory rate, improving oxygenation, reducing hypercapnia, and may symptomatically improve dyspnea. A recent meta-analysis of 14 published randomized control trials showed a lower incidence of endotracheal intubation (relative risk [RR] 0.39) and hospital mortality (RR 0.52) among patients who received NIPPV versus standard therapy alone. RR is a ratio of the probability of the event occurring in the exposed group versus a nonexposed group. Patients who received NIPPV in addition to standard therapy are about 2½ times less likely to need intubation (1 divided by 0.39) and about 2 times less likely to die (1 divided by 0.52) compared to patients receiving standard therapy only. If the two groups were exactly identical, the RR would be 1. Thus, NIPPV, in conjunction with standard therapy (bronchodilators and steroids), is the first-line therapy for COPD patients in moderate-to-severe respiratory distress.

In congestive heart failure (CHF) patients presenting with acute pulmonary edema, a combination of pulmonary vasculature congestion, interstitial edema, and alveolar edema causes hypoxemic respiratory failure. Positive pressure ventilation recruits alveoli units, decreases both cardiac preload and afterload, improves oxygenation, corrects hypercapnia, and decreases dyspnea. In a prehospital trial consisting of approximately 220 patients presenting with acute pulmonary edema, subjects receiving standard treatment only were more likely to be intubated (odds ratio [OR] 4.04) and more likely to die (OR 7.48) than those receiving CPAP in addition to standard therapy. The OR is the ratio of the odds of an event occurring in one group to the odds of it occurring in another group, so patients in the control group were about 4 times more likely to be intubated and about 7½ times more likely to die than the patients in the experimental group. If the incidence of intubation and mortality were the same in both groups, the OR would be 1. Similarly, in a meta-analysis including 20 relevant randomized control trials involving patients presenting with cardiogenic pulmonary edema, treatment failure (defined as endotracheal intubation and hospital mortality) was significantly lower for patients receiving CPAP (RR 0.23). Along with nitrates, positive pressure ventilation is the first-line treatment for patients presenting with pulmonary edema.

The benefits of staving off endotracheal intubation are innumerable. Complications of intubation can include ventilator-associated pneumonia, vocal cord dysfunction, increased length of hospital stay, and the need for an ICU setting. Patients requiring endotracheal intubation often need sedation, which has its own inherent risks and complications. Additionally, intubated patients lose the ability to speak and eat. Data have shown that CPAP is equally as effective as BiPAP. Given that CPAP is more accessible, is easier to operate, and will not significantly prolong scene time or transit time in the prehospital setting, it is an ideal intervention for patients in moderate-to-severe respiratory distress.

While positive pressure ventilation has been used in patients with pneumonia, status asthmaticus, and acute respiratory distress syndrome (ARDS) with varied success, there is less compelling evidence for using NIPPV for patients in these clinical settings. Fortunately, there are relatively few drawbacks to placing a patient on a trial of NIPPV. Patients who benefit from NIPPV often improve within the first few minutes of therapy. Be wary if the patient is looking worse on positive pressure. The most crucial mistake is starting NIPPV on a patient who truly needs to be intubated. The prehospital provider may do harm by delaying or failing to recognize an inevitable intubation. The patient needs to be alert, responsive, and able to protect his/her airway. Because the airway is not protected by a cuffed tube in the trachea, aspiration continues to remain a risk. If the patient is actively vomiting or not handling secretions, do not use NIPPV. Additionally, there is a subset of patients who are preload dependent (e.g., those with a large pulmonary embolism, aortic stenosis, pulmonary hypertension, or right-ventricular failure) who will deteriorate on NIPPV. In this subset of patients, positive pressure will reduce preload and may precipitate acute hypotension. Be prepared to respond with intravenous fluid resuscitation if this happens. Finally, and perhaps most importantly, successful noninvasive ventilation requires a cooperative patient. The prehospital provider may need to spend significant time coaxing and counseling an air-hungry patient into wearing a constricting mask and working with the machine.

In summary, consider noninvasive ventilation early in a patient's course!

SELECTED READINGS

Bolton R, Bleetman A. Non-invasive ventilation and continuous positive pressure ventilation in emergency departments: Where are we now? *Emerg Med J.* 2008;25:190–194.

Ho KM, Wong K. A comparison of continuous and bi-level positive airway pressure noninvasive ventilation in patients with acute cardiogenic pulmonary oedema: a meta-analysis. *Crit Care.* 2006;10:R49.

Hubble MW, Richards ME, Jarvis R, et al. Effectiveness of prehospital continuous positive airway pressure in the management of acute pulmonary edema. *Prehosp Emerg Care.* 2006;10:430–439.

Keenan SP, Sinuff T, Burns K, et al. Clinical practice guidelines for the use of noninvasive positive-pressure ventilation and noninvasive continuous positive airway pressure in the acute care setting. *CMAJ.* 2011;183(3):E195–E214.

Lightowler JV, Wedzicha JA, Elliot M, et al. Non invasive positive pressure ventilation to treat respiratory failure resulting from exacerbations of chronic obstructive pulmonary disease: Cochrane systematic review and meta-analysis. *BMJ.* 2003;326:185–189.

5

CANNULAS AREN'T JUST FOR SUPPLEMENTAL OXYGEN ANYMORE: THE USE OF EtCO$_2$ FOR DIFFERENTIATING CAUSES OF RESPIRATORY DISTRESS

JONATHAN WENDELL, MD

The real-time monitoring of the partial pressure of end-tidal carbon dioxide (PEtCO$_2$), either as a number (capnometry) or as a waveform (capnography), is no longer limited to the operating room. What started in the 1940s as a simple CO$_2$ measuring device has now become a multipurpose patient assessment tool. Current capnometers are capable of providing real-time, noninvasive visual assessment of a patient's respiratory, metabolic, and cardiac status. As this amazing technology progresses, it permits the skilled provider to immediately recognize and intervene on critical conditions. This chapter provides an overview on the use of PEtCO$_2$ to differentiate various causes of respiratory distress.

In order to understand the changes in PEtCO$_2$ with respiratory distress, we should first review the normal findings. Your body's normal value of CO$_2$ is between 35 and 45 mm Hg. Multiple studies show that with standard perfusion, your PEtCO$_2$ corresponds very closely with blood levels, typically differing only 2 to 5 mm Hg. PEtCO$_2$ > 45 mm Hg (hypercapnia) can indicate hypoventilation or increased metabolic activity. Values <35 mm Hg (hypocapnia) may be caused by hyperventilation, decreased cardiac output, or poor pulmonary perfusion.

When we graph PEtCO$_2$ during normal exhalation, there are four distinct phases. During phase I, the beginning of exhalation, there is no CO$_2$, accounting for the physiologic "dead space" where no gas is exchanged. Phase II, or the ascending phase, corresponds with CO$_2$ from the alveoli mixing with dead space air causing a rapid rise in the amount of CO$_2$ detected. Phase III is the plateau phase, where there is a synchronous emptying of CO$_2$ from the alveoli. During this phase there is a slight positive slope reflecting the continuous gas exchange. The descending phase IV is due to the beginning of inhalation, where CO$_2$ levels quickly drop. The individual characteristics of the PEtCO$_2$ waveform, including frequency, rhythm, height, baseline, and shape, should be similar in humans with healthy lungs. Any deviations from the expected capnography could alert the clinician to potential physiologic or pathologic problems *(Fig. 5.1)*.

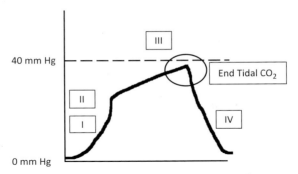

FIGURE 5.1. End-tidal carbon dioxide waveform.

MONITORING VENTILATION

Continuous graphing of $PEtCO_2$ allows providers to monitor a patient's respiratory status over time. Therefore, it can be understood as an early warning system for impending respiratory crisis. Hyperventilation can be an indication of metabolic (diabetic ketoacidosis [DKA], overdose), respiratory (pulmonary embolism, edema), cardiac, psychiatric (anxiety, mania), or infectious pathology. This will appear as frequent waves due to the increase in respiratory rate, but with diminished height of the plateau phase as the CO_2 concentration drops.

Hypoventilation will appear as a decreased respiratory rate with larger waves consistent with increased CO_2 levels, which could be indicative of medication overdose, sedation, intoxication, postictal states, head trauma, or respiratory failure. When monitoring ventilation, it is more important to follow the trend, rather than the actual number. A steadily rising $PEtCO_2$ in conjunction with hypoventilation is a better indication of respiratory compromise than a single elevated $PEtCO_2$ reading, which could be baseline for some chronic obstructive pulmonary disease (COPD) patients. In fact, when used to monitor sedated patients in the emergency department, capnography has repeatedly been shown to detect respiratory depression prior to pulse oximetry and clinical examination.

DIAGNOSING OBSTRUCTIVE PATHOLOGY

For those patients in severe respiratory distress, it is important to look for indications of obstruction in your capnography tracing. With obstructive airway disease (asthma and COPD), the slope of the alveolar plateau increases due to asynchronous emptying of the alveoli and delayed rise in CO_2 from poorly ventilated areas. This has often been described as a "shark-fin" appearance. Moreover, analysis of these waves has been shown to correlate with peak expiratory flow rate (PEFR) and forced expiratory volume in one second (FEV1). This provides a direct and effort-independent measure of the degree of bronchospasm, which is extremely beneficial in young patients or those with altered mental status. Continuous monitoring of waveform during and after treatment with bronchodilators can show decreased sloping and normalization of the plateau phase. These changes can suggest improvement in respiratory condition, as well as assist in further treatment decisions.

DIFFERENTIATING CHF FROM OTHER CAUSES OF RESPIRATORY DISTRESS

It is often difficult to discern COPD from congestive heart failure (CHF) in the severely dyspneic patient. Routine use of bronchodilators for undifferentiated respiratory distress is common in emergency medical services (EMS). However, looking for the characteristic "shark-fin" of obstructive disease may prevent the unnecessary administration of tachycardia–inducing bronchodilators in patients with no bronchospasm. Furthermore, some studies have shown that, although not diagnostic, patients with a $PEtCO_2$ > 37 mm Hg had a decreased likelihood of pulmonary edema/CHF as the cause of the respiratory distress.

METABOLIC CAUSES

Lastly, metabolic conditions, such as DKA, must be considered when a patient presents with respiratory distress. Again, monitoring $PEtCO_2$ with the right clinical situation can help diagnose DKA. In a 2002 study of diabetic children presenting to the emergency department, 95% of patients with a $PEtCO_2$ < 29 mm Hg were in ketoacidosis, whereas no ketoacidosis was present if the $EtCO_2$ > 36 mm Hg.

BOTTOM LINE/SUMMARY

Have a low threshold for the early application of capnography. This modality provides the clinician with clues to hyper- or hypoventilation. A "shark-fin" appearance of the waveform is consistent with an obstructive problem like COPD. Patients with a $PEtCO_2$ > 37 mm Hg are less likely to have pulmonary edema and CHF as a cause of their respiratory distress. Accordingly, $PEtCO_2$ values >36 mm Hg are unlikely to be found in patients suffering from DKA. Familiarity with waveform interpretation will help you deliver evidence-based and cutting-edge respiratory care.

SUGGESTED READINGS

Brandt PA. Measuring live and breathe: the benefits of capnography in EMS. *JEMS*. 2010; (suppl):4–9.

Brown LH, Seim G, Seim R. Can quantitative capnometry differentiate between cardiac and obstructive causes of respiratory distress. *Chest*. 1998;113:323–326.

Fearon DM, Steele DW. End-tidal carbon dioxide predicts the presence and severity of acidosis in children with diabetes. *Acad Emerg Med.* 2002;9(12):1373–1378.

Kupnik D, Skok P. Capnometry in the prehospital setting: are we using its potential? *Emerg Med J.* 2007;24:614–616.

Kurt OK, Alpar S, Sipit T, et al. Diagnostic role of capnography in pulmonary embolism. *Am J of Emerg Med.* 2010;28:460–465.

Nagler J, Krauss B. Capnography: a valuable tool for airway management. *Emerg Med Clin North Am.* 2008;26(4):881–897.

6

Errors in difficult airway assessment: Always assess the anatomy first

Jonathan Wenk, MD

Studies have demonstrated that between 1% and 3% of all patients will have anatomic properties that make endotracheal intubation difficult. Since the establishment of a patent airway in critically ill patients is of paramount importance, it is essential that prehospital providers familiarize themselves with rapid assessment. Providers should recognize anatomic features that signal a difficult intubation. That said, every intubation attempted in the field has its own unique set of challenges and obstacles. Consider that every airway has the potential for difficulty. Fortunately, there are some easy-to-use tools that can assist the provider in reliably predicting a difficult intubation. One such tool is a mnemonic called, "LEMON." This chapter reviews the components of the commonly utilized LEMON tool *(Table 6.1)*.

L → Look at the Airway

A common mistake made during airway management is to proceed directly to attempts at intubation without first assessing the patient's anatomy. A seasoned airway manager should first look for characteristics that predict a challenging intubation. Prospectively identifying a difficult airway may help stave off multiple intubation attempts. Repeated attempts traumatize the airway and cause complications such as bleeding, swelling, and tracheal wall injury. To avoid this pitfall, providers should conduct a brief, visual airway inspection. Predictors of a difficult airway include:

- Craniofacial trauma or congenital abnormality
- Short, fat neck
- Micrognathia (small chin)
- Tongue swelling or enlargement
- Prominent incisors

Another telltale sign in some patients is a scar on the anterior neck from prior tracheostomy.

E → Evaluate the "3-3-2" Rule

Another error health care providers experience is failure to fully assess the mouth and oral cavity. First, providers should be able to place three fingers between the patient's upper and lower teeth, as well as three fingers under the chin. Two-finger widths should fit in the space between the

TABLE 6.1	CHARACTERISTICS OF A DIFFICULT EMERGENCY AIRWAY
Look externally	■ Large tongue ■ Large incisors ■ Trauma ■ Receding jaw
Evaluate the 3-3-2 rule	■ Mouth opening distance in fingers ■ Hyoid-mental distance in fingers ■ Thyroid to floor-of-mouth distance
Obstruction	■ Abscess, foreign bodies, trauma, or other conditions that may impair visualization of the airway
Neck mobility	■ Cervical spine injury ■ Cervical collar

thyroid notch and the floor of the mouth. Less than three-finger widths between the incisors correlate with increasing intubation difficulty. A three-finger distance beneath the chin will reliably predict successful intubation. It is important to note that morbidly obese individuals will not have this distance due to redundant soft tissue in the anterior neck. A small mouth will provide reduced visibility, and emergency care providers should consider smaller-sized laryngoscopes to help maximize visibility. Dentures, if present, should be removed during inspection of the oral cavity.

M → MALLAMPATI: WORTH ASSESSING?

This rapid and easy-to-use scoring system has been used by anesthesiologists in the evaluation of preoperative patients. The examiner asks the patient to open their mouth and fully extend their tongue. Visualization of the soft palate and uvula corresponds with a less challenging intubation. Conversely, a patient in whom only a portion of the soft palate is seen is classified as a Mallampati 3 or 4. There are several problems with the Mallampati score as it pertains to an emergency department or prehospital patient population. First, patients must be able to sit up and obey commands. Patients presenting in extremis may have alterations in mental status that obviate cooperation. In addition, multi-trauma patients and individuals placed in spinal immobilization will not be able to cooperate with the Mallampati test. A study by Reed et al. conducted in 2005 showed no association between a high Mallampati score and the presence of a difficult airway. In 2010, a prospective single-center study identified several barriers to completion of the Mallampati assessment. Lack of patient cooperation and patient instability were cited as primary obstacles. The Mallampati score, therefore, has limited applicability in the critically ill emergency department patients who require urgent intubation.

O → OBSTRUCTION

Prehospital providers often forget that airways may become obstructed by food, vomitus, dentures, teeth, or blood. Avoidance of this pitfall centers on access to reliable suctioning equipment. Providers should also have ample lighting for visualizing the oral cavity. Equipment for removal of obstructing objects should be readily available. If intubation is occurring outside of the ambulance, portable suction should be readied and positioned close to the patient's side.

N → NECK MOBILITY

Many patients are unable to extend their necks. This is particularly important to remember when treating the elderly patient. Degenerative joint disease or rheumatoid arthritis can sometimes cause the cervical spine to be locked into a high degree of flexion, making direct laryngoscopy quite difficult. If the patient's neck is immobilized in a cervical collar, this will also make intubation challenging. The best practice for direct visualization of the airways employs a two-person technique; one provider maintains manual in-line stabilization while the other performs laryngoscopy. Remember to remove the cervical collar while inspecting the airway. The collar may obscure important findings such as neck trauma or a rapidly expanding hematoma that threatens airway patency.

One final pitfall is failure to have a backup plan. Not every difficult airway can be anticipated. After one or two concerted attempts to establish the airway are unsuccessful, a backup option should be employed.

Emergency medical service providers should have an intimate familiarity with rescue airway devices including supraglottic devices (i.e., laryngeal mask airway), dual lumen devices (i.e., easy tube), oro/nasopharyngeal airways, and surgical airway equipment. In addition, good bag-valve mask ventilation technique can be life-saving in cases of failed airway encounters and should be a fully developed skill in the prehospital provider armamentarium.

SUGGESTED READINGS

Bair AE, Caravelli R, Tyler K, et al. Feasibility of the preoperative mallampati airway assessment in emergency department patients. *J Emerg Med.* 2010;38(5):677–680.

Caplan RA, Benumof JL, Berry FA, et al. Practice guidelines for management of the difficult airway: a report by the American Society of Anesthesiologists Task Force on Management of the Difficult Airway. *Anesthesiology.* 1993;78:597–602.

Crosby ET, Cooper MR, Douglas MJ, et al. The unanticipated difficult airway and recommendations for management. *Can J Anesth.* 1998;45:757–776.

Mallampati SR, Gatt SP, Guigino LD, et al. A clinical sign to predict difficult tracheal intubation: a prospective study. *Can Anaesth Soc J.* 1985;32:429–434.

Reed MJ, Dunn MJG, McKeown DW. Can an airway assessment score predict difficulty at intubation in the emergency department? *Emerg Med J.* 2005;22:99–102.

Walls RM, Barton ED, McAfee AT, for the National Emergency Airway Registry Investigators. 2,392 emergency department intubations: First report of the ongoing National Emergency Airway Registry Study (NEAR 97). *Ann Emerg Med.* 1999;34:S14.

Walls RM, Luten RC, Murphy MF, et al. *Manual of Emergency Airway Management.* Philadelphia, PA: Lippincott Williams & Wilkins; 2000.

7

PROBLEMS ENCOUNTERED WITH MOVEMENT AND AIRWAY MANAGEMENT: CONFIRM AND RECONFIRM ENDOTRACHEAL INTUBATION

SCOTT H. WHEATLEY, BS, NREMT-P

We all have been there at 3 o'clock in the morning. We respond to the patient located in the third-story mini apartment where there is no space to move. The next thing you know, the patient has gone into cardiac arrest and landed between the toilet and the bathtub. There's no space to walk in and turn around, and certainly less than adequate room for work and life-saving treatments. Emergency medical care has as much to do with resuscitation as it does with keeping our interventions safe. The delivery of expert care is synonymous with checking and double-checking the success of our treatments. With respect to endotracheal intubation, it is imperative that providers remain vigilant for the possibility of dislodgement during patient movement and transport.

The necessity of tube confirmation has been drilled into the brains of prehospital providers. Tube dislodgement may have disastrous consequences such as hypoxia and cardiac arrest. There are many different strategies for the accomplishment of a single goal. However, confirmation needs to be thought of as an ongoing task. That is to say, an endotracheal tube is constantly at risk for dislodgement. Head flexion, rotation, and extension cause migration of the endotracheal tube. Patient movement during actual transport and the delivery of chest compressions may further increase the risk of dislodgement. Dr. Paul Matera's study suggests that routine application of a cervical collar may guard against this particular hazard. So, what else is necessary after the tube is confirmed, a collar is secured, and a commercial tube holder is applied?

Traditionally, providers have relied on pulse oximetry, auscultation, and other methods to ensure that the tube remains in the correct location. The National Association of EMS Physicians (NAEMSP) position statement affirms that "confirmation of tube placement is a dynamic process." The NAEMSP recommends that providers re-verify tube location after a patient is moved or at any time when dislodgement is suspected. Unfortunately, the familiar methods of confirmation may be less than adequate in the prehospital setting. Direct visualization may be impossible after a commercial tube holder is applied and is less reliable when vocal cords are obscured. The presence of "chest rise" is similarly deceiving. Conditions such as chronic obstructive lung disease and morbid obesity may obviate visualization of chest wall movement. Lung sounds also have the potential to deceive. Listening to breath sounds at both axillae "may result in misdiagnosis of up to 15% of all esophageal intubations." Pulse oximetry has also been held up as a method for endotracheal tube confirmation. Unfortunately, desaturation does not occur immediately following tube displacement. By the time hypoxia is detected, several minutes may have elapsed. Pulse oximetry also requires an adequate perfusing rhythm. Shock states, hypothermia, and peripheral vasoconstriction may limit oximetry's utility.

What is the best method to continually confirm and reconfirm proper placement? Though any comprehensive strategy for confirmation should incorporate multiple methods, the analysis of the carbon dioxide waveform provides the most reliable reassurance. A study by Langhan et al. compared pulse oximetry to capnography for the detection of dislodged endotracheal tubes. Senior paramedic students were given a simulated scenario during which the endotracheal tube became misplaced. Students in the capnography group recognized and corrected the event approximately 2 minutes earlier than their counterparts in the pulse oximetry group. Despite a loss of both breath sounds and chest rise, only 12% of providers in the study group without capnography accurately diagnosed tube dislodgement. Silvestri et al. conducted a study that examined the impact of waveform capnography on the rate of unrecognized esophageal intubation. The study enrolled a total of 153 patients; 93 of them were monitored with continuous end-tidal carbon dioxide. No unrecognized esophageal intubations occurred in the treatment group that utilized continuous capnography. The sensitivity of end-tidal carbon dioxide, coupled with its ability to rapidly detect tube malfunction, makes it an ideal supplement for clinical judgment. It is simply not enough to confirm that the tube has traversed the laryngeal opening. After successful intubation, providers must secure the tube and guard against further movement. Frequent patient assessment plus the objective measurement of end-tidal carbon dioxide provides the best assurance against inadvertent dislodgement. If ever in doubt, confirm and re-confirm!

Properly securing an endotracheal tube requires careful and continuous attention to detail. Utilize a commercially available tube holder whenever possible. Apply a cervical collar to all intubated patients and implement waveform capnography to guard against unrecognized tube dislodgment. Finally, reconfirm tube placement following the transfer or turnover of patient care.

SELECTED READINGS

Langhan ML, Ching K, Northrup V, et al. A randomized controlled trial of capnography in the correction of simulated endotracheal tube dislodgement. *Acad Emerg Med.* 2011; 18(6):590–597.

Matera P. Anchor the airway. *JEMS.* 1997;22(2):24–25.

O'Connor RE, Swor RA. Verification of endotracheal tube placement following intubation. Position paper of the National Association of Emergency Medical Services Physicians. *Prehosp Emerg Care.* 1999;3(3):248–250.

Silvestri S, Ralls GA, Krauss B, et al. The effectiveness of out of hospital use of continuous end tidal carbon dioxide monitoring on the rate of unrecognized misplaced intubation within a regional emergency medical services system. *Ann Emerg Med.* 2005;45(5): 497–503.

8

HIGH PRESSURE AIRWAY?
LAY OFF THE CRICOID!

BENJAMIN J. LAWNER, DO, EMT-P, FAAEM

Cricoid pressure has been incorporated into the heads of many airway managers. For decades, emergency medical service personnel have pushed down on the cricoid cartilage in hopes of getting a better view of the cords. Interestingly enough, cricoid pressure was never intended to optimize laryngeal view. The technique has its roots in the attempt to prevent aspiration. In early studies of cricoid pressure, Sellick infused saline into the esophagus of an anesthetized patient. It was thought that downward pressure would occlude the esophagus and prevent liquid from filling up the oropharynx. A review of the evidence indicates that cricoid pressure does not result in a better view. Furthermore, the technique may not guard against aspiration or regurgitation as was previously thought.

CRICOID COMPLICATIONS

"Mashing down" on the cricoid cartilage is not a benign procedure. Studies and case reports have documented several complications including esophageal rupture and fracture of the cricoid cartilage. In other cases, downward pressure results in complete occlusion of the airway. Also of interest is the fact that there is no consensus on how much force is required to prevent insufflation of the stomach. Sellick himself advocated for the application of "firm" pressure, and the exact amount of force is a continued matter of debate. The current clinical environment does not permit a reliable measurement of applied force. Given the lack of consensus and the presence of documented complications, caution should be used whenever force is applied to the cricoid cartilage.

CRICOID AND THE CORDS

In addition to the theoretical benefit of preventing gastric aspiration, providers commonly apply cricoid pressure in an attempt to get a better view. Studies demonstrate that cricoid pressure does not improve an intubator's look at the glottic opening. It seems intuitive that downward pressure exerted by a provider who is blind to the laryngoscopist's view might not result in visualization. Clearly, it is the LARYNGEAL cartilage which must be manipulated in order to bring cords into view. Maneuvers such as "BURP" (backward, upward, and rightward pressure) and ELM (external laryngeal manipulation) have gained traction as evidence-based strategies for improving intubation. Levitan et al. compared all three methods (cricoid, BURP, and ELM) in a cadaveric study. He found that cricoid pressure consistently worsened an intubator's view. Furthermore, BURP was also found inferior to ELM with respect to the POGO, or percentage of glottic opening score. Simply put, movement of the larynx results in better intubating views. This makes sense because the vocal cords are housed within the cage of the laryngeal cartilage. Simple strategies such as ELM have the potential to improve the view of the cords at laryngoscopy.

Cricoid and Insufflation

In theory, the application of cricoid pressure during positive pressure ventilation guards against excessive inflation of the stomach. A few studies demonstrated that cricoid use was beneficial during mask ventilation. However, these studies were conducted at a time when providers ventilated patients at faster rates and at higher tidal volumes. A better understanding of respiratory physiology and an almost universal adaptation of a lower tidal volume ventilation strategy may be sufficient enough to prevent gastric distention. Providers may be justified in the decision to apply gentle cricoid pressure in order to avoid inflation of the stomach.

Best Practices

A review of available evidence indicates that cricoid manipulation is not without complications. Furthermore, the technique may not reliably guard against aspiration. These conclusions resulted in a modification to the recent American Heart Association guidelines. Providers must gauge the potential benefit of any intervention applied to their patients; the positive effects from cricoid pressure are less than robust. Whether or not cricoid prevents against gastric insufflation is another question altogether. There is no evidence to suggest that gentle cricoid pressure results in harm. Cautious application of pressure may have a role in reducing the amount of airflow into the stomach during positive pressure ventilation. However, it is increasingly clear that cricoid pressure should not be synonymous with an optimized view of the cords. The next time you are faced with a challenging airway, use that intubating right hand to grasp the LARYNGEAL cartilage. Move the cartilage around until the cords or other landmarks (arytenoids) come into view. Learn about external laryngeal manipulation and take the next step toward an evidence-based approach to emergency airway management. Be cautious with cricoid pressure!

Suggested Readings

Ellis DY, Harris T, Zideman D. Cricoid pressure in emergency department rapid sequence tracheal intubations: a risk benefit analysis. *Ann Emerg Med*. 2007;50(6):653–665.

Hartsilver EL. Airway obstruction with cricoid pressure. *Anaesthesia*. 2000;55(3):208–211.

Heath KJ. Fracture of the cricoid cartilage after Sellick's manoeuvre. *Br J Anaesth*. 1996; 76(6):877–878.

Levitan RM, Kinkle WC, Levin WJ, et al. Laryngeal view during laryngoscopy: a randomized trial comparing cricoid pressure, backward-upward-rightward-pressure, and bimanual laryngoscopy. *Ann Emerg Med*. 2006;47(6):548–555.

Neumar FR, Otto CW, Link MS, et al. Part 8: Adult cardiovascular life support: 2010 American Heart Association guidelines for cardiopulmonary resuscitation and emergency cardiovascular care. *Circulation*. 2010;122:S729–S767.

Sellick BA. Cricoid pressure to control regurgitation of stomach contents during induction of anesthesia. *Lancet*. 1961;2:404–406.

9

DON'T BE SO QUICK TO THROW YOUR BATTERY OPERATED LARYNGOSCOPE AWAY!

Benjamin J. Lawner, DO, EMT-P, FAAEM

There's little question that newer technologies have revolutionized the way prehospital providers literally "look" at an airway. Next-generation video laryngoscopes feature high-definition screens and cutting-edge optics to furnish the intubator with a near-perfect view of a glottic opening. The relative ease of learning may encourage some emergency medical services systems to rapidly adopt these video laryngoscopes and cast off the poor old battery-powered laryngoscopes. However, be very cautious about letting direct laryngoscopy skills go to waste. Technology, like everything else, is never perfect. Remaining proficient at prehospital airway management means maintaining your skillset in a perpetual degree of readiness. This chapter will discuss the Glidescope video laryngoscope (GVL) and concerns specific to its operation.

GLIDESCOPE CONSIDERATIONS AND COMPLICATIONS

The Glidescope facilitates endotracheal intubation through superior visualization of the glottic opening. The intubating handle is bent at an acute handle so that the anterior larynx is easily brought into view. Similarly, the Glidescope includes a rigid stylette designed to direct the endotracheal tube through the cords. Indeed, video laryngoscopy is not the same as direct laryngoscopy with a traditional handle and blade. In addition to learning the nuances of these devices, providers should be conscious of possible complications.

Recent literature has documented several untoward events including dental injury and damage to laryngeal nerves. Lip lacerations and gum injures may also occur. More serious complications linked to use of the GVL include tissue perforation and tracheal injury. Studies suggest that the Glidescope is an easy device to learn, but like any other device or technology, its use requires practice and adequate familiarization. Emergency airway management literature is also filled with tips and tricks designed to avoid side effects such as injury or improper visualization. Any training program involving optical or video laryngoscopes should take these device-specific pointers into consideration. For example, disengaging the endotracheal tube from the Glidescope's rigid metal stylette involves a different technique than the withdrawal of the usual malleable stylette.

Glidescope's Success and Failures

The success of the Glidescope is well documented in the literature. Aziz et al. (2011) studied over 2,000 GVL intubations at two academic medical centers. Over 142 attending level anesthesiologists used the GVL for 2004 intubations. A success rate of over 96% was reported in the predicted difficult airway. However, the study identified several factors predictive of Glidescope failure. Even with its superior rates of success, the authors concluded that "providers should maintain their competency with alternate methods of intubation." Traditional indicators of a difficult airway, like the Mallampati score, did not always apply for the GVL patient population. Similarly, obesity alone (determined by body mass index) was not linked to failed GVL intubation. The authors documented the presence of neck pathology as a factor associated with failure instead. Specifically, previous radiation, scarring, or anatomical alteration predicted failed or difficult GVL intubations. Limited cervical motion also factored into unsuccessful video laryngoscopy attempts. "Technical difficulties" such as excessive fogging and the lack of video output occurred in a few GVL failures.

The Bottom Line

The data suggest that video laryngoscopes facilitate visualization of the opening. Though many studies are conducted in the operating room setting, it seems reasonable that the GVL and systems like it may mitigate some of the difficulty associated with direct laryngoscopy. There are several barriers to widespread adoption of the GVL, however. The equipment itself is associated with significant costs, and there is the need for initial and ongoing training. The higher success rates should encourage EMS providers and administrators to at least examine the use of the GVL. However, it is important to realize that there is no one device that provides all of the solutions to the challenges posed by prehospital endotracheal intubation. This rather large study cited a number of factors linked to failed video laryngoscopy. Though failures were rare, they nevertheless reiterate a time-honored and tested principle of emergency airway management: Be prepared! Technical difficulties like power failure and fogging may occur during emergency intubation. Patient anatomy may also impair visualization with the GVL.

As these new and exciting devices make their way into the prehospital arena, it is important to remain vigilant about maintaining skills. Your old battery-powered handle should never be too far away from any difficult airway!

FACTORS THAT PREDICT A DIFFICULT GLIDESCOPE INTUBATION

- Limited cervical motion
- Neck pathology
  - Scar
  - Mass
  - Radiation
- Short thyromental (TM) distance <6 cm

SELECTED READINGS

Aziz MF, Healy D, Kheterpal S, et al. Routine clinical practice effectiveness of the Glidescope in difficult airway management. *Anesthesiology.* 2011;114(1):34–41.

Kramer DC, Osborn IP. More maneuvers to facilitate tracheal intubation with the Glidescope. *Can J Anaesth.* 2006;53:737.

Leong WL, Lim Y, Sia H. Palatopharyngeal wall perforation during GlideScope® intubation. *Anaesth Intensive Care.* 2008;36(6):870–874.

Nouruzi-Sedeh P, Schumann M, Groeben H. Laryngoscopy via Macintosh blade versus GlideScope: Success rate and time for endotracheal intubation in untrained medical personnel. *Anesthesiology.* 2009;110:32–37.

10

Drop that tube! Alternative airways in the prehospital setting

Stephen C. Andrews, BA, MSN, CCEMT-P, ACNP

You are called to respond to a 69-year-old female complaining of 4 days of exertional dyspnea, chest pain, nausea, and vomiting. Upon your arrival, you find the patient seated in a chair with audible rales, expiratory wheezing, respiratory extremis (rate = 32), sinus tachycardia, and a SpO_2 of 82% on room air. She is conscious, alert, follows commands but is very anxious. Your initial impression is acute respiratory distress and hypoxia. You must now provide an appropriate clinical intervention. Many prehospital providers would argue that this patient should be immediately sedated, paralyzed, and intubated. I would caution you against reflexively intubating this patient and ask you to "drop that tube."

In other words, drop it, put it down, and step away from it. Think about how many intubations you perform in a week, month, or even a year? Does that number comfort or frighten you? What is your end goal with intubation? Hopefully, you want a secure airway that is simple to insert, does not cause further clinical deterioration, reduces complications, and does not take time away from other interventions. Your ultimate goal is to provide proper ventilation and subsequent perfusion safely and effectively with a minimum of interruption. Each of us has been taught that endotracheal intubation (ETI) is the optimum method for airway management. I would counter that unless the provider intubates regularly, they will not be facile enough to perform the procedure quickly and with minimal interruptions in the delivery of clinical care.

A variety of studies have been performed, which call into question the viability of ETI for a variety of prehospital scenarios. Stewart et al. (1984) studied 122 paramedics intubating 763 patients in a 27-month period and found that they had a 90.3% success rate. Conversely, this represents a 9.7% failure rate. The most common complication was prolonged intubation. Anesthesiologists performing ETIs in the stable environment of the operating suite sometimes have difficulty with placing the tube properly. Russi et al. (2008) compared the speed with which paramedics were able to successfully intubate a simulated difficult airway patient. On average, it took 91.3 seconds to place an endotracheal tube and 27.0 seconds for the King LT airway. Katz and Falk (2001) studied 108 patients who were intubated in the field and found that 25% of the endotracheal tubes were placed in the esophagus. These esophageal intubations were directly attributed to improper provider assessment of tube placement as well as failure to utilize $ETCO_2$ as a postintubation and continuing airway assessment. Given that many prehospital providers do not have the opportunity to perform ETI in situations other than annual recertification or training, perhaps another option for managing critical airways should be considered.

Approved for use by the FDA in 2003, the King LT airway provides an excellent alternative to ETI in a variety of clinical applications. This supraglottic airway devise is being utilized in the operating room and the prehospital environment with excellent success and patient outcomes. Hagberg et al. (2006) studied the use of a variety of alternative airway devices among them the laryngeal mask airway (LMA) and the King Airway. They found that the King Airway was superior in the ease of insertion (less than 5 seconds in 90% of the cases), delivery of proper ventilations and tidal volumes. In a study of a rural EMS system, the King LT was placed without difficulty in all but one case. The discomfort that many providers have is that we have all been trained that ETI is the "gold standard" for airway management in virtually all clinical scenarios. The major issue for providers is the supposed protection that ETI provides from aspiration. ETI is not a benign procedure. Improperly performed ETI can result in further patient hypoxia (due to prolonged intubation) and pulmonary infections due to contaminated tubes. While we as providers do not like to think or admit that it takes us very long to intubate, the reality is it can take up to 91 seconds. This delay coupled with the potential of infection can be disastrous to the patient's overall morbidity and mortality.

According to the National Association of EMS Physicians (NAEMSP), "Although paramedics in the United States are trained to perform ETI, the intervention is often unsuccessful," with failure "rates ranging from 8% to over 30%." The authors further describe the types of situations where an alternative airway device, such as the King Airway, may need to be the primary airway device selected. Conditions judged to be "difficult" airways are often subjective and rely on the operator's level of experience and comfort with the clinical scenario and ETI. In a perfect world, a provider would have the opportunity to take a full medical and surgical history while fully assessing the patient's airway. This is not often practical or the case in the field. As with any psychomotor skill, our perceived level of difficulty is directly proportional to the number of repetitions and situations we have performed that skill. If the provider's assessment of the difficulty of ETI exceeds their experience of skill, then ETI should be deferred and an alternative airway placed. While the NAEMSP position paper does not recommend one particular device over another, their message is clear. Do not attempt an

ETI if your comfort level and experience will further prolong the placement of an ETT. Consider an alternative airway.

Returning to our initial case presentation, there is no doubt that the patient requires aggressive and immediate intervention. Should the application of PPV fail and the patient require a more permanent and secure airway, the King Airway can be considered as the primary airway. Proper placement of the airway theoretically decreases the risk of aspiration via the inflation of distal and proximal occluding cuffs. Keep in mind that ETI does not protect from aspiration 100%, and repeated ETI attempts increase the risk of vomiting and subsequent aspiration. In fact, studies have shown that there is no more risk of aspiration with a King Airway than traditional ETI. Frascone et al. (2009) studied the use of the King LTS-D airway in medication-assisted intubation rapid sequence intubation (RSI) scenarios and reported only one case of aspiration. Additionally, the King LTS-D allows for the passage of suction catheters (up to 18Fr) without difficulty. The King Airway's proximal tip supports connection with $ETCO_2$ monitoring devices. Finally, many EMS agencies are authorized to administer antiemetics. It would be reasonable to consider consultation for antiemetic administration after King Airway placement.

Even if you feel you can intubate quickly and efficiently, can you reliably anticipate all of the complications associated with ETI? Do your patients and your stress level a favor, place the King Airway. You will achieve quick and proper placement, effective ventilation, and oxygenation without increased risk of tube misplacement and further hypoxemia due to a prolonged intubation attempt. You can suction and monitor $ETCO_2$ with the King just as effectively as with ETI. Upon arrival at the ED, the King can easily be switched out for ETI, should the case require it. You owe it to your patient and yourself in critical airway situations to consider the use of an alternative airway.

SELECTED READINGS

Brainard C. (2010). Airway Encounters in JEMS.com. Extracted July 21st, 2011.

Frascone RJ, Wewerka SS, Griffith KR, et al. Use of the King LTS-D during medication assisted airway management. *Prehosp Emerg Care.* 2009;13(4):541–545.

Guyette FX, Greenwood MJ, Neubecker D, et al. Alternate airways in the prehospital setting (Resource Document to NAEMSP Position Statement). *Prehosp Emerg Care.* 2007; 11(1):56–61.

Hagberg C, Bogomolny Y, Gilmore C, et al. An evaluation of the insertion and function of a new supraglottic airway, the King LT, during spontaneous ventilation. *Anesth Analg.* 2006;102(2):621–625.

Katz SH, Falk JL. Misplaced endotracheal tubes by paramedics in an urban emergency medical services system. *Ann Emerg Med.* 2001;37(1):32–37.

Russi CS, Buresh CT. A pilot study of the King LT supralaryngeal airway use in a rural Iowa EMS system. *Int J Emerg Med.* 2008;1(2):135–138.

Russi CS, Miller L, Hartley MJ. A comparison of the King-LT to endotracheal intubation and Combitube in a simulated difficult airway. *Prehosp Emerg Care.* 2008;12(1):35–41.

Soo Hoo GW. Ventilation, Noninvasive in eMedicine.com. Extracted July 7th, 2011.

Stewart RD, Paris PM, Pelton GH, et al. Effect of varied training technique on field endotracheal intubation success rate. *Ann Emerg Med.* 1984;13(11):1032–1036.

Stone K, Humphries R. (eds.) *Principles of Intubation in Current Diagnosis and Treatment: Emergency Medicine.* McGraw-Hill; 2008.

11

IT'S NOT ALL ABOUT INTUBATION: NEW PERSPECTIVES ON PREHOSPITAL AIRWAY MANAGEMENT

KEVIN G. SEAMAN, MD, FACEP

Remember when you first learned to intubate in paramedic class? Did you think, "Wow, now I can perform endotracheal intubation, a rare skill allowed for doctors and a few select EMS providers." In fact, doesn't it seem like intubation is THE most prized procedure? Don't make the mistake of tying your self-worth to a single procedure. Paramedics provide excellent care that does make a difference for patients, and as a paramedic you need to be open to learning throughout your career. The topic of airway management has experienced many changes in the past few years. In this chapter we'll explore the most important changes and provide an updated perspective focusing on errors to avoid.

IS AN ENDOTRACHEAL INTUBATION A FALSE GOLD STANDARD?

In the 21st century, the lens has been focused very tightly on prehospital intubation. A study from Orlando documented a missed ET tube (not in the trachea) rate of 25%. Of the missed intubations, one-third were in the pharynx, above the cords, and two-third were in the esophagus. A similar study done in Los Angeles looked at outcomes for pediatric patients with field airway management. The authors found less complications in patients managed via BVM compared with pediatric patients that were intubated. In fact, the same authors surveyed EMS services in California in 2010 and found that 22 of 25 services had not changed their protocols regarding pediatric intubation despite the evidence that BVM ventilation was as effective with fewer complications. It's clear that prehospital attempts to manage the airway must be done quickly, accurately, and correctly and that confirmation and continuous monitoring must include waveform capnography.

The recently published 2010 American Heart Association (AHA) Guidelines for Cardiopulmonary Resuscitation and Emergency Cardiovascular Care address some of the controversies associated with intubation. It is more clear than ever that chest compressions are one of the few interventions in cardiac arrest that are tied to improved survival. Intubation attempts frequently result in excessively long pauses in compressions. These interruptions decrease coronary perfusion and the responsiveness of the heart to defibrillation. In addition, if the intubation is successful, overventilation is common and decreases venous return to the heart, decreasing coronary perfusion, cardiac output, and, ultimately, survival. The AHA guidelines deemphasize intubation in the period immediately following cardiac arrest and encourage providers to focus on those interventions most closely linked to survival.

So, Given What You've Told Me, What Should I Do?

It's not uncommon, when a patient presents an opportunity for an intubation, that the intubator, feeling some adrenaline, grabs the laryngoscope, inserts it in the mouth, and attempts intubation without creating the optimal conditions to succeed at intubation (read the chapter on "Glottic Visualization: Making the First Pass the Best Pass"). There are good reasons to optimize intubating conditions during the first attempt: safety and success. Studies in the airway literature consistently demonstrate that the first pass at intubation is always the best pass. Each subsequent attempt has incrementally less success and causes complications that can create problems, some small but some significant. Thus, patient safety is maximized if we prepare well and succeed on the first attempt to intubate.

If we succeed at successful placement initially, confirm the tube, secure the tube, and connect hook the tube up to waveform capnometry. If we don't succeed initially, consider allowing one additional attempt. The perspective on the subsequent attempt should be, what factors can I change to improve my chance of success? (see "Don't Attempt Intubation without Having a Plan")

What About Managing the Airway in Cardiac Arrest?

Certainly the priority in cardiac arrest is CPR with effective chest compressions. Patients who were breathing just before arrest have some minutes of oxygen reserve, allowing chest compressions to take precedence. If the patient can be oxygenated and ventilated using BVM, that should continue while both CPR and defibrillation are accomplished. In your judgment, if the priority tasks are accomplished, you may attempt intubation; make sure chest compressions continue during your attempt. If you must interrupt chest compressions to intubate, make sure you limit your intubation attempt to 10 seconds. New technologies (video laryngoscopes) can facilitate intubation while chest compressions are ongoing.

What if the Attempts at Intubation Do Not Succeed?

Remember that the prehospital environment is chaotic and unpredictable. Intubation is a technically difficult procedure that requires adequate preparation, training, and resources. Successful prehospital airway management is quite simply the establishment and maintenance of a patent airway. Paramedics have many tools at their disposal, and it is clear that there are several ways to secure an airway. Utilization of a bag valve mask or successful placement of a supraglottic airway should not be considered a failure! Keep in mind that tracheal intubation is not always the goal of airway control.

SUMMARY

Pearls

- Don't rush or make your ET intubation attempt without optimizing conditions, giving yourself the best chance at success.
- In cardiac arrest, don't necessarily hurry to intubate if BVM ventilation is providing effective oxygenation.
- In cardiac arrest, intubate while compressions are continuing; don't interrupt CPR for your intubation attempt.
- In cardiac arrest, when you successfully intubate, avoid overventilation as it counteracts the life-saving effects that CPR has on coronary perfusion.
- If you don't succeed with your first or second intubation attempt, rather than repeat a third intubation attempt, consider placing a rescue airway (King Airway, Combitube, or LMA).
- Consider successful placement of a rescue airway as a success.

SELECTED READINGS

Gausche M, Lewis RJ, Stratton SJ, et al. Effect of out-of-hospital pediatric endotracheal intubation on survival and neurological outcome: a controlled clinical trial. *JAMA*. 2000;283:783–790.

Katz SH, Falk JL. Misplaced endotracheal tubes by paramedics in an urban emergency medical services system. *Ann Emerg Med*. 2001;37:32–37.

Neumar RW, Otto CW, Link MS, et al. Part 8: adult advanced cardiovascular life support: American Heart Association Guidelines for Cardiopulmonary Resuscitation and Emergency Cardiac Care. *Circulation*. 2010;122(suppl 3):S729–S767.

Youngquist ST, Gausche-Hill MA, Squire BT, et al. Barriers to adoption of evidence-based airway practices in California. *Prehosp Emerg Care*. 2010;14:505–509.

12

GCS LESS THAN 8? DON'T AUTOMATICALLY INTUBATE!

BENJAMIN J. LAWNER, DO, EMT-P, FAAEM

The head-injured patient represents significant challenges for the pre-hospital provider. These patients often present with a depressed level of consciousness, combativeness, and intact airway reflexes. Blood and vomitus may obstruct the oropharynx, and there are significant concerns with respect to airway control. As rapid sequence intubation (RSI) techniques have matured, emergency departments and trauma centers have adopted RSI as the standard of care for the intubation of critically ill, head-injured patients. Accordingly, some prehospital systems have adopted RSI as their modality of choice for securing an airway. However, RSI is not without complications. Patients undergoing RSI in the field are at higher risk for aspiration, worsened neurologic outcome, and death. Furthermore, it remains unclear as to whether or not endotracheal intubation should be thought of as the gold standard for prehospital care with respect to combative, head-injured patients.

Though it is true that RSI is associated with higher rates of first-pass success, RSI involves much more than placing a piece of plastic through the glottic opening. Indeed, paramedics in the landmark San Diego study demonstrated endotracheal intubation success rates of over 99%. However, the RSI study was halted due to increased patient mortality. Though the success rates were impressive, patients arrived at the hospital with dangerously low carbon dioxide levels. It is hypothesized that the hyperventilation contributed to worsened neurologic outcome. Furthermore, a majority of patients in the RSI group demonstrated at least one episode of hypoxia. Vital sign abnormalities indicate an extremely poor prognosis. Even an isolated episode of hypotension or hypoxia in the brain-injured patient may significantly increase mortality rates. The analysis of the San Diego study demonstrated quite clearly that RSI is a complex and controlled process that requires meticulous attention to detail. Slipping an endotracheal tube through the vocal cords is only ONE part of the ongoing airway management process. Paramedics must guard against pre-intubation hypoxia and maintain near-normal levels of end-tidal carbon dioxide.

Technological advances have addressed many concerns that surfaced during the original San Diego study. Pulse oximetry is now standard on most all ambulances, and there is greater availability of both waveform and colorimetric carbon dioxide measurement devices. However, the ability to proficiently paralyze and intubate patients is directly related to skill maintenance. Indeed, paramedics authorized to use neuromuscular blocking agents should receive comprehensive initial and ongoing training in airway management. Operating room time and other supervised intubation training is difficult to secure but extremely vital to maintaining a high level of intubation expertise. Simply put, proficiency in intubation relates to practice.

Head-injured patients encountered in the prehospital setting are at risk for poor outcomes. Furthermore, the ones that undergo endotracheal intubation, with or without paralytics, are an especially sick group. Intubation itself is certainly not the cure-all. The procedure itself can worsen intracranial pressure and stimulate vomiting. It can induce laryngospasm in patients with an intact gag reflex. Even if intubation goes without a hitch, these patients must have their end-tidal carbon dioxide levels carefully scrutinized in order to avoid hyperventilation. The imperative of transport to definitive care, coupled with the complexities inherent in any intubation attempt, merits serious consideration of rapid transport.

The debate about prehospital intubation and RSI will continue into the future and extend far beyond the pages of this textbook. It is extremely important for practicing prehospital providers to remember that patients must be carefully selected and prepared for RSI. The intervention, like any other treatment, may cause serious complications and side effects. Head-injured patients represent a unique and critically ill patient population. They benefit from carefully controlled interventions and treatment, which may be difficult to administer in the often chaotic out-of-hospital environment. Though it is true that some emergency medical services (EMS) have successfully implemented RSI protocols, these programs usually incorporate intensive physician oversight and ongoing intubation training.

The bottom line is that prehospital RSI for head-injured patients remains a risky and controversial topic. RSI may not be the gold standard for every system; providers should instead focus on the time-tested principles of noninvasive airway support. Supportive maneuvers may help avoid aspiration and prevent unnecessary spikes in intracranial pressure. If intubation is attempted without the assistance of sedatives and paralytics, providers must remain vigilant to avoid hyperventilation and hypoxia. A GCS of less than 8, especially for those patients with head injuries, does not always mean intubate! Initial, noninvasive attempts at airway control may lessen the risk of complications and result in better neurologic outcomes.

SELECTED READINGS

Davis DP, Ochs M, Hoyt DB, et al. Paramedic administered neuromuscular blockade improves prehospital intubation success in severely head injured patients. *J Trauma.* 2003;55(4):713–719.

Dunford JV, Davis DP, Ochs M, et al. Incidence of transient hypoxia and pulse rate reactivity during paramedic rapid sequence intubation. *Ann Emerg Med.* 2003;42(6):721–728.

Jeremitsky E, Omert L, Dunham CM, et al. Harbingers of poor outcome the day after severe brain injury: hypothermia, hypoxia, and hypoperfusion. *J Trauma Inj Crit Care.* 2003;54:312–319.

Warner KJ, Carlborn D, Cooke CR, et al. Paramedic training for proficient prehospital endotracheal intubation. *Prehospital Emerg Care.* 2010;14(1):103–108.

13

I can't see cords! What to do when you're already in too deep

BENJAMIN J. LAWNER, DO, EMT-P, FAAEM

Prehospital providers pride themselves on the ability to drop a difficult tube. The ability to conquer a difficult airway represents both skill and experience. Intubation is a technically difficult skill, and the literature is clear that EMS providers can DO BETTER with respect to success rates. Training in intubation is often minimized, and few providers can take advantage of ongoing practice sessions with live patients or cadavers. An eventual encounter with a difficult airway is unavoidable; this chapter will discuss some techniques that you can use the next time you find yourself peeking down the blade of a laryngoscope ... without a cord in sight.

LAY OUT THE GLOTTIC "WELCOME MAT" (PATIENT POSITIONING, MOUTH OPENING AND TONGUE CONTROL)

As previously mentioned, preparation and training are key components of airway success. Remember that patients should ideally be positioned in an "ear to sternal notch" configuration. That configuration aligns the airway axes in order to achieve a "straight to cords" view. The process of intubation starts with opening of the mouth. Use your thumb and index finger in a scissors-like motion to force the mandible downward and maximize mouth opening. Keep your eyes on the blade as you progress toward the epiglottis. Another strategy to maximize your first-pass attempt is to ensure that the tongue is swept completely to the left of the oropharynx. A large tongue or one that "straddles" the laryngoscope blade will obscure the glottic opening. An experienced laryngoscopist can insert the blade at a 90-degree angle into the mouth. As the handle is turned upright, the flange of a Macintosh blade displaces the tongue to the left. The Macintosh blade should also fit firmly into the vallecula. Ensuring that the blade is well placed will achieve indirect elevation of the vallecula and maximize glottic exposure.

PEARLS

- Intubation starts with opening of the mouth.
- Open the mouth widely with a scissors-type technique.
- Ensure that the patient's tongue is swept completely to the left side of the mouth.
- "Seat" a curved blade firmly into the vallecula.

EXTERNAL LARYNGEAL MANIPULATION

This simple technique, described by Levitan, involves the use of the laryngoscopist's right hand. With the intubating blade in position, take your right hand and maneuver the laryngeal cartilage until familiar landmarks come into view. Frequently, external laryngeal manipulation (ELM) will help bring at least a portion of the glottic opening into your line of sight. Once a satisfactory view is achieved, replace your hand with one of your assistant's. Now, you are free to guide the tube into the opening. If available and skilled in its use, consider placement of an endotracheal tube introducer (flex guide or bougie). According to Levitan's study of first year emergency medicine residents, the ELM maneuver improved the percentage of glottis opening score in all study cases. The study described an improvement in view by an average of 57%.

CALL FOR H.E.L.P.!

During truly difficult intubations, you may be confronted with an "epiglottis-only" view. If you've adequately prepared and positioned, few options remain for this challenging scenario. The presence of additional rescuers has been shown to reduce complications associated with intubation. Now is the time to actually call for help and summon the most senior airway managers to the bedside. An ear nose and throat physician, anesthesiologist, or another experienced emergency physician may provide additional expertise. Finally, "HELP" is an acronym for the head elevated laryngoscopy position. With your blade in position, have your assistant raise the patient's head off of the stretcher. If there is little suspicion for cervical spine injury, elevation of the head may further align the airway axes and bring familiar glottic airway anatomy into better view. HELP also induces a significant degree of neck flexion. In another cadaveric study conducted by Levitan, the HELP strategy increased POGO scores from 31% to 64%.

CONCLUSIONS

Intubation is a technically complex technique that requires training and adequate preparation. Before any attempt, ensure adequate patient positioning. The patient's external auditory meatus should line up horizontally with the sternal notch. Whenever possible, the presence of additional intubators (paramedics or physicians) may help reduce complications. Pay particular attention to maximizing opening of the patient's mouth. Follow the laryngoscope blade down to the epiglottis. Seat a curved blade firmly in the vallecula and use external laryngeal manipulation to bring glottic landmarks into view. Finally, the "HELP" maneuver may optimize alignment of the airway axes. These simple, low-cost tips will assist novice and expert intubators in their management of the difficult airway.

SELECTED READINGS

Levitan RM, Mickler T, Hollander JE. Bimanual laryngoscopy: A videographic study of external laryngeal manipulation by novice intubators. *Ann Emerg Med.* 2002;40(1):30–37.

Levitan RM. Head elevated laryngoscopy position: improved laryngeal exposure during laryngoscopy by increasing head elevation. *Ann Emerg Med.* 2003;41(3):322–330.

Jaber S. An intervention to decrease complications related to endotracheal intubation in the intensive care unit: a prospective, multiple-center study. *Intensive Care Med.* 2010; 36(2):248–255.

14

Pediatric airway management: don't underestimate the value of a step-wise approach

Spencer C. Smith, MD

Most emergency medical services (EMS) have limited experience with pediatric patients, let alone advanced pediatric airway management. It is estimated that only 13% of EMS responses are for pediatric patients. Of these, many are of a respiratory nature. Yet the need and level of airway management for these patients can be quite variable. For example, the majority of pediatric cardiac arrests are due to respiratory failure. Therefore, competency in pediatric airway management is of vital importance to the prehospital provider.

There are many tools and techniques to assist with management of the pediatric airway. Importantly, one should not underestimate the calming presence of a parent or a caregiver. Sometimes, putting an already anxious and agitated infant or toddler on the lap or in the arms of a familiar family member may be enough to adequately ease a child experiencing respiratory distress. Even when additional interventions are needed, a provider would be wise to take advantage of a parent's presence. Oxygen, if needed, can frequently be given as "blow by." This is done by placing a source of oxygen flow near a patient's face without it actually touching the child. This avoids giving a non-cooperative child the sensation of being smothered by a face mask. If needed, a nasal cannula or face mask should be of appropriate size to allow for greatest comfort and cooperation. Of course, this idea applies to the delivery of nebulized medical therapies as well.

Aggressive airway management is required for the pediatric patient in respiratory failure or respiratory arrest. However, aggressive management is not always synonymous with more invasive skills and techniques. Correct placement of oral and nasal airway adjuncts is important during the delivery of bag valve mask (BVM) ventilations. When a BVM is implemented, correct positioning is vital as well as use of the correct size bag and face mask. A two-person ventilation technique is preferred if practical. Rate and volume should be adjusted according to the size of the patient. In addition, providers should be familiar with the risks of gastric distention, vomiting, and aspiration. Use of a BVM in children is a skill that all providers should master as the standard in airway management.

The difficulty of emergent endotracheal intubation of a pediatric patient is compounded by the uncontrolled setting of the field environment.

Fortunately, it is rare that a child will require intubation. Because of the relatively infrequent presentation of such patients and the rarity of pediatric intubations by any one EMS provider, the potential exists for more harm to be done than good. Providers may not have the opportunity to maintain profiecy in pediatric intubation. Pediatric prehospital intubation is a rare occurrence and the rate of successful placement is unacceptably low. Considering the harm of delayed oxygenation during intubation attempts, the delay to definitive care, the dangers of misplacing the endotracheal tube, as well as other complications of endotracheal intubation, it has been suggested that intubation of the pediatric patient may not be the best option; and that basic life support (BLS) airway management with BVM may be the appropriate course of action.

Studies comparing prehospital pediatric intubation to BVM fail to demonstrate the superiority of endotracheal intubation with respect to survival or neurologic outcome (REF). Complications also plague pediatric prehospital intubation attempts. Therefore, it makes sense to consider alternatives to endotracheal intubation. Laryngeal mask airways (LMAs) are designed for blind insertion and come in a variety of sizes. Combitubes are designated for patients greater than 4 feet tall and have limited pediatric use. The King Airway, another blind insertion airway, is limited to children greater than 12 kg. If the child is of sufficient size and these options are used, special attention should be given to securing the device to prevent tube migration with patient movement.

Experience with pediatric airway management varies greatly, depending on the demographics of a given jurisdiction. While some providers may be comfortable with their intubating skills, others may not feel so confident. Because of the enormous variability in providers' intubating skill and given the research demonstrating questionable benefit, intubation of the pediatric patient should not be taken lightly. And perhaps even more fundamental EMS providers should never underestimate the benefit of BVM ventilation. This technique is the primary means of airway management.

SELECTED READINGS

Babl F, Vinci R, Bauchner H, et al. Pediatric pre-hospital advanced life support in an urban setting. *Ped Emerg Care.* 2001;17(1):5–9.

Gausche M, Lewis RL, Stratton SJ, et al. Effect of out-of-hospital pediatric endotracheal intubation survival and neurologic outcome. *JAMA.* 2000;283:783–790.

Shah MN, Cushman JT, Davis CO, et al. The epidemiology of emergency medical services use by children: An analysis of the National Hospital Ambulatory Medical Care Survey. *Prehosp Emerg Care.* 2008;12(3):269–276.

Youngquist S, Gausche-Hill M, Burbulys D. Alternative airway devices for use in children requiring prehospital airway management: update and case discussion. *Ped Emerg Care.* 2007;23(4):250–258.

15

INTUBATION PRACTICE MAKES PERFECT: THERE'S NOT ENOUGH PRACTICE

JESSICA MANKA, NREMT-P
CYNTHIA SHEN, DO, FACOEP, FACEP

Emergency medical service (EMS) providers are obligated to maintain their education and hone the important skills necessary to manage a wide variety of airway emergencies.

A paramedic's initial training includes airway maintenance, airway monitoring, and effective oxygen delivery. A portion of this training includes learning the technique for endotracheal intubation via direct laryngoscopy. Among advanced prehospital providers, endotracheal intubation is considered the gold standard for airway control. The National Registry of Emergency Medical Technicians (NREMT) standard for live intubations for a paramedic to complete their initial training program is five intubations in the operating room. The American Heart Association has recommended that paramedics should have 6 to 12 intubations a year for "regular field experience." Strote et al. suggest that 15 to 240 intubations are required to reach "minimum proficiency" by the paramedic. One study suggests that there is only a 33% success rate in the prehospital setting when there is not a required endotracheal intubation minimum per year. Furthermore, Wang et al. conclude that endotracheal intubation success improves with live experience. It logically follows that increased training opportunities will correlate with better success rates.

Using this line of reasoning, several jurisdictions have imposed more rigid training requirements for their paramedics. Seattle requires students in the "Medic One" program to perform 20 live intubations, including two pediatric patients during training. After their initial training, Seattle medics are required to perform 12 field intubations a year. If this standard is not met, they are returned to the operating room for further remediation. These stringent requirements surely contribute to Seattle's Medic One prehospital endotracheal intubation success rate of 98.4%.

Paramedics are faced with many obstacles in real life, which are not encountered during their initial training. These challenges include poor lighting, trauma, blood, food, variable patient size, and the stress and anxiety associated with the uncontrolled chaos of a prehospital resuscitation. While these variables are impossible to recreate in the classroom setting, it is imperative that paramedics are given as many opportunities as possible to intubate a live patient. In reality, prehospital providers aren't always able to get enough field experience in endotracheal intubation. Accordingly, it is immensely important that providers take responsibility for improving their skill at endotracheal intubation. A suitable airway continuing education program might incorporate lectures, workshops, conferences, and dedicated "operating room time."

Practice does make perfect. Unfortunately, it is often necessary to obtain that experience in places other than the field. Providers should not settle for minimum airway training requirements and associate airway expertise with ongoing education. There is simply no clear-cut, minimum number of intubations required for success; EMS providers, training officers, and medical directors should take advantage of any opportunity for ongoing skills practice.

SELECTED READINGS

Burton JH, Baumann MR, Maoz T, et al. Endotracheal intubation in a rural EMS state: Procedure utilization and impact of skills maintenance guidelines. *Pre Hospital Emergency Care.* 2003;7(3):352–356.

Strote J, Roth R, Cone D, et al. Prehospital endotracheal intubation: the controversy continues. *Am J Emerg Med.* 2009;27:1142–1147.

Wang HE, Abo BN, Lave JR, et al. How would minimum experience standards affect the distribution of out-of-hospital endotracheal intubations? *Ann Emerg Med.* 2007;50(3): 246–252.

16

RSI WITHOUT PARALYTICS?
JUST DON'T DO IT

BENJAMIN J. LAWNER, DO, EMT-P, FAAEM

Without question, rapid sequence intubation (RSI) is associated with high rates of successful tracheal tube placement. Multiple studies and a wealth of emergency department experience confirm that the combination of sedation and neuromuscular blockade provides optimum intubating conditions. Dropping a tube through the cords, however, is only one part of the drug-assisted intubation puzzle. RSI has an excellent track record and has been used for decades to proactively manage at-risk airways. It is less clear, however, that the same strategy for airway control can be extended into every prehospital setting. An effective RSI program involves active medical direction, ongoing quality improvement, and a significant amount of initial and continuing education. RSI protocols, therefore, may be impractical for systems with limited advanced life support resources and oversight. Nevertheless, providers and medical directors alike struggle with the question of how best to manage the airway of a patient with intact reflexes. The patient who is combative from a head injury or who has a "clenched" jaw represents a unique challenge to prehospital providers who do not have RSI at their disposal.

If RSI remains too complex for implementation in a prototypical ALS EMS system, then why not consider the use of drugs like midazolam or etomidate? These drugs are short acting, widely available, and relatively inexpensive. Providers might wonder why they aren't authorized to administer a dose of midazolam to help "facilitate" endotracheal intubation in the semiawake patient. The administration of sedatives without paralytics is a strategy known as "sedation-facilitated intubation." Though gaining popularity in some EMS systems, it is a dangerous strategy without proven mortality benefit. RSI is the gold standard for managing the at-risk airway in a patient with intact protective reflexes. The use of sedatives as a single intubation agent introduces more risk and complexity into an already difficult situation.

WHY NOT JUST GIVE 'EM A DOSE OF VERSED?
Midazolam is a rapid-onset, short-acting benzodiazepine. It causes sedation when administered in the usual intravenous dose of 2 to 5 mg. It may relax patients sufficiently to permit orotracheal intubation and has been studied as a single agent in both prehospital and emergency department

sedation-facilitated intubation. However, midazolam has some important side effects. In one study, (15/77) or 19.5% of patients receiving midazolam for the purpose of intubation developed significant hypotension. The authors defined hypotension as a "decrease in systolic blood pressure (SBP) below 90 mm Hg or a decrease of more than 20% within five minutes" following intubation. Hypotension occurred more frequently in patients younger than 70 years of age. Another study by Davis et al. corroborates the association between midazolam, hypotension, and drug-assisted intubation. The authors postulate, however, that the degree of hypotension may be dose related. It is commonly accepted that even a single episode of hypotension in the brain-injured patient is associated with a poorer prognosis. Furthermore, it is unclear whether or not single-dose midazolam results in higher rates of successful tube placement. Using conservative estimates, success rates for emergency physicians and paramedics who are sufficiently experienced in RSI are estimated at upward of 95%. Pooled intubation success rates for paramedics vary considerably, but a study by Wang et al. estimates success at 80% to 90%. Ideally, the addition of a drug to any intubation algorithm should result in either improved success or fewer complications. Midazolam has performed poorly in the prehospital setting. In a prospective study by Jacoby et al., the overall intubation success rate for midazolam is reported at 75%. Wang examined the use of midazolam as a "pharmacologic adjunct" to endotracheal intubation and described success rates of 62.5%. The bottom line here is that midazolam is not a "magic bullet" for intubation. Though the drug may help ablate protective airway reflexes, its utilization does not result in success rates similar to those achieved with standard RSI medications. Furthermore, hypotension may occur even at small doses (2 to 4 mg) used for sedation.

WHAT ABOUT ETOMIDATE?

Etomidate is another short-acting sedative medication that rapidly induces unconsciousness. It is regarded as a hemodynamically "friendly" drug in that it is less likely to cause cardiovascular instability or hypotension. Many emergency physicians are familiar with this agent and incorporate it into emergency department-based protocols for RSI. Several authors have examined etomidate as a single agent for prehospital intubation. The Jacoby trial, which prospectively randomized patients to receive either etomidate or midazolam for intubation, reported a 76% success rate. Interestingly, 7/55 (13%) of patients vomited following etomidate administration. None of the patients in the midazolam group experienced emesis. Bozeman and Young described success rates of 89% when etomidate was administered by aeromedical providers. Etomidate-associated masseter muscle spasm occurred in 3/5 patients for whom intubation was unsuccessful. Etomidate is a valuable addition to the intubation arsenal but has important limitations when employed as a single agent.

IS THERE A ROLE FOR SEDATION-FACILITATED INTUBATION?

Generally speaking, there is insufficient evidence to recommend the use of sedatives alone to facilitate intubation in the prehospital setting. When used as a sole agent, neither midazolam nor etomidate result in improved success or better patient outcomes. Even more concerning is the fact that hypotension has been linked to single-dose midazolam administration. Though these drugs may induce sedation and relax a clenched jaw, they may not sufficiently relax the vocal cords. Inducing unconsciousness in a critically ill patient is a risky practice. If the goal is placement of an endotracheal tube, then it makes sense to create the best possible changes for first-pass success. Sedation without paralysis may place your patient at risk for a failed intubation.

SELECTED READINGS

Bozeman WP, Young S. Etomidate as a sole agent for endotracheal intubation in the prehospital air medical setting. *Air Med J.* 2002;21(4):32–35.

Choi YF, Wong TW, Lau CC. Midazolam is more likely to cause hypotension than etomidate in emergency department rapid sequence intubation. *Emerg Med J.* 2004;21:700–702.

Davis DP, Kimbro TA, Vilke GM. The use of midazolam for prehospital rapid sequence intubation may be associated with a dose-related increase in hypotension. *Prehosp Emerg Care.* 2001;5(2):163–168.

Jacoby J, Heller M, Nicholas J, et al. Etomidate versus midazolam for out of hospital intubation: a prospective, randomized trial. *Ann Emerg Med.* 2006;47(6):525–530.

Wang HE, Kupas DF, Paris PM, et al. Multivariate predictors of failed prehospital endotracheal intubation. *Acad Emerg Med.* 2003;10(7):717–724.

17

TANTALIZINGLY TANGIBLE TECHNIQUES
FOR TELEGRAPHING THE TOUGH TUBE

P. MARC FISCHER, MBA, NREMT-P
KEVIN G. SEAMAN, MD, FACEP

Managing the airway of a high-acuity patient is a critically important skill for an EMS provider to master, and the exceptional EMS provider remains mindful of the following tips to avoid being surprised by a difficult airway:

- Not evaluating the airway prior to advanced life support (ALS) airway management
- Not using a simple/easy system to predict and plan for difficult airways
- Proceeding to RSI in either the predicted or not predicted difficult airway

According to the American Society of Anesthesiology, the difficult airway can be divided into two subsets:

- *Difficulty with mask ventilations (or failure to ventilate)*—measured by the provider's inability to maintain an SpO_2 of greater than 90% using a bag valve mask (when the patient's initial O_2 saturation was normal)
- Difficulty with intubation (difficult laryngoscopy, difficult ET tube placement, and/or failure to intubate)—as measured by the provider's inability to place an endotracheal tube within 10 minutes or three attempts. *(This benchmark has been established for anesthesiologists in a controlled environment for elective procedures. This is likely to be an unrealistic expectation for EMS providers attempting emergency airway management procedures for a patient who is decompensating.)*

How does a prehospital provider telegraph the difficult airway? There are several different assessment models to evaluate the patient's airway and to predict with great accuracy the difficulty associated with managing that airway, but airway management experts have focused on a select few methods as the "gold standard" for classification/identification of potential airway catastrophes.

During the initial response and the first few moments of patient care, the exceptional EMS provider should quickly and thoroughly evaluate any factors that could negatively impact the patient's airway. For example, the provider should have a "high index of suspicion" that patients who have respiratory burns, anaphylaxis, vomitus, hemorrhage, reactive airway diseases and a host of other ailments and injuries are highly likely to possess a difficult airway. In addition, patient factors (such as obesity, advanced age, presence of facial hair [beard or goatee], lack of teeth, and history of snoring) also predict a difficult airway. The EMS provider will prepare accordingly to manage a difficult airway—long before the patient begins to deteriorate.

As part of that assessment, the EMS provider should develop the habit of evaluating the oropharyngeal structures of all of his/her patients, but especially of those who are (or have the potential to become) high-acuity patients. The most commonly used method to assess the patient's oropharynx is the Mallampati classification, a simple, non-invasive predictive scheme in which the provider evaluates the size and position of the patient's tongue in relationship to the other airway structures and then assigns one of four gradations to predict the difficulty of managing the patient's airway. The process is straightforward: Ask the patient to open his/her mouth and observe the oropharynx to sort the patient into one of the four classes. Intubation is predicted to be progressively more difficult from Mallampati Class I to IV *(Fig. 17.1)*.

In the prehospital environment, it may not be possible to evaluate the patient using the Mallampati classification system because this assessment tool requires an awake, cooperative patient. Furthermore, there are questions about the score's applicability to the emergency medicine and prehospital setting. In many cases, the EMS provider may encounter a patient in extremis who requires immediate ALS intervention. In those situations, the first opportunity to recognize the difficult airway will occur under direct laryngoscopy just prior to intubation. Cormack and Lehane use a similar four-class evaluation system to evaluate the glottic opening, and

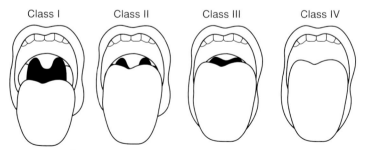

| Class I | Class II | Class III | Class IV |

FIGURE 17.1. Samsoon and Young modification of Mallampati classification, evaluating relative size of oropharyngeal structures in order to predict difficulty in laryngeal exposure during direct laryngoscopy. Higher class number suggests greater difficulty in glottic exposure (reprinted with permission by Blackwell Science, Ltd. (9)).

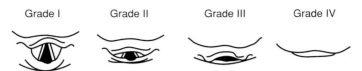

FIGURE 17.2. Grades of laryngeal exposure (reprinted with permission by Blackwell Science, Ltd. (9)).

this grading system also correlates directly with intubation success—the lower the classification, the easier the intubation *(Fig. 17.2)*. The Cormack and Lehane evaluation technique is further defined in the article "Glottic Visualization: Making the First Pass the Best Pass."

More recently, the "percent of glottic opening" (POGO) evaluation method has been introduced as a proposed enhancement of the original Cormack and Lehane model. This method also requires the provider to visualize the glottic opening under direct laryngoscopy in order to evaluate the patient's POGO score. The measurements fall under one of four classifications:

- Grade I: Full visualization of the patient's glottic opening—very common—easily managed by the competent provider
- Grade II: Partial visualization of the patient's glottic opening—very common—managed by the competent provider, sometimes with the assistance of intubation adjuncts (like a bougie)
- Grade III: Almost no visualization of the patient's glottic opening—uncommon—difficult intubation
- Grade IV: No visualization of the patient's glottic opening—uncommon—very difficult intubation

In those cases where advanced airway management is likely to be required, the patient should also be evaluated using the "Rule of Threes," another noninvasive way to predict the difficulty of the potential intubation. With this technique, the provider uses the width of three fingers to measure three critical airway dimensions:

- The distance between the upper and lower teeth with the patient's mouth open as wide as possible
- The distance between the hyoid bone and the mandibular genu (essentially from the top of the neck to the chin on the underside of the patient's lower jaw)
- The distance between the sternal notch and the thyroid cartilage

Direct laryngoscopy is more likely to result in success when the critical dimensions total three or more finger widths.

Using these evaluation techniques, the EMS provider is equipped/prepared to predict the difficult airway—long before the laryngoscope and ET tube are prepared for use. However, the exceptional EMS provider should remain vigilant—even when all of the predictors indicate otherwise—for the difficult airway, and he/she should be prepared with the equipment and training to manage even the most challenging airway in the emergency setting.

SELECTED READINGS

Caplan RA, Benumof JL, Berry FA, et al. Practice guidelines for management of the difficult airway: a report by the ASA task force on the management of the difficult airway. *Anesth.* 1993;78:597–602.

Cormack RS, Lehane J. Difficult tracheal intubation in obstetrics. *Anaesthesia.* 1984;39:1105.

Levitan RM. Salvaging the difficult airway – a practical approach. http://www.femf.org/education/ClinCon01/Levitan.htm.

Levitan R, Ochtroch EA, Kush S. Validation of the percentage of glottic opening (POGO) Score. *Acad Emerg Med.* 1998;5:482.

Mallampati SR. Clinical signs to predict difficult tracheal intubation (Hypothesis). *Can Anaesth Soc J.* 1983;30:316–318.

Orebaugh SL. Difficult airway management in the emergency development. *J Emerg Med.* 2002;22:31–48.

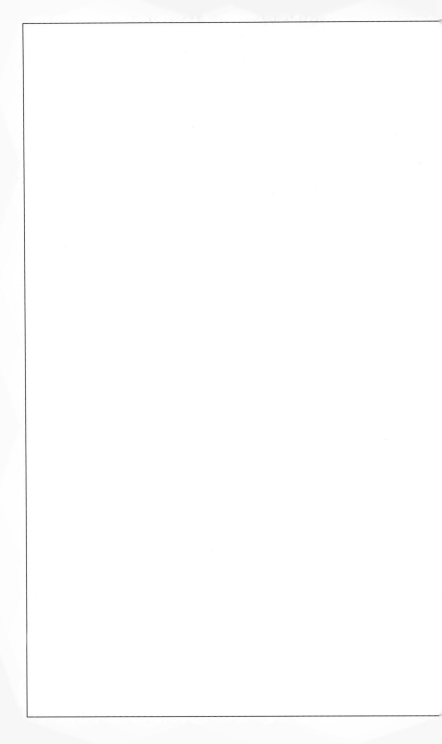

18

Avoid becoming a patient when transporting one

Jeremy Brywczynski, MD
Jared J. McKinney, MD

Prehospital providers are specially trained to care for, manage, and treat a variety of medical illness under less than ideal conditions on a daily basis. Most enter this profession in order to selflessly provide the earliest care and first contact with the community's sickest patients. However, providers must remember that personal protection and safety are paramount and should never be compromised. Whenever you are transporting a patient with cough, fever, or other respiratory symptoms, you must take all steps necessary to avoid exposure to common pathogens and becoming a patient yourself.

Perhaps the most important action that should be taken by any paramedic responding to the scene of a medical emergency with potential infectious disease exposure is the utilization of appropriate personal protective equipment (PPE) to prevent accidental exposure to contaminated patients. Approach every patient as if they are a potential reservoir for transmission of illness by coughing or sneezing. Proper training, fit testing, and storage of equipment such as particulate filtering (N-95) masks, gloves, powdered respirators, gowns, hoods, and eye protection are essential, as these items will likely be utilized in cases of infectious outbreaks.

Accidental exposure is a very high risk whenever you are transporting patients with respiratory illness. The coughing or sneezing patient often warrants nebulizations, suctioning, oxygen application, and possibly advanced airway procedures that are performed with virtual direct contact with the patient's secretions. In addition, most procedures are performed in the back of a moving ambulance, making exposure to droplets and other respiratory secretions much more common. When in doubt, always wear an N-95, eye protection, and gloves when treating these patients. Remember, the paramedic serves as a role model for other members of the healthcare team. Less experienced EMS providers may erroneously think that being splashed by blood or coughed upon is a "badge of honor." Ensure that this does not occur and always stress personal safety first.

There are many serious and potentially life-altering or life-ending diseases that have the potential to be spread to providers during treatment and transportation. Tuberculosis (TB) is one of the greatest threats to public health in the United States. Worldwide, there are 2 billion people infected, with 3 million deaths a year attributable to active TB. TB is caused by the bacterium *Mycobacterium tuberculosis*, which is spread by respiratory droplets. Symptoms of pulmonary TB include fever, weight loss, hemoptysis, and night sweats. TB should always be suspected in patients with these symptoms and PPE used for the entire patient contact and treatment. Prevention is as simple as wearing a NIOSH-approved (National Institute for Occupational Safety and Health) N-95 particulate filter mask. EMTs and paramedics can also decrease their chances of an occupational exposure developing into a full-blown illness by undergoing yearly PPD skin testing in accordance with local health provider statutes.

Another serious illness in which the paramedic must prevent personal exposure is that of meningococcal meningitis. This disease is caused by the bacterium *Neisseria meningitidis* and causes a devastating infection of the central nervous system (CNS) called meningitis. Meningococcus is also spread by respiratory droplets and colonizes the mucosa of the oropharynx. This illness develops quickly with sudden onset of fever, headache, neck stiffness, rash, shock, and death. Patients suspected of this illness must immediately be isolated. Facemask and shields should be worn. If exposed to the secretions of the patient with suspected meningitis, notify your healthcare representative immediately as prophylactic antibiotics are mandatory.

The most common respiratory pathogen that EMS personnel will be exposed to while caring for a patient is influenza. It is also spread by respiratory droplets but can survive on surfaces for hours. Symptoms of influenza include fever, rhinorrhea, cough, myalgias, nausea, and possibly vomiting. Typically, elderly patients and the very young are at increased risk of complications including pneumonia, sepsis, and death. This viral outbreak usually occurs yearly in the winter months extending into the early fall. Some strains are more severe than others, and changes in the virus characteristics can lead to mutation causing more severe outbreaks on occasion. Paramedics should be wary of influenza during the winter months and should practice universal precautions, including wearing facemasks, when contacting patients suspected as having influenza. If a patient is suspected of having influenza, nebulizer use should be minimized to decrease disease spread. Due to survival of the virus on surfaces, disinfection of the ambulance will also be necessary after transport of the patient. Yearly, the Centers for Disease Control (CDC) produces a vaccine that attempts to predict the strain that will be most prominent that season and cause the most illness. It is imperative that paramedics and all prehospital providers get vaccinated against influenza every year.

In conclusion, the paramedic places himself or herself in the line of potential exposure to communicable respiratory diseases such as TB, meningococcus, and influenza on a daily basis. The provider must remember that personal protection always comes before any patient care, and ignoring the use of PPE in the line of duty is not acceptable.

SUGGESTED READINGS

Centers for Disease Control. Prevention and Control of Meningococcal Disease: Recommendations of the Advisory Committee on Immunization Practices (ACIP). *Morbidity and Mortality Weekly Report: Surveillance Summaries*. 1997;46(RR-5):1–21.

Centers for Disease Control and Prevention. Epidemilogy and Prevention of Vaccine-Preventable Disease. Pp. 173–192. Atkinson W, Wolfe S, Hamborsky J, eds. 12th ed. Washington DC: Public Health Foundation, 2011.

Chapleau W, Burba A, Pons P, Page D. *The Paramedic*. McGraw-Hill Higher Education; 2009.

Dye C, Scheele S, Dolin P, et al. Consensus statement: global burden of tuberculosis: estimated incidence, prevalence, and mortality by country. WHO Global Surveillance Monitoring Project. *JAMA*. 1999;282(7):677–686.

Kyle SN. NHTSA releases EMS pandemic influenza guidelines. *EMS Mag*. 2007;36(11):52.

Rebmann T, Coll B. 2009 APIC Emergency Preparedness Committee. Infection prevention at points of dispensing. *Am J Infect Control*. 2009;37(9):695–702.

Tippett VC, Watt K, Raven SG, et al. Anticipated behaviors of emergency prehospital medical care providers during an influenza pandemic. *Prehosp Disaster Med*. 2010;25(1):20–25.

19

KNOW THE DOWNFALLS OF HYPERVENTILATION AND POSITIVE PRESSURE IN THE INTUBATED PATIENT

JEFFREY M. GOODLOE, MD, NREMT-P, FACEP

An essential concept to both understand and apply in the field revolves around the importance of avoiding hyperventilation in an already intubated patient. It is the mark of an EMS novice to believe that if a patient is intubated, they must have a serious enough illness or injury to require as much oxygenation and ventilation as possible. One can make the assumption that if normal people increase their minute ventilation and tidal volume with exertion and stress, so should the ill patient in respiratory failure requiring intubation. This is a false assumption.

Avoiding hyperventilation in the intubated patient does not make obvious sense until you think about the key words being "inhale" and "blow," and the significant differences between them in describing how air and oxygen are transported into the lungs. More specifically, it's the difference in the pressure effect of inhaling as compared to blowing that makes hyperventilating the intubated patient an error to avoid.

When one inhales, air travels fairly easily into the lungs from the atmosphere due to the negative pressure created in the chest when the diaphragm contracts. This air, which contains 21% oxygen, naturally flows from spaces with higher pressures (outside the body) to spaces with lower pressures (inside the thoracic cavity) when the diaphragm contracts. This is why ventilation and oxygenation at rest, or even at exercise, occurs without conscious thought.

When a prehospital provider "inhales" for someone else by applying ventilations via bag valve mask (BVM) or endotracheal tube, the negative pressure of a normal inhalation is replaced by positive pressure ventilation. Thus, it's not the increase in oxygen we want to avoid in the intubated patient; it's the excessive positive pressure and aggressive ventilations.

In the confined space of the thoracic cavity, positive pressure compresses compressible structures including veins. The vena cava itself can be compressed by overinflated lungs. Reliable scientific studies demonstrate that the faster, harder, and longer patients are ventilated, the more venous return decreases to the heart and lungs. The more the patient is ventilated, the higher the pressure within the lungs. This high intrathoracic pressure will impair venous return to the central circulation and lower cardiac output along with the patient's blood pressure. A simple "pump" rule applies here; the heart can't push out what the heart doesn't receive in. This applies to all forward-flow circulation, even in the coronary arteries where this may cause a decrease in coronary perfusion pressure. Any decrease in coronary artery blood flow can be dangerous as it is now well established that optimizing coronary perfusion pressure is a critical element in successfully resuscitating victims of sudden cardiac arrest.

Whenever one is dealing with a critically ill patient, it is imperative to remember that both ventilation and perfusion are inter-related. If the EMS provider is dealing with a patient in either cardiac arrest or shock, perfusion is already severely compromised or totally absent. One must carefully balance needed oxygenation with unneeded pressure effects accompanying that oxygen in these patients.

The prehospital provider must realize that it is not just the rate of ventilation that has to be controlled; it's also the duration and amount of each of those ventilations. For example, if one ventilates a patient in respiratory failure at 8 to 10 breaths per minute and takes 3 seconds to deliver each of those ventilations, almost half of every minute working to improve circulation is compromised by the positive pressure itself. If not enough time is devoted to allowing a full exhalation, "breath stacking" occurs and may cause auto-peep. That is, if 400 mL of air is "pushed" into the lung during each ventilation and only 390 mL is exhaled, then 10 mL will be added to the patient's lung residual volume. Within 10 breaths, 100 mL of extra air will accumulate in the lungs, and within 5 to 10 minutes an extra 500 to 1,000 mL may cause hypotension, inability to bag easily, a tension pneumothorax, or even cardiac arrest.

It is a careful and delicate balance that the paramedic must be aware of in the treatment of the intubated patient or one being ventilated by a BVM apparatus. Avoiding hyperventilation may sound simple, but as the provider's adrenaline levels increase, so does the rate of ventilations. Avoiding this error requires "thinking it through" before the call and focusing on accurate ventilation rates during the resuscitation.

SUGGESTED READINGS

Aufderheide TP. The problem with and benefit of ventilations: should our approach be the same in cardiac and respiratory arrest? *Curr Opin Crit Care.* 2006;12(3):207–212.

Berg RA, Hemphill R, Abella BS, et al. Part 5: adult basic life support: 2010 American Heart Association Guidelines for Cardiopulmonary Resuscitation and Emergency Cardiovascular Care. *Circulation.* 2010;122(18 Suppl 3):S685–S705.

Pepe PE, Raedler C, Lurie KG, et al. Emergency ventilatory management in hemorrhagic states: elemental or detrimental. *J Trauma.* 2003;54:1048–1057.

20

HEMOPTYSIS: BE CAREFUL OF JUST A LITTLE BLOOD!

BENJAMIN W. WEBSTER, MD

Hemoptysis, or the coughing of blood from below the vocal cords, is a reason for people to seek emergency care by activating the emergency response system. Hemoptysis can range from minor to massive, with massive hemoptysis defined as anywhere from greater than 100 mL to 600 mL of blood over a 24-hour period. While massive hemoptysis only accounts for a minority of cases, it carries a mortality rate of 80% and must be treated expertly and expeditiously. There are many causes of hemoptysis, and the most common varies widely based on region, socioeconomics, and age. However, hemoptysis from an underlying infectious or inflammatory process like pneumonia or bronchitis accounts for most cases (60% to 70%). Lung cancer accounts for about 20%, with other miscellaneous causes such as heart failure, pulmonary embolism, cocaine-induced pulmonary hemorrhage, trauma, and coagulopathies (e.g., anticoagulant use, advanced liver disease) comprising the remaining. Although the patient may state he or she coughed up the blood, it is important to consider other sources of bleeding, such as gastrointestinal sources, a nose bleed, or from bleeding gums, all which can easily be mistaken for hemoptysis.

When caring for a patient with hemoptysis in the prehospital arena, there are three basic tenets to always remember: (1) protect yourself, (2) prepare for the worst, and (3) communicate with the team.

First, *always protect yourself*. While universal precautions should always be employed, it is of utmost importance when caring for a patient with hemoptysis. Infection is the leading cause of hemoptysis, and patients with HIV infection are susceptible to a number of the causative infections. Although bronchitis and common bacterial pneumonias are still more common in patients with HIV infection and those with AIDS, other agents such as tuberculosis and fungal infections also occur and can infect the EMS provider. Patients may also have hemoptysis secondary to an underlying coagulopathy or bleeding disorder that has developed from liver dysfunction from hepatitis. The underlying hepatitis is a potential blood and body fluid exposure risk to the provider.

It is very important to remember that when evaluating a patient with hemoptysis, always wear gloves, cover broken skin, and wear a face shield that adequately protects your mouth, nose, and eyes. In 2010, the Center for Disease Control and Prevention and the National Institute for Occupational

Safety and Health presented data from a survey of more than 2,600 paramedics regarding exposure to blood. More than 80% of paramedics had access to safety goggles and masks, yet those reporting exposure failed to use the provided gear. Even more alarming, less than half of those exposed reported the exposure to their medical supervision and therefore did not receive appropriate medical care. If you do not have access to the appropriate protective equipment, demand it. If you have access to protective gear, use it. If you are exposed, report it. Keep yourself safe.

Second, *prepare for the worst.* While as little as 5% of patients with hemoptysis have massive life-threatening bleeding, the distinction is very subjective and difficult to quantify early in the course of patient care and transport. What appears as minor bleeding at any given point in time can rapidly progress to florid hemorrhage without warning. Do not make the mistake of being ill-prepared should a patient begin to deteriorate and begin to cough up larger quantities of blood and develop airway compromise. Make sure to have good suction set-up and readily available. Obtain early IV access, preferably two large bore lines. In massive hemoptysis, however, patients typically die from asphyxiation, not exsanguination. As patients aspirate blood into other areas of the lung, they become progressively hypoxemic. In this situation, the priority is oxygenation. Provide high-flow oxygen via non-rebreather mask. Prepare for a difficult airway. Have all airway adjuncts immediately available (e.g., oropharyngeal airway, LMA, King LT^{TM}) for use until a definitive airway can be established. If these measures fail and endotracheal intubation becomes necessary, a large bore endotracheal tube (8.0) should be used to facilitate oxygen delivery and emergent bronchoscopy once at the hospital.

Lastly, *communicate with the hospital.* The critically ill hemoptysis patient is not only difficult to manage in the field, but very complex and complicated in the emergency department. Often, advanced airway equipment is required and definitive management requires prompt radiographic evaluation and a multidisciplinary approach involving the emergency, pulmonary, thoracic surgery, and interventional radiology teams. Early communication with the receiving hospital allows the staff to begin mobilizing resources and locating the appropriate teams.

When evaluating, treating, and transporting a patient with hemoptysis, remembering these three tenets will help to provide focused, safe, and effective care. Always protect yourself first. Do not become a patient from an avoidable exposure. Always prepare for the worst. Be careful of just a little blood as a patient can deteriorate at any time. Always communicate with the team. Ultimate care of a patient with hemoptysis requires advanced technology and a multidisciplinary approach.

SELECTED READINGS

Bidwell J, Pachner R. Hemoptysis: diagnosis and management. *Am Fam Physician.* 2005;72:1253–1260.

Brown CA. Chapter 31: hemoptysis. In: Marx JA, Hockberger RS, Walls RM, et al., eds. *Rosen's Emergency Medicine: Concepts and Clinical Practice.* 7th ed. Philadelphia, PA: Mosby Elsevier; 2010.

Hirshberg B, Birna I, Glazer M, et al. Hemoptysis: etiology, evaluation, and outcome in a tertiary referral hospital. *Chest.* 1997;112:440–444.

Johnson JL. Manifestations of hemoptysis: how to manage minor, moderate, and massive bleeding. *Postgrad Med.* 2002;112(4):101.

Nelson JE, Forman M. Hemoptysis in HIV-infected patients. *Chest.* 1997;110:737–743.

Preventing exposures to bloodborne pathogens among paramedics. Department of Health and Human Services. DHHS (NIOSH) Publication No. 2010-139. http://www.cdc.gov/niosh/docs/wp-solutions/2010-139/.

Young JE. Chapter 66: hemoptysis. In: Tintinalli JE, Stapczynski JS, Cline DM, et al. eds. *Tintinalli's Emergency Medicine: A Comprehensive Study Guide.* 7th ed. China: McGraw-Hill; 2011.

21

FEAR THE TRACHEOSTOMY PATIENT!

CHRISTOPHER B. COLWELL, MD

A tracheostomy is a surgical procedure in which an opening is created between cartilaginous rings in the trachea and a tube is inserted, usually for the purpose of long-term airway management. Most tracheostomy tubes will have an inner and outer cannula and are inserted through the opening in the neck called the stoma. The removable inner cannula allows secretions to be cleared from the lumen without removing the entire tube from the trachea.

Patients with tracheostomy tubes come to the attention of prehospital providers for a variety of reasons. Some of the more common reasons include obstruction, dislodgement, and bleeding at the tracheostomy site. It is helpful to know the reason the patient has a tracheostomy and how long it has been in place whenever possible. Patients who have undergone a laryngectomy, or who have tumors or scarring that occlude the upper airway, cannot be orally intubated, which is crucial information to have. If the tracheostomy is new, particularly 3 days old or less, the stoma has a much greater chance of closing if the outer cannula is removed. This also increases the probability of replacing the cannula into a "false lumen," or into the subcutaneous tissues as opposed to the airway itself. If the tracheostomy is older and "mature" (months to years), the stoma opening may become smaller over time, and a smaller tracheostomy tube or endotracheal tube may be necessary.

Obstruction of the tracheostomy tube can occur, most commonly due to mucous plugging. For a number of reasons, patients with tracheostomy tubes will often have an increase in the production of mucous in the airway. When excess dried mucous is produced and not cleared, the accumulation can develop into a plug and occlude the airway. The approach to the patient who may have an occluded tracheostomy tube will be similar to the approach with any patient with respiratory complaints. When assessing the airway, if there is inadequate air exchange or a complete obstruction, you will need to insert a suction catheter and attempt to suction the airway, or remove the inner cannula of the tracheostomy tube. Removal of the inner cannula will often resolve an obstruction problem as it is this inner cannula that is most commonly clogged. If this does not resolve the problem, the next step is to deflate the cuff. This alone may allow for passage of air through the upper airway. If the problem is still not corrected, you will need to remove the outer cannula as well. To remove the outer cannula, be sure the balloon is completely deflated and cut the tracheal tie, which will allow you to then easily remove the tracheostomy tube. This can be replaced with another tracheostomy tube if available (have the same size tube and the next smaller size if possible) or an endotracheal tube that will generally have to be half a size smaller than the tracheostomy tube that was removed. Tracheostomy tubes should only be removed in emergent situations as it may be difficult to insert a new airway. This is most especially true when dealing with newly performed tracheostomies.

Displacement of a tracheostomy tube may be handled in a very similar manner. Forceful coughing, pulling of the ventilator tubing, patient movements, obese necks, and low stoma placement can all lead to displacement of tracheostomy tubes. If the patient has a patent upper airway, supplemental oxygen should be delivered by non-rebreather mask while placing an occlusive dressing over the tracheal stoma. Intubating the upper airway may be necessary. If the patient has an obstructed upper airway, the tracheostomy tube will need to be replaced. In the meantime, you can ventilate the stoma using a neonatal or pediatric mask attached to a bag-mask device. Again, when replacing a tracheostomy tube, be prepared to use the next smaller size if necessary. If you do not have a tracheostomy tube available, some patients will have a backup tracheostomy tube set at home for these types of emergencies. Once again, an endotracheal tube is an option to use in these situations as well. Blind, forceful attempts at tracheostomy tube reinsertion, particularly in newer tracheostomies, can result in the creation and intubation of a false lumen.

Bleeding at the tracheostomy site is another problem you may encounter in the field. In most cases, bleeding results from erosion of tissue around the tracheostomy tube, but can also be caused by erosion of the internal end of the tube into major vessels in the neck. What may appear to be minor or insignificant bleeding can be a warning of a major, life-threatening bleed that is about to occur. It is important to recognize the potential for serious bleeding in tracheostomy patients and transport all patients with bleeding complaints to the hospital whenever possible. Slow bleeding originating from the stoma may be controlled by packing the site with saline-soaked gauze. In extreme situations, bleeding within the trachea can sometimes be temporarily controlled by placing an endotracheal tube either through the stoma or orally, and then inflating the cuff at the site of the bleeding.

A good rule of thumb when caring for patients with tracheostomy tubes is to leave the tube alone whenever possible. When your patient's situation requires intervention, it will be important to know the essentials discussed here in order to provide the appropriate care. Always contact medical control as soon as possible to advise the receiving hospital of the nature of the tracheostomy problem.

SUGGESTED READINGS

Casserly P, Lang E, Fenton JE, et al. Assessment of healthcare professionals' knowledge of managing emergency complications in patients with a tracheostomy. *Br J Anaesth.* 2007;99:380–383.

Theodore PR. Emergent management of malignancy-related acute airway obstruction. *Emerg Med Clin North Am.* 2009;27(2):231–241.

Zeitouni A, Kost K. Tracheostomy: a retrospective review of 281 patients. *J Otolaryngol.* 1994;23:61–66.

22

DON'T ASSUME THE PULSE OXIMETER IS PERFECT!

KAREN WANGER, MD

Oxygen saturation is frequently referred to as the "5th vital sign" in the growing list of what prehospital providers measure and assess in their course of patient care. Pulse oximeters are ubiquitous, and while the O_2 saturation measurements are very useful, these machines have limitations, and thus, there are important pitfalls to avoid. Good decisions based on the "pulse ox" reading come from an understanding of how an oximeter functions and what the reading indicates.

Standard pulse oximeters emit red and infrared light. The frequencies correspond to those absorbed by deoxyhemoglobin (unbound) and oxyhemoglobin (bound with O_2). The oximetry unit measures the relative absorption of the two frequencies of light across the digit and calculates the oxygen saturation. This calculation is based on reference values obtained from a healthy volunteer study; this limits the accuracy and utility of oximetry once a patient's O_2 saturation falls below 70%. There are multiple other factors that can affect the O_2 reading such as abnormal hemoglobins, the presence of nail polish (especially blue, green, and black), hypotension, hypothermia, vasoconstriction, and fluorescent or xenon lamps. It is also important to be able to distinguish an accurate waveform from one that is seen with motion artifact—a common cause of error which can lead to inappropriate patient management.

As mentioned above, abnormal hemoglobin can cause inaccurate pulse oximeter readings. Remember that the machine *calculates* the oxygenation saturation; it doesn't directly measure it, and it does the calculation based on the absorption of red and infrared light. Abnormal hemoglobins absorb similar frequencies of light, which can lead to falsely high- or low-oxygen saturation readings that can lead a prehospital care provider down a dangerous path of assuming the patient is less ill than they truly may be. Carboxyhemoglobin absorbs the same frequency as oxyhemoglobin, or "normal" hemoglobin. Thus, carbon monoxide–poisoned patients have falsely elevated oxygen saturation readings when the patient is actually oxygen deprived and hypoxic at the tissue level.

EMS providers must remember that even with high carbon monoxide levels, a normal or near-normal oxygen saturation may be displayed on the monitor.

Methemoglobinemia, a result of abnormal iron oxidation in the heme ring of hemoglobin, absorbs the same frequency as oxy and deoxyhemoglobin and will also cause inaccurate pulse oximetry readings. Many over-the-counter and prescription drugs can predispose a patient to this condition. Methemoglobinemia will cause falsely low pulse oximetry readings (which do not improve with supplemental oxygen administration), which often display around 85% to 88%. This condition is easily treatable if one remembers how pulse oximetry readings interpret and display this condition.

Another significant potential pitfall in the interpretation of O_2 saturation readings is to assume it provides accurate information on patient ventilation status. Oxygen saturation can remain high as ventilation deteriorates and the pCO_2 silently rises, especially in patients who are receiving supplemental oxygen. This is very important to remember with respect to disease processes affecting ventilation but not oxygenation, such as asthma and COPD. Young healthy asthmatics with otherwise normal lungs can progress far into ventilatory failure before their O_2 saturation starts to fall. The falling O_2 saturation is a late occurrence and signals impending respiratory failure.

A final potential pitfall in the use of pulse oximetry is using it to determine a patient's heart rate. It's tempting, but the machines are not designed to perform this assessment accurately. The pulse reading that is performed by the oximeter is only designed to assess if the machine is picking up a pulse accurately enough for the saturation reading to be reliable.

The patient's pulse has to be taken manually; a pulse oximeter is not a substitute.

As an example, in extreme tachycardias there can be variable cardiac output, with the oximeter picking up only every few beats. A reading of 75 might actually be reflecting the real atrial flutter rate of 150 or even 300. In those cases where the pulse oximeter is picking up the same pulse rate as the manual reading, it can be used as a monitor, with changes manually verified.

In conclusion, while pulse oximetry is an incredibly useful tool for patient monitoring, it is important to understand how to appropriately interpret the O_2 saturation in the context of the patient's clinical presentation. Providers must be knowledgeable of oximetry's limitations when assessing a patient needing prehospital provider care and transport.

SELECTED READINGS

Limmer D, Mistovich JJ, Krost WS. Beyond the basics: respiratory assessment & diagnosis. *Emerg Med Serv.* 2006;35(2):67–73.

McMorrow RC, Mythen MG. Pulse oximetry. *Curr Opin Crit Care.* 2006;12(3):269–271.

Sinex JE. Pulse oximetry: Principles and limitations. *Am J Emerg Med.* 1999;17(1):59–67.

23

BEWARE THE INTUBATED PATIENT!

JARED J. MCKINNEY, MD
JEREMY BRYWCZYNSKI, MD

Paramedics must be expert at intubation as it is a critical intervention that is not often performed by most health care providers. Airway and intubation expertise involves not only the process of ventilating and then passing the endotracheal tube (ETT), but also managing the patient who is now intubated. This specifically includes the ability to rapidly identify causes of decompensation after intubation in a rapid, stepwise approach. Failure to do so will quickly result in a hypoxic arrest and potentially a dead patient. A quick pneumonic to remember when evaluating a crashing intubated patient is **DOPE: D**isplaced ETT, **O**bstructed ETT, **P**neumothorax, and **E**quipment failure.

One of the biggest errors during intubation and the postintubation period is the failure to recognize a misplaced or dislodged endotracheal tube. Intubation in the prehospital environment is often done under suboptimal conditions. Commonly used clinical findings to confirm ETT placement include visualization of the tube passing through the vocal cords, fogging or misting in the tube, chest rise, and bilateral breath sounds with no sounds over the epigastrium are not accurate enough to prevent esophageal placement and are often difficult in the field where there is poor lighting and significant background noise. It has been shown in multiple studies that 5% to 10% of endotracheal tubes placed in the field are esophageal, with some studies demonstrating as high as a 25% misplaced ETT rate. The difficulty with intubation in the field does not stop there. Once intubated, patients undergo multiple moves from the scene to the stretcher, stretcher to the ambulance, and then again when patients are placed on the hospital gurney. Each time a patient is moved there is a potential for dislodgement of the ETT. Worse yet, tube displacement may go unrecognized until the patient acutely decompensates. Both of the above errors can be mitigated by the use of $ETCO_2$ monitoring. This can be done with colorimetric $ETCO_2$ detectors or continuous $ETCO_2$ waveform capnography.

Two other complications that can occur in the intubated patient that must be rapidly recognized include tube obstruction and pneumothorax. Obstruction of the endotracheal tube can occur as a result of a kink or plugging. A clue to the presence of an obstruction is increasing resistance with manual ventilation. Attempts can be made to clear the obstruction by placing a suction catheter. If the obstruction cannot be relieved, it may be necessary to pull the ETT and ventilate with a bag valve mask. Pneumothorax is also a risk whenever patients are ventilated with positive pressure. Patients with COPD and asthma are of particular concern as they often have increased intrathoracic pressure as a result of air trapping. EMS providers must quickly assess breath sounds in the crashing intubated patient as a unilateral absence of breath sounds is a clue to the presence of a pneumothorax. Other physical findings that may be seen with a pneumothorax include increased resistance with bagging and tracheal deviation, which unfortunately is often a very late and near-terminal finding.

A final potential error to be avoided in intubated patients who suddenly decompensate is failure to evaluate for equipment failure. As simple as it may seem, paramedics must be sure that if a bag is being used, it is connected to the oxygen supply and there are no kinks in the tubing. If a transport ventilator is being employed, providers should immediately disconnect it and initiate manual ventilation with a bag.

If endotracheal intubation is going to be performed in the prehospital setting, paramedics must be expert in the indications for the procedure, confirmation of tube placement, as well as management of patients after successful ETT placement. Intubated patients may suddenly and unexpectedly decompensate, and paramedics must be able to rapidly identify the cause for deterioration, as failure to do so will lead to the patient's demise. Do not become complacent after you successfully pass an endotracheal tube.

SELECTED READINGS

Colwell CB, Cusick JM, Hawkes AP, et al. A prospective multicenter evaluation of prehospital airway management performance in a large metropolitan region: Denver Metro Airway Study Group. *Prehosp Emerg Care.* 2009;13(3):304–310.

Jemmett ME, Kendal KM, Fourre MW, et al. Unrecognized misplacement of endotracheal tubes in a mixed urban to rural emergency medical services setting. *Acad Emerg Med.* 2003;10(9):961–965.

Katz SH, Falk JL. Misplaced endotracheal tubes by paramedics in an urban emergency medical services system. *Ann Emerg Med.* 2001;37(1):32–37.

24

DON'T UNDERESTIMATE WAVEFORM CAPNOGRAPHY IN THE INTUBATED PATIENT

JEFFREY M. GOODLOE, MD, NREMT-P, FACEP

"What's all this discussion about continuous waveform capnography? Once we see the endotracheal tube pass through the vocal cords, how does continuous waveform capnography really add anything to assuring that the tube is in the right position? Besides, when someone requires field intubation, they must be significantly ill or injured; if not already clinically dead...we've got far more important things to do than look at some respiratory waveform. Besides, we got pulse oximetry, why do we need capnography, too?"

These are understandable questions, but waveform capnography, though no longer a novel concept in EMS, is still relatively new in terms of its implementation. Underestimating its vital importance in the intubated patient is an error that all prehospital providers must avoid.

It is an interesting and sobering fact that as humans we sometimes "see" events that are not quite reality on further inspection. If you have ever intubated a patient and "knew" the endotracheal tube passed through the vocal cords only to subsequently see a rising abdomen on bag-valve ventilations, you are not alone. The reality is that visualization alone cannot be trusted as a means to verify correct initial and ongoing endotracheal tube placement. Paramedics should never make the mistake of relying on their observations alone to confirm correct endotracheal tube placement. Scientific review also concludes that the same limitation applies to auscultating breath sounds, as well as to observing condensation in the tube. A continuous capnography waveform, specifically one showing rhythmic rise and fall with exhalation and ventilation respectively, is the best validated method for confirming correct placement of an endotracheal tube.

Do not underestimate the importance of ongoing use of capnography in the management of the intubated patient. Mobility of care is both a hallmark and a challenge in EMS. Anytime the intubated patient is moved, the prehospital provider must focus on waveform capnography; any loss of typical rise and fall of the capnography will immediately pick up accidental endotracheal tube dislodgement. Do not just rely on oxygen saturations as it will take several minutes before the pulse oximetry demonstrates hypoxia. Sudden loss of normal capnography demands sudden reassessment and corrective action to whatever occurred that compromised oxygenation and ventilation.

Many intubated patients may be in cardiac arrest and will have low-amplitude waveforms with end-tidal carbon dioxide values of 20 mm Hg or less. Do not solely rely on displayed low capnography numbers to make any decisions. Because many of the currently available capnography monitors cannot display numerical values less than 8 mm Hg, direct capnograph evaluation of the waveform is critical to determine tube location. This characteristic of continuous waveform capnography provides useful to overall resuscitation assessment. When waveforms with low amplitude and no numerical value are displayed, it can be assumed that the patient has no spontaneous circulation. If during quality CPR, there is a spontaneous rise in capnography amplitude and $ETCO_2$ levels, one can assume that the patient may have a perfusing rhythm and a pulse assessment should be performed.

Despite our best efforts, many patients in cardiac arrest stay in cardiac arrest. Though not as well validated as other termination criteria, many large, urban EMS systems stipulate at the time of termination decision that the end-tidal carbon dioxide level must be less than 20 mm Hg, again indicating lack of spontaneous circulation. This helps us avoid terminating the resuscitation of a patient that is perfusing, yet too hypotensive for us to appreciate it by palpation alone.

In summary, failure to utilize continuous waveform capnography in the intubated patient is a critical error that must be avoided.

SELECTED READINGS

Neumar RW, Otto CW, Link MS, et al. Part 8: Adult advanced cardiovascular life support: 2010 American Heart Association Guidelines for cardiopulmonary resuscitation and emergency cardiovascular care. *Circulation.* 2010;122:S729–S767.

Silvestri S, Ralls GA, Krauss B, et al. The effectiveness of out-of-hospital use of continuous end-tidal carbon dioxide monitoring on the rate of unrecognized misplaced intubation within a regional emergency medical services system. *Ann Emerg Med.* 2005;45(5):497–503.

Warner KJ, Cuschieri J, Garland B, et al. The utility of early end-tidal capnography in monitoring ventilation status after severe injury. *J Trauma.* 2009;66(1):26–31.

25

KNOW THE PROS AND CONS
OF NITROGLYCERIN IN ACUTE
RESPIRATORY DISTRESS

JAMES V. DUNFORD, MD

NITROGLYCERIN IS A VERY IMPORTANT DRUG IN PREHOSPITAL CARE AND ALL PARAMEDICS SHOULD BE EXPERT IN ITS USE

The OPALS study demonstrated that prehospital treatment of heart failure (HF) with combinations of sublingual nitroglycerine (NTG), noninvasive positive pressure ventilation, inhaled albuterol, and advanced airways improved survival. By preferentially dilating veins particularly in the lower extremities, NTG quickly reduces blood return to the heart (preload) and improves pulmonary congestion. However, when NTG is administered to patients who require increased (not reduced) preload, patient care is compromised. Patients with disease such as pneumonia may initially look like they have HF. Without the ability to do an X-ray and perform biomarkers in the back of an ambulance, paramedics need a "sixth sense" to discriminate HF from its clinical mimics. Here are a few suggestions to help determine when and how NTG should be given.

THINK LIKE SHERLOCK HOLMES—LOOK FOR IMPORTANT CLUES

Serious diseases including acute decompensated heart failure (ADHF) often leave vivid memories. Ask patients if they recognize their current symptoms as due to HF. When people are too sick to speak, their medications often tell the story. Identifying current bottles (especially when empty) of diuretics, antihypertensives (particularly ACE inhibitors, angiotensin receptor blockers, and beta blockers), NTG, aspirin, clopidogrel, warfarin, digoxin, and dysrhythmics are powerful evidence of heart dysfunction. Physical evidence of a prior sternotomy or automated internal cardiac defibrillation (ACID) coupled with atrial fibrillation or a paced rhythm builds a case for HF as does a history of a missed dialysis appointment. Since patients rarely develop asthma or COPD late in life (whereas it is relatively common in the elderly), new wheezing and dyspnea in the absence of prior pulmonary conditions or medications (short- or long-acting bronchodilators, ipratropium, inhaled or oral corticosteroids, antibiotics, leukotriene modifiers, allergy shots, aminophylline, chronic oxygen requirement, etc.) are great clues to new-onset HF.

PRIMUM NON NOCERE—THAT IS, DON'T MAKE THINGS WORSE

Never administer NTG when preload actually needs to be increased. Dyspneic conditions that can mimic HF include pneumonia, pulmonary embolus, pneumothorax, and cardiac tamponade, all which may require fluid administration, not preload reduction. Consequently, assume elderly patients with fever, cough, and shortness of breath are dehydrated until proven otherwise. This is especially true for individuals in skilled nursing facilities at risk of aspiration. Similarly, cancer and other immunocompromised patients without known cardiovascular disease should not receive empiric NTG for shortness of breath.

The initial systolic blood pressure (SBP) provides a useful guide to field treatment. SBP > 140 mm Hg suggests preserved left ventricular (LV) function. During the so-called "flash pulmonary edema," an upwardly spiraling blood pressure triggers acute LV dysfunction, pulmonary hypertension, interstitial edema, hypoxia, and anxiety. While prehospital vital signs in ADHF are somewhat variable, most patients are initially hypertensive (SBP > 160 mm Hg) and hypoxic. Medics should not wait for the development of audible rales and frothy blood-tinged sputum to initiate NTG.

Dyspneic HF patients with SBP 100 to 140 mm Hg have impaired LV function, and their symptoms generally come on more gradually. Signs of fluid overload (such as edema) are more common. NTG may be employed carefully when SBP > 110 mm Hg. Patients with SBP < 100 mm Hg typically have severe LV dysfunction with or without shock and NTG is contraindicated. Finally, acute coronary syndromes manifesting with isolated right HF should not receive NTG. Approximately 15% of inferior wall myocardial infarctions are complicated by hemodynamically significant right ventricular infarction. These patients have impaired right-sided filling and require fluid administration, not NTG, which will exacerbate hypotension.

Finally, patients taking phosphodiesterase inhibitors (e.g., Viagra) for erectile dysfunction or pulmonary hypertension should not receive NTG since dramatic venodilation and hypotension can result. These patients have enough problems already.

DON'T BE SHY USING NTG WHEN IT'S INDICATED

NTG and oxygen are first-line medications for suspected acute pulmonary edema and ADHF. While prior use of NTG can attenuate the potency of future doses (patients on long-acting nitrates only take them once a day so enzyme systems can reset), fresh NTG will always deliver benefit. NTG spray administers 400 mcg per dose and should be administered every

3 to 5 minutes. Spray is preferable to tablets since the latter frequently don't dissolve in the dry mouths of hyperventilating patients. Transcutaneous forms of NTG (patch or paste) should also be avoided due to decreased skin perfusion and inconsistent absorption in pulmonary edema. Tachycardia and hypertension will begin to resolve as dyspnea improves. Be aggressive with repeat nitroglycerin as long as the patient's BP remains elevated, and be sure to repeat vital signs often.

Summary

In summary, pitfalls in the use of NTG are commonly due to: (1) failure to elicit a careful cardiac-focused history and physical exam; (2) failure to identify mimics of HF in whom NTG is potentially deleterious; and (3) failure to dose NTG aggressively in hypertensive pulmonary edema patients who are the patients with the greatest potential gains to be had.

Selected Readings

Mebazza A, Gheorghiade M, Pina IL, et al. Practical recommendations for prehospital and early in-hospital management of patients presenting with acute heart failure syndromes. *Crit Care Med.* 2008;36(suppl 1):S129–S139.

Mosesso VN Jr, Dunford J, Blackwell T, et al. Prehospital therapy for acute congestive heart failure: state of the art. *Prehosp Emerg Care.* 2003;7(1):13–23.

Sporer KA, Tabas JA, Tam RK, et al. Do medications affect vital signs in the prehospital treatment of acute decompensated heart failure? *Prehosp Emerg Care.* 2006;10:41–45.

Stiell IG, Spaite DW, Field B, et al. for the OPALS Study Group. Advanced life support for out-of-hospital respiratory distress. *NEJM.* 2007;356(21):2156–2164.

26

FEAR THE ELDERLY PATIENT WITH NEW ONSET WHEEZING

MARC ECKSTEIN, MD, MPH, FACEP

It has often been said that "not all wheezing is due to asthma." This is an important "clinical pearl" for the prehospital provider when encountering an elderly patient with shortness of breath and wheezing.

You are called to respond to a patient with difficulty breathing. Upon arrival, you find an 80-year-old female in moderate respiratory distress. She is sitting in the tripod position, is only able to speak a few words at a time, and has obvious intercostal and supraclavicular accessory muscle usage. She has a history of hypertension and COPD. Her vital signs are BP 168/94, HR 118, RR 28, SpO_2 94% on room air. Upon auscultation of her lungs, you hear diffuse expiratory wheezes in all fields.

You immediately administer a dose of albuterol via nebulizer and place the patient on the cardiac monitor. She is in sinus tachycardia with no obvious signs of myocardial ischemia. You establish a saline lock. The patient is not responding very well to the albuterol with continued wheezing, dyspnea, and severe retractions. In conjunction with medical control, you administer epinephrine, 0.3 mg of a 1:1,000 concentration intramuscularly. The patient appears to have some improvement during transport, but she begins to complain of severe crushing and substernal chest pain. She is becoming increasingly tachycardic and diaphoretic. You repeat a 12-lead ECG, and it now shows an ST elevation myocardial infarction (STEMI). After transferring care to the emergency physician at the nearest STEMI Receiving Center, the doctor questions you as to your decision to administer epinephrine. You state that the patient was experiencing a severe COPD exacerbation, which was confirmed by the presence of wheezes on examination. The physician explains that this patient had an STEMI with resultant acute cardiogenic pulmonary edema. Her wheezing was due to interstitial lung edema, and not from a COPD or airway problem. He also informs you that epinephrine was contraindicated on this patient due to her age and history of hypertension, and in fact, it may have actually caused her to have an acute myocardial infarction. What went wrong?

The prehospital provider cannot assume that all wheezing is due to asthma or reactive airway disease.

In the early stages of congestive heart failure, one may only hear wheezing on lung auscultation. Not uncommonly, after the administration of a beta agonist such as albuterol, the paramedic will then hear the classic rales on examination. The efficacy of administering a beta agonist to a patient with congestive heart failure is somewhat controversial. While there is concern that the beta effects can increase myocardial oxygen demand due to increased chronotropy and inotropy, some experts believe that there may be some component of bronchospasm that should be treated initially, and the increased myocardial oxygen demand is nominal.

The mainstay of therapy for wheezing due to congestive heart failure is administration of nitrates. Nitrates decrease venous return and allow a compromised myocardium to be less stressed resulting in increased cardiac output and decreased pulmonary congestion. Once nitrates are administered, noninvasive positive pressure ventilation (CPAP) may be very helpful for patients in moderate-to–severe respiratory distress. Epinephrine should always be used with caution for any patient, especially when the patient is older, has known or suspected cardiac disease or hypertension, or if the wheezing may actually be due to "cardiac asthma" of congestive heart failure. Although epinephrine is an excellent bronchodilator in asthma and is lifesaving in the wheezing patient with anaphylaxis, it has no role in COPD patients due to its lack of proven benefit in patients with irreversible lung disease and its high potential for cardiac toxicity in elderly patients with heart and lung disease. When any doubt exists as to the cause of new audible wheezing in the elderly, always consider a cardiac etiology. If the patient has new onset wheezing in conjunction with fever, cough, sputum production, weakness, or lethargy, also consider that this might be infectious and be prepared to treat hypotension with volume in conjunction with alerting medical control to a possible septic patient. The safest prehospital approach is to administer oxygen to patients with wheezing. If you believe that the patient has pulmonary edema as the cause of the wheezing, then oxygen, nitrates, and CPAP, in that order, should be used to treat the patient. If you believe that the patient has wheezing from the bronchospasm of lung disease, then bronchodilators can be added. Regardless of the etiology or therapy used, it is essential that you stay vigilant and closely monitor the patient's vital signs and other associated symptoms (e.g., chest pain) and frequently reassess your patient's condition and response to therapy. New wheezing in the elderly is often due to myocardial dysfunction and pulmonary edema, be careful in these high-risk patients.

SUGGESTED READINGS

Jorge S, Becquemin MH, Delerme S, et al. Cardiac asthma in elderly patients: incidence, clinical presentation and outcome. *BMC Cardiovasc Disord.* 2007;7:16.

Hubble MW, Richards ME. Effectiveness of prehospital continuous positive airway pressure in the management of acute pulmonary edema. *Prehosp Emerg Care.* 2006;10:430–439.

O'Brian JF, Falk JL. Heart failure. In: *Rosen's Emergency Medicine: Concepts and Clinical Practice.* 7th ed. Philadelphia, PA: Mosby; 2009.

27

THE PERILS AND PITFALLS OF NEEDLE DECOMPRESSION

JULLETTE M. SAUSSY, MD, FACEP

A pneumothorax is defined as a collection of air within the pleural cavity between the chest wall and the lung. This air collection externally "presses" on the lung causing a reduction in vital capacity and an increase in intrathoracic pressure. Some pneumothoraces warrant needle decompression in the second intercostal space in the midclavicular line on an immediate basis. EMS providers must know when emergency needle decompression is indicated and the potential complications of this invasive procedure.

A pneumothorax can be spontaneous with no true underlying cause, or more commonly as a result of blunt or penetrating trauma. They can also result from iatrogenic barotrauma secondary to positive pressure ventilation from CPAP, BiPAP, or overzealous ventilation after endotracheal intubation. Any airway intervention that increases intrathoracic pressure places patients at increased risk for a pneumothorax.

Trauma-induced pneumothoraces are caused by blunt or penetrating mechanisms resulting in puncture of the lung parenchyma, most commonly from a rib. These are often accompanied by blood and air in the pleural space which can expand over time, leading to a patient in extremis from tension physiology. A spontaneous pneumothorax should be considered in patients with asthma, COPD patients who have air-filled blebs (seen on CXR), and patients with Marfan syndrome. Many patients may inform you they have suffered from a pneumothorax in the past, and they will usually be treated with a small catheter placed into the pleural space once in the emergency department.

A "simple" pneumothorax is diagnosed by X-ray or CT scan once at the hospital. Simple pneumothoraces do not compromise the hemodynamic status of the patient because the air in the pleural space is either not large enough to cause pressure on the great vessels or there is a mechanism for the air to escape following the injury. Generally, pneumothoraces of less than 40% do not cause hemodynamic compromise. A pneumothorax should always be suspected when a patient develops acute pleuritic shortness of breath with mild respiratory compromise.

EMS providers must know the differences between a simple pneumothorax and a tension pneumothorax. A "tension" pneumothorax is just as it implies; the lung parenchyma is being forced against the mediastinal structures creating tension and both impeding venous return and obstructing aortic outflow. This loss of preload and increase in afterload causes a marked decrease in cardiac output and results in the clinical picture that characterizes a patient who has a life-threatening pneumothorax. These very ill patients are almost always tachypneic, hypotensive, and hypoxic; they may sometimes have distended neck veins due to the pressure on the mediastinum. Decreased, tubular, or absent breath sounds will be auscultated on the affected side as the trachea shifts away from the side under tension and the patient continues to decompensate. EMS providers should not make the mistake of depending on the findings of distended neck veins or tracheal deviation to diagnose a tension pneumothorax. These are unreliable findings and may only appear after the patient has become agonal or is in complete cardiac arrest.

The prehospital provider must recognize this life-threatening condition and treat it promptly. A large-gauge IV catheter should be placed in the second intercostal space in the midclavicular line. The needle should be inserted just above the rib to avoid injuring the neurovascular bundle. Cutting the finger of a glove and placing the needle and catheter through prior to insertion can create a simple "flutter valve." This prevents re-entry of air into the thoracic cavity and allows a "one-way" valve to exist. Needle decompression should result in return of hemodynamic stability if the patient was truly suffering from a tension pneumothorax. Definitive treatment for a tension pneumothorax will be a large bore chest tube inserted in the emergency department.

There is no clinical indication for needle decompression in the prehospital setting for patients who are hemodynamically stable and who are oxygenating adequately. Decreased breath sounds and shortness of breath are not in themselves indications for needle decompression.

Decompressing a patient's chest for a suspected pneumothorax without demonstrating tension pathology (tachycardia, tachypnea, hypoxia, and hypotension) is a critical error that can damage vital thoracic structures and force a patient to undergo insertion of a chest tube as a result of the paramedic's erroneous intervention. Tube thoracostomy is associated with a significant increase in patient morbidity. Thus, needle decompression should only be performed if absolutely indicated. Paramedics should be aware that studies in the past have shown an unacceptably high rate of needle decompression in patients who ultimately did not have a pneumothorax.

In a patient truly in extremis from a suspected tension pneumothorax, choosing an appropriate length needle has been studied and suggests that at least a 4.5 cm (approximately 3 inches) needle is necessary to penetrate the chest wall and enter the pleural space. Many EMS systems only carry

1.5 to 2.5 inch IV catheters, and providers must understand that these shorter needles may be inadequate to successfully relieve trapped air in the pleural cavity. A significant failure rate of decompression (65%) has been seen with the use of a shorter catheter.

Failure to identify chest landmarks appropriately and not correctly puncture in the second intercostal space, midclavicular line, above the rib, may result in unnecessary penetration of the neurovascular bundle and cause arterial bleeding into the chest cavity, worsening an already emergent condition. The needle must be inserted into the affected lung. Decompressing the wrong side is a pitfall that common sense and good training can help the medic avoid.

Take the time to assess your patient; it may make the difference between life and death. Be sure to only consider needle decompression in patients whose clinical history is consistent with the development of a tension pneumothorax, and only in those patients who have refractory hypoxemia in association with shortness of breath and/or hypotension.

SELECTED READINGS

Ball C, Wyrzykowski A. Thoracic needle decompression for tension pneumothorax: clinical correlation with catheter length. *Can J Surg.* 2010;53(3):184–188.

Blavias M. Inadequate needle thoracostomy rate in the prehospital setting for presumed pneumothorax: an ultrasound study. *J Ultrasound Med.* 2010;29:1285–1289.

Eckstein M, Suyehara D. Needle thoracostomy in the prehospital setting. *Prehosp Emerg Care.* 1998;2:132–135.

Harcke H, Pearse LA, Levy AD, et al. Chest wall thickness in military personnel: implications for needle thoracentesis in tension pneumothorax. *Mil Med.* 2007;172:1260–1263.

28

DON'T FORGET CPAP IN PREHOSPITAL RESPIRATORY DISTRESS

KATHLEEN SCHRANK, MD, FACEP, FACP

Paramedics and other prehospital providers are often skeptical when first learning the skills needed for CPAP administration, but based on the results they soon see, prehospital providers can quickly become believers. CPAP can provide rapid and often dramatic relief for patients in respiratory distress due to acute cardiogenic pulmonary edema. The initial research and application of CPAP in emergency care focused on heart failure, and that is where noninvasive positive pressure ventilation (NPPV) has had its most impressive effects. Because of this, many EMS programs restrict CPAP use and only allow it to be specifically used in patients with heart failure. However, many patients in the EMS CPAP studies were misdiagnosed as "acute CHF" when they actually had another cause of respiratory distress such as COPD or pneumonia. It is essential to remember that diagnosing the cause of acute shortness of breath and/or respiratory distress may be very difficult in the prehospital setting. This is especially true in patients who have both heart and lung disease. In fact, in these patients, physicians may require both X-ray and blood testing to determine the true cause of a patient's respiratory issues. However, regardless of the underlying cause, most patients improved with CPAP, and most impressively there clearly was no harm from CPAP use. Remember that because CPAP helps in almost all causes of respiratory distress, restricting its use to cardiogenic pulmonary edema is almost always unnecessary. Because CPAP works so well, some patients who were in extreme distress on initial EMS assessment will be so improved by the time of ED arrival that the nurse or doctor will want to discontinue CPAP at transfer of care. Don't let the ED staff be fooled into taking off that mask too soon—paint a clear picture of how sick the patient was. If they elect to abruptly discontinue CPAP support, move the patient over to the ED stretcher with CPAP still on, and let those in the ED take off the mask.

Although CPAP can provide dramatic relief to patients in respiratory distress, it is of paramount importance to remember that CPAP alone is not enough to treat acute cardiogenic pulmonary edema or bronchospasm secondary to asthma or COPD. CPAP supplements, and can work synergistically, with the primary therapies of each of these diseases. Always administer nitroglycerin for heart failure and use nebulized bronchodilators for wheezing in conjunction with NPPV; never just use CPAP alone in these patients. It is also important to remember that CPAP only works if a patient is breathing adequately on his/her own, and this therapy is not to be used in patients who have tired to the point of respiratory failure and decreased mental status. Providers must remember also that CPAP application may lead to vomiting and forced aspiration, and the mask should be rapidly removed and suction ready if a patient begins to complain of nausea or vomits. In addition, CPAP masks don't fix an obstructed airway. Patients sick enough to need CPAP need to be watched closely. If a patient doesn't improve, or gets worse, then BVM support and endotracheal intubation are indicated. Declining mental status, low or falling oxygen saturation, and very high $ETCO_2$ readings are just some of the indicators that CPAP is not working.

Finally, be careful with CPAP usage in the hypotensive patient. Don't forget that all forms of positive pressure breathing including CPAP mask, BVM, and endotracheal ventilation can cause a drop in blood pressure by decreasing preload and venous return to the heart. With normal breathing, the negative pressure in the chest pulls air and blood into the thorax. Positive pressure breaths push air into the lungs but reduce blood return into the central circulation. The drop in blood pressure will be the worst in hypovolemic patients and if treating patients with borderline systolic blood pressures, reassess the BP often during CPAP administration.

There were some early concerns about potential barotrauma and lung tissue damage from CPAP, and all claims have proved groundless. "Best practice" education reminds us to reassess breath sounds for a developing pneumothorax if a patient deteriorates on CPAP; however, there are no reports of pneumothorax from EMS or emergency department CPAP use.

Given the clear benefit to the application of CPAP in the patient with acute respiratory distress, coordination with the receiving hospital is paramount. Alert the hospital by radio during transport of a CPAP patient, so that the staff can assure rapid availability of hospital CPAP or BiPAP for transfer of care. If an emergency department must depend upon calling respiratory therapy to set up CPAP upon arrival, there may be a time delay that prolongs EMS turnaround time and transfer of care. CPAP devices that require no generator can be turned over more quickly by hooking those CPAP masks to wall oxygen in the ED. When an EMS provider is implementing a new CPAP program, let the area hospitals know before it starts. Encourage them to streamline their system for rapid turnover of care. Some departments have bought their own simple CPAP devices, which can be used until definite machine arrival.

With more CPAP products on the market for EMS care, the cost has come down. However, if your EMS system cannot afford to add CPAP, consider approaching the hospitals for support. Speak with emergency physicians and critical care providers and note that CPAP is a major benefit not only to the patient, but to decreasing healthcare costs. Avoiding endotracheal intubation avoids all the complications of ventilator care including pneumonia, sepsis, and barotrauma, and CPAP use decreases hospital length of stay. Several cities have worked out funding for CPAP from their hospitals or local philanthropic foundations.

In summary, the use of early CPAP in prehospital respiratory distress is a safe practice that can decrease the progression to intubation or complete respiratory failure in a patient who received this treatment early in the course of transport. Although there are few contraindications to CPAP, it should be one of the first-line treatments for many patients with extreme dyspnea and respiratory complaints.

SELECTED READINGS

Baird JS, Spiegelman JB, Prianti R, et al. Noninvasive ventilation during pediatric interhospital ground transport. *Prehosp Emerg Care.* 2009;13:198–202.

Hubble MW, Richards ME, Jarvis R, et al. Effectiveness of prehospital continuous positive airway pressure in the management of acute pulmonary edema. *Prehosp Emerg Care.* 2006;10:430–439.

Hubble MW, Richards ME, Wilfong DA. Estimates of cost-effectiveness of prehospital continuous positive airway pressure in the management of acute pulmonary edema. *Prehosp Emerg Care.* 2008;12:277–285.

Kallio TK, Kuisma M, Alaspää A, et al. The use of prehospital continuous positive airway pressure treatment in presumed acute severe pulmonary edema. *Prehosp Emerg Care.* 2003;7:209–213.

Masip J, Roque M, Sánchez B, et al. Noninvasive ventilation in acute cardiogenic pulmonary edema. *JAMA.* 2005;294:3124–3130.

Seupaul RA. Should I consider treating patients with acute cardiogenic pulmonary edema with noninvasive positive-pressure ventilation? *Ann Emerg Med.* 2010;55:299–300.

29

USE MORPHINE WITH CAUTION IN THE TREATMENT OF ACUTE CARDIOGENIC PULMONARY EDEMA

NEAL RICHMOND, MD, FACEP
JESSE YARBROUGH, EMT-P

The clinical presentation of acute pulmonary edema (APE) is commonly associated with exacerbations of congestive heart failure, and it represents one of the more challenging management problems encountered by prehospital emergency medical providers.

PATHOPHYSIOLOGY

APE results from a variety of causes that may be divided into two broad categories: cardiogenic and noncardiogenic *(Table 29.1)*.

In the setting of cardiogenic APE, cardiac dysfunction is either precipitated or worsened by any number of factors, leading to increased pulmonary capillary pressure and leakage of fluid into the alveoli of the lungs. A vicious cycle is created whereby peripheral vascular resistance increases due to impaired ventricular contractility, thereby elevating diastolic pressure and left-ventricular (LV) workload. The result is an elevation in pulmonary venous pressure, with fluid leak into the surrounding interstitial lung tissue and alveolar gas-exchange units. As oxygen diffusion and saturation are decreased in the face of reduced alveolar gas exchange, the already impaired ventricular function may be compromised even further, and the cycle continues.

In the scenario of noncardiogenic APE, there is also inappropriate redistribution of intravascular fluid into the lungs, but it is caused by increased pulmonary capillary permeability and not from intrinsic ventricular dysfunction *(Table 29.1)*.

DIAGNOSIS

Although the underlying etiologies are different, both cardiogenic and noncardiogenic pulmonary edema may present with a similar constellation of clinical findings, including anxiety, dyspnea, tachypnea, rales, diaphoresis, and signs of right-sided heart failure including lower-extremity edema and jugular venous distention. As a result, it may be difficult to distinguish between the two on the basis of such symptoms and signs alone.

In many cases, prehospital personnel may find it extremely difficult, or even impossible, to distinguish between APE, chronic obstructive pulmonary disease (COPD), pneumonia, and other acute respiratory disorders

TABLE 29.1	PRECIPITATING/AGGRAVATING FACTORS IN ACUTE PULMONARY EDEMA
CARDIOGENIC	**NONCARDIOGENIC**
Myocardial ischemia/infarction	Systemic/pulmonary infection
Acute dysrhythmia	Trauma
Medication noncompliance	Sepsis
Dietary indiscretion	Toxic inhalation
Hypertensive crisis	Aspiration

in the back of an ambulance. Although accurate field diagnosis and proper prehospital treatment has proven to decrease morbidity, mortality, and hospital length of stay in patients with APE, be aware that retrospective studies have calculated EMS misdiagnosis rates to be as high as 32%.

A thorough but directed past medical history focusing on any prior heart disease, cardiac catheterization, or surgery, noncompliance with medication and dietary restriction (reduced salt intake), or any recent illness, can significantly increase the accuracy of diagnosis. Patients with cardiogenic APE may have a history of uncontrolled or poorly controlled hypertension and present with new onset or worsening chest pain, dyspnea on exertion, orthopnea, or lower-extremity edema. Physical exam findings such as rales, wheezes, or rhonchi on lung auscultation may be helpful but of potentially limited value in sorting out COPD from APE. Similarly, ancillary tests like pulse oximetry may reveal decreased oxygen saturation in the face of hypoxemia from a variety of causes. Rhythm analysis and 12-lead EKG interpretation may demonstrate dysrhythmias or possible signs of ischemia/infarction, but these are typically nonspecific and may be prone to misinterpretation. APE tends to be more acute than the exacerbations of COPD. A history of increasing lower-extremity edema, sleeping on more pillows at night, or suddenly waking up short of breath (PND) should make APE due to heart failure more likely, while increasing cough and sputum production may lead one to assume COPD as the cause of respiratory distress.

TREATMENT

Prehospital and emergency department treatment of the patient with suspected APE includes reducing pulmonary capillary pressure, redistributing fluid in the pulmonary vasculature, and optimizing forward cardiac flow. These goals may be accomplished by treating the underlying cause, by pharmacologically reducing LV preload and afterload with nitroglycerin, and by initiating supplemental oxygen as well as inotropic and ventilatory support—particularly with noninvasive positive pressure ventilation (CPAP or Bi-PAP). Most care providers often learned the pneumonic "MONA" (morphine, oxygen, nitroglycerin, and aspirin) for the treatment of chest pain and APE. Be careful though and understand that before we began using evidence-based medicine, simple mnemonics often guided treatment without question of their validity.

While oxygen and nitroglycerin are indeed mainstays of care in APE, morphine continues to be used for the treatment of known or suspected APE despite a total lack of any clinical evidence to support either its efficacy or safety in this setting.

A recent retrospective study on the management of APE in the emergency department actually found an association between morphine use and an increased frequency of endotracheal intubation, hospital length of stay, ICU admission rates, and mortality. Another study did a prospective prehospital evaluation of morphine in conjunction with nitroglycerin and/or furosemide. This study showed no increased benefit of adding morphine or furosemide to nitroglycerin in comparison to using nitrate therapy alone. On the other hand, patients who received morphine and furosemide in the absence of nitroglycerin were more likely to experience clinical deterioration. Such potential adverse effects secondary to respiratory and central nervous system depression are of particular concern when an illness like COPD may be easily misdiagnosed as APE.

In the absence of any clear advantage, and in the face of a potential deleterious effect, there is no evidence to support the use of morphine in the prehospital management of APE. Moreover, the potentially destabilizing hemodynamic and respiratory depressant effects of morphine, especially in the setting of its overzealous use, may actually serve to limit the use of the one drug—nitroglycerin—that has been shown to provide any substantial benefit. Be careful; only use therapies that have proven value.

SELECTED READINGS

Caroci A, Laureau S. Descriptors of dyspnea by patients with chronic obstructive pulmonary disease versus congestive heart failure. *Heart Lung.* 2004;33:102–110.

Francis GS, Greenberg BH, Hsu DT, et al. ACCF/AHA/ACP/HFSA/ISHLT 2010 clinical competence statement on management of patients with advanced heart failure and cardiac transplant: a report of the ACCF/AHA/ACP Task Force on Clinical Competence and Training. *Circulation.* 2010;122:644–672.

Hoffman JR, Reynolds S. Comparison of nitroglycerin, morphine, and furosemide in treatment of presumed prehospital pulmonary edema. *Chest.* 1987;92:586–593.

Jaronik J, Mikkelson P, Fales W, et al. Evaluation of prehospital use of furosemide in patients with respiratory distress. *Prehosp Emerg Care.* 2006;10:194–198.

Mosesso Jr VJ, Dunford J, Blackwell T, et al. Prehospital therapy for acute congestive heart failure: State of the art. *Prehosp Emerg Care.* 2003;13–24.

Saccheti A, Ramoska E, Moakes ME, et al. Effect of ED management on ICU use in acute pulmonary edema. *Am J Emerg Med.* 1999;17(6):571–574.

Weintraub NL, Collins SP, Pang PS, et al. Acute heart failure syndromes: emergency department presentation, treatment, and disposition: current approaches and future aims: a scientific statement from the American Heart Association. *Circulation.* 2010;122:1975–1996.

30

TO PE OR NOT TO PE? DON'T FORGET EMBOLISM IN THE PATIENT WITH SHORTNESS OF BREATH!

NEAL RICHMOND, MD, FACEP
JESSE YARBROUGH, EMT-P

INTRODUCTION

Pulmonary embolism (PE) occurs when a deep-venous thrombosis (DVT) or clot forms, typically in the calf veins, and then travels into the pulmonary vascular tree. Once in the lungs, it creates a mismatch between ventilation and perfusion as alveoli are ventilated but, due to the clot, there is no blood flow to that area of the lung. This will usually result in hypoxemia, and if a large enough embolus, diminished cardiac output, hypotension, and eventual death if not diagnosed and treated early.

PE is diagnosed in over 600,000 people each year, resulting in up to 200,000 deaths. Mortality may be as high as 30% in untreated patients. A high index of suspicion for PE by EMS can help increase the likelihood of a timely workup in the hospital. This is extremely important as early diagnosis and treatment of a pulmonary embolus can reduce mortality to less than 10%.

RISK FACTORS

The majority of patients with PE have at least one risk factor that fits into the classic Virchow's triad of (1) venous stasis; (2) hypercoagulability; and (3) vascular endothelial damage *(Table 30.1)*. Remember, however, that some patients may have no predisposing conditions. Patients may also be entirely unaware of any such underlying condition (e.g., a hypercoagulable state 2° to an as yet undiagnosed cancer), with as many as 50% presenting with no evidence of any underlying risk at all *(Table 30.1)*.

SYMPTOMS AND SIGNS

Patients with PE present with a variety of nonspecific symptoms and signs and may therefore provide a significant diagnostic challenge to the prehospital provider. A PE may be entirely asymptomatic, or it may present with signs of severe hypoxemia, right-ventricular insufficiency, hemodynamic collapse, or sudden death. To make matters worse, the classic triad of clinical findings—hemoptysis, dyspnea, and chest pain—appears together in less than 20% of cases.

TABLE 30.1   **RISK FACTORS FOR PULMONARY EMBOLUS**

- Age >40
- History of prior PE or DVT
- Recent surgery
- Prolonged immobilization
- CHF
- Cancer (may be occult)
- Trauma (pelvis, femur, tibia)
- Obesity
- Pregnancy/recent delivery
- Hormones (including oral contraceptives)

Patients are also often misdiagnosed, especially when exacerbations of heart disease or COPD may mimic PE, something that may result in a four- to sixfold increase in mortality.

The most common symptom across all age groups is dyspnea, but it may be absent in more than 25% of patients with a known diagnosis of PE. When present, it should raise a red flag, especially when lung sounds are normal, when the EKG shows no ischemia or infarction, or when nothing points to another diagnosis like pneumonia or COPD. The most common EKG finding in a patient with an acute PE is sinus tachycardia.

Only about half of patients have chest pain, and even fewer describe it as being pleuritic. To confuse matters further, the chest pain may be reproducible to palpation. The presence of tenderness or the absence of chest pain altogether does not rule out the diagnosis of pulmonary embolus in the patient with shortness of breath.

When present, findings such as tachypnea and tachycardia may be helpful, but just over 50% of patients have a significantly elevated respiratory rate (>20), while substantially fewer have a heart rate above 100 (<25%). Most ironic perhaps, is that while the majority of emboli result from calf vein DVT, less than half will have lower extremity signs of edema, erythema, tenderness, or a palpable cord.

Also potentially confusing, one-third of patients may have a cough and almost half may present with temperatures >100.4°F (though temperatures >102.5°F are unusual), either or both of these potentially suggesting alternative diagnoses like bronchitis or pneumonia.

Hemoptysis is not common, appearing in no more than about one-third of cases, so other diagnoses, e.g., bronchitis, should be considered, especially when other findings associated with PE are not present. Finally, keep in mind that a PE can initially point to entirely different diagnoses—5% to 8% of patients with PE, for example, present with syncope, seizure-like activity, or confusion.

DIAGNOSTIC ADJUNCTS

The 12-lead EKG is abnormal in most cases (>85%), but findings are typically nonspecific. Tachycardia, followed by ST-T wave changes, is most commonly seen. An S1-Q3-T3 pattern (S in I, and Q and inverted-T in III) may be seen with a massive PE, but this is uncommon (<15%). Oxygen saturation is also normal in most cases, so it too should never be used to rule out PE.

TREATMENT

While definitive therapy for PE is provided in the emergency department or after admission to the hospital, prehospital providers can initiate patient stabilization in the field. Supplemental oxygen is indicated for hypoxemia, and mechanical ventilation should be provided for respiratory failure. Intravenous fluids may be given for hypotension, but with attention to worsening the performance of a potentially already compromised right ventricle, and vasopressors may be administered for shock. At a minimum, any patient in whom a PE is suspected should be transported, and refusal of treatment or transport is never a reasonable alternative. Always communicate to the receiving physician your concerns and findings that lead you to believe your patient may have a PE.

BOTTOM LINE

EMS providers should unlearn the classic clinical triad for PE but suspect this diagnosis in *any* patient with symptoms or signs of respiratory compromise, especially when they appear to be unexplained. A high index of suspicion in the field can set the course for a focused and timely workup in the hospital, thereby reducing patient mortality. Finally, avoiding the use of drugs such as furosemide and morphine in the wrong clinical setting, e.g., for misdiagnosed congestive heart failure, can prevent any potentially deleterious effects of these agents. Always consider the diagnosis of PE in unexplained dyspnea, especially if the patient has any risk factors for PE.

SELECTED READINGS

Fedullo PF, Tapson VF. The evaluation of suspected pulmonary embolism. *N Engl J Med.* 2003;349:1247–1256.

Ferrari E, Imbert A, Chevalier T, et al. The ECG in pulmonary embolism: Predictive value of negative T waves in precordial leads - 80 case reports. *Chest.* 1997;111(3):537–543.

Harrigan RA, Jones K. ABC of clinical electrocardiography: Conditions affecting the right side of the heart. *BMJ.* 2002;324(2002):1201–1204.

Kline JA, Courtney DM, Kabrhel C, et al. Prospective multicenter evaluation of the pulmonary embolism rule-out criteria. *J Thromb Haemost.* 2008;6:772–780.

Le Gal G, Righini M, Roy PM, et al. Differential value of risk factors and clinical signs for diagnosing pulmonary embolism according to age. *J Thromb Haemost.* 2005;3:2457–2464.

Pineda LA, Hathwar VS, Grant BJ. Clinical suspicion of fatal pulmonary embolism. *Chest.* 2001;120(3):791–795.

Stein PD, Beemath A, Matta F, et al. Clinical characteristics of patients with acute pulmonary embolism: data from PIOPED II. *Am J Med.* 2007;120:871–879.

31

Avoid overzealous use of furosemide

Jullette M. Saussy, MD, FACEP

When a patient says, "I can't breathe," what does that really mean? One of the most difficult EMS dilemmas and one ripe for mistakes is assessing and diagnosing the cause of dyspnea. COPD patients have a long history of shortness of breath and are often on many medications to help them breathe better. They may complain of increased cough and sputum production. Patients suffering from pneumonia usually present with fever (or hypothermia in the elderly or immunocompromised), tachypnea (RR >20), some degree of hypoxia (pulse ox <94%), as well as a productive cough. Acute respiratory distress from a congestive heart failure (CHF) includes tachypnea, jugular venous distention (JVD), extremity swelling, and hepatojugular reflux (if right heart failure has been induced by left heart failure and your patient has hepatic congestion) as well as "crackles" or "rales" can be heard. These patients, unless end stage, will usually present hypertensive, tachycardic, and often hypoxic.

It is extremely difficult for the paramedic to distinguish the cause of shortness of breath and hypoxia in the brief time assessing and treating the patient. Moreover, establishing whether the patient needs volume resuscitation or diuresis is even more complicated.

Furosemide (commonly known by its brand name Lasix), a diuretic traditionally used for diuresis in the patient with fluid overload, results in decreased preload and lowers blood pressure. Historically, it also has been used for the treatment of hypertension and CHF, mostly in combination with other medications. Many prehospital providers have attempted to use their initial history and physical examination to determine whether the patient presenting with shortness of breath is secondary to CHF (possibly requiring diuresis), or possible other etiologies such as pneumonia or COPD. Deciding whether your patient with respiratory distress is indeed "fluid overloaded" rather than euvolemic or hypovolemic remains difficult even in the emergency department. Ancillary tests such as a BNP (B–type natriuretic peptide) level and a simple chest radiograph can often help the healthcare provider in the emergency department.

Several studies and articles have been written about the use of furosemide in the prehospital setting dating back to 1992. One retrospective study looked at 493 patients diagnosed with CHF or pulmonary edema and found furosemide administration by EMS was associated with 11% overall mortality. There was no decrease in length of hospital stay, and the study's results showed an increase in mortality in patients misdiagnosed as having heart failure. This increased mortality was likely due to the erroneous administration of cardiac medications, such as furosemide, to patients not in CHF.

Subsequently, another study done a few years later found that paramedics misdiagnosed their patients as having pulmonary edema due to CHF 42% of the time, and that the use of furosemide was indeed "harmful" in 17% of those misdiagnosed. This is not because the paramedic is poorly skilled in patient assessment and treatment; it implies that the patient is extremely complex with a combination of multiple factors causing dyspnea that is nearly impossible to distinguish on initial patient assessment in the prehospital arena.

So, how does the prehospital provider match the correct treatment with the most likely diagnosis and avoid giving furosemide to the wrong patient? All that wheezes is not asthma, and all that crackles is not heart failure. Protocols, while a guideline, tend to steer medics to put patients in a diagnosis "box" or "algorithm" and that is often very dangerous. Because furosemide has been used in the wrong patients repetitively, there has been a lot of discussion about either greatly limiting its use or not using this agent at all in the prehospital setting.

WHEN IN DOUBT, AVOIDING FUROSEMIDE IS THE BEST CHOICE

While the task of recognizing the etiology of your patient's shortness of breath may seem daunting, this abbreviated focus must point to developing a systematic approach to medical decision making and critical thinking during respiratory emergencies. The days of making a patient's complaint fit a protocol so a therapy can be administered are over. Less may actually be more, and always do no harm.

SELECTED READINGS

Dobson T, Jensen J. Correlation of paramedic administration of furosemide with emergency medicine physician diagnosis of congestive heart failure. *J Emerg Prim Health Care.* 2009;7(3):Article no. 990378.

Jaronik J, Mikkelson P. Evaluation of prehospital use of furosemide in patients with respiratory distress. *Prehosp Emerg Care.* 2006;10(2):194–197.

McKinney J, Brywczynski J, Slovis C. The declining roles of furosemide, morphine and beta blockers in the prehospital setting. State of the Science, 2009.

Tintinalli JE. *Emergency Medicine: A Comprehensive Study Guide.* 6th ed. New York: McGraw-Hill; 2003:1113, 1368.

Wuerz RC, Meador SA. Effects of prehospital medication on mortality and length of stay in congestive heart failure. *Ann Emerg Med.* 1992;21(6):669–674.

32

Shortness of breath: remember that it's not always the lungs!

Corey M. Slovis, MD

Shortness of breath (SOB) is usually due to a pulmonary problem, but there are other causes that must always be considered. Essentially, all of the causes of SOB can be divided into five major causes: (1) pulmonary, (2) cardiac, (3) neuromuscular–skeletal, (4) CNS, and (5) blood.

The pulmonary causes of SOB are multiple and include common etiologies such as asthma and COPD, infectious causes like viral upper respiratory infections (URIs) and pneumonia, to rarer causes like pulmonary fibrosis. Cardiac causes of SOB include congestive heart failure along with myocardial ischemia and infarction. Neuromuscular–skeletal causes range from neurologic diseases like myasthenia and Guillain–Barre syndrome to skeletal problems like rib fractures and flail chest. CNS causes include anxiety, CNS stimulants like cocaine, and Kussmaul ventilations due to an underlying metabolic acidosis. Finally, blood abnormalities like anemia, sickle cell disease, and carbon monoxide may cause SOB.

All patients with SOB should be assumed to be seriously ill until both the cause and severity of the SOB have been carefully evaluated. A rapid cardiopulmonary exam should be performed with attention to respiratory rate, ventilating efforts, and quality of air exchange. Unless there is an obvious reason not to, all patients should be given oxygen, placed on an oxygen saturation monitor, and have continuous ECG monitoring. If the patient is potentially seriously ill, at least one IV line should be started, and any patient at risk for myocardial ischemia or infarction should have a 12-lead ECG performed.

Paramedics should never immediately assume that the patient has SOB due to anxiety. Anxious patient may also be seriously ill, even with relatively normal vital signs and clear lung fields. Having an anxious patient try to breath slowly into a paper bag, or non-rebreather with no concomitant oxygen being administered, can be fatal in SOB patients in diabetic ketoacidosis (DKA) or in those who have a severe metabolic acidosis due to sepsis. Even potentially fatal aspirin overdoses may present initially with just anxiety, hysteria, hyperventilation, and SOB.

Although most myocardial infarctions present with chest pain, some may present with only the chief complaint of SOB. This is especially true in the elderly where up to 40% of elder patients may deny chest pain and merely complain of new-onset SOB. Similarly, it may be impossible to separate a COPD exacerbation from pulmonary edema in patients who have both a history of heart and lung disease. Thus, always be suspicious and perform a 12-lead ECG in new-onset SOB patients who are above 40 years old, and in anyone with a history of ischemic heart disease. Conversely, doing an electrocardiogram in a stable young healthy patient with asthma is wasting time and effort.

Physicians and paramedics often relax when an SOB patient has equal and clear lung sounds, no wheezes, and has an O_2 saturation in the mid-90s. However, "Beware PE" should always be considered in SOB patients who have any risk factors for a pulmonary embolus. Virchow's triad, a group of major risk factors for embolism formation, is: stasis, injury, and hypercoagulability. So any SOB patient who has been on bed rest, had a leg immobilized, or who recently completed a long drive or flight is at increased risk for PE. So too are those who have recently had a knee injury or who were kicked in the leg or calf. Finally, hypercoagulable patients are at increased risk for PE, including those who smoke, who use birth-control pills, or who have a history (or family history) of blood clots. Diagnosing a pulmonary embolus is sometimes difficult, but considering it in the differential diagnosis of a hyperventilating patient is easy.

Unexplained SOB can be secondary to the patient's blood not being able to carry or unload oxygen in a normal fashion. Even if a patient is saturating at 100%, unexplained SOB patients should receive high-flow O_2 if there is any chance they have severe anemia, acute blood loss, sickle cell disease, or have been exposed to carbon monoxide or cyanide. Providing 100% O_2 by non-rebreather or CPAP to patients with carbon monoxide exposure or anemia can allow more oxygen to be delivered to tissues as higher quantities of O_2 dissolve into the blood. This is very important, as severely anemic patients may not have enough hemoglobin to carry enough oxygen to adequately supply the heart and brain.

SOB patients with neuromuscular and skeletal abnormalities may be very challenging to treat. Patients with respiratory muscle weakness may appear stable until they have a sudden respiratory arrest. Patients with myasthenia, Guillain–Barre syndrome, ALS (Lou Gehrig's disease), or any neuromuscular disease should receive 100% O_2 by CPAP if possible and be monitored closely for respiratory effort and rate. Paramedics should have a bag valve mask and endotracheal tube ready should a sudden change in the patient's status occur.

Please don't forget these final five points:

■ Treat SOB with respect and always search out a cause.
■ Never initially assume SOB is due to anxiety.

- Remember that SOB may be the sole presenting sign of a myocardial infarction, especially in older patients.
- Never use a paper bag or a non-rebreather without oxygen in an anxious patient unless you are 100% sure nothing else is wrong with the patient.
- SOB patients with clear lungs and high O_2 saturations may have carbon monoxide, cyanide, or a pulmonary embolus as the cause.

SELECTED READINGS

Brieger D, Eagle KA, Goodman SG, et al. Acute coronary syndromes without chest pain, an underdiagnosed and undertreated high-risk group: insights from the Global Registry of Acute Coronary Events. *Chest.* 2004;126:461–469.

Kao LW, Nanagas KA. Carbon monoxide poisoning. *Emerg Med Clin N Am.* 2004;22:985–1018.

Murphy P, Colwell C, Pineda G, et al. Shortness of breath: A review of select conditions. *EMS Mag.* 2009;38(7):51–52, 54–61.

Slovis CM, McKinney J, Brywczynski J, et al. Shortness of breath prehospital treatment of respiratory distress. *JEMS.* 2010;35(5):56–63.

Susec O Jr, Boudrow D, Kline JA. The clinical features of acute pulmonary embolism in ambulatory patients. *Acad Emerg Med.* 1997;4:891–897.

33

Be vigilant for stridor in adults

Jeff Beeson, DO, EMT-P

Stridor is an abnormal upper-airway sound resulting from air moving through a partially obstructed upper-airway structure. Prehospital providers are often educated that stridor is a whistling sound heard in pediatric patients that have the potential to become very ill from infectious causes or ingestion of a foreign body. Most EMS test questions describing an ill-appearing 2-year-old found in a tripod position, drooling, are often asking about epiglottitis. There is, however, little to no discussion of stridor in adults because the incidence is rare. The adult trachea and glottic opening are significantly larger than that of a pediatric patient and can tolerate more swelling or other pathology before critical narrowing of upper-airway structures occurs and stridor is heard. EMS providers should be aware that stridor presents in the adult patient more than we realize and may be missed by EMS assessment because the provider is not expecting it. Remember, "The eye doesn't see what the mind doesn't know."

Stridor is a symptom and not a diagnosis. As with any complaint prehospital providers confront, a thorough history and physical exam must be paramount. When stridor is heard, the provider should recognize the airway anatomy is distorted. Common causes of stridor in adults include acute anaphylaxis, retropharyngeal or peritonsillar abscesses, foreign bodies, epiglottitis, congenital diseases or masses, and chemical or thermal injuries. Patient presentations can vary from a foreign body sensation with difficulty swallowing to the inability to talk with extreme shortness of breath.

With the success of pediatric vaccination programs, epiglottis in the pediatric patient population is rarely seen. Epiglottitis in adults is now more common but often missed. Epiglottis can evolve rapidly and cause abrupt changes in symptoms. The most common complaints are sore throat, difficulty swallowing, and a muffled voice. Stridor is a late sign and often indicates severe supraglottic swelling. It is felt that President George Washington may have died from epiglottis as he woke up from sleep with a sore throat and was dead by nightfall.

When obtaining a history, it is important to identify how rapidly the symptom onset occurred and what the patient had been doing. If the symptom onset is within a few minutes or hours, you are often dealing with a more time-sensitive process than one with an onset over several days.

Stridor Indicates the Impending Loss of an Airway

The patient will often be found in an upright position extending the neck. It is important to evaluate if the patient is able to maintain their own secretions or is drooling or spitting out saliva. Difficulty swallowing often indicates a more supraglottic process. Caution should be used when attempting to evaluate the pharynx if stridor is present to prevent laryngospasm from direct contact of pharyngeal structures. Tidal volume and respiratory rate are important clues to the patient condition since stridor is more often heard on the inspiratory phase. Waveform capnography is an important tool when evaluating the effectiveness of ventilation. The anxious or panicking patient indicates impeding airway collapse.

An important point for the prehospital provider to embrace is to let the patient position themselves. They will most always assume a position of comfort, sitting upright and leaning forward. This is the patient that you do not want to lie supine on the cot; they will not tolerate this and may decompensate. Provide the patient with a rigid suction device and allow them to suction themselves. This provides an additional way to monitoring the patient's condition.

Rarely, the patient may require a definitive airway; the prehospital environment is not the ideal location to do this very high-risk procedure. These patients are frequently taken to the operating room and receive a definitive airway by a surgeon utilizing general anesthesia. Although it is important to have your equipment available during transport if the patient decompensates, remember the airway anatomy is always abnormal and often unrecognizable even to the most experienced intubator. It may be impossible to pass an endotracheal tube from the supraglottic approach and most supraglottic devices will be unsuccessful in ventilating these patients; therefore, if the patient is ventilating themselves, let them! Performing a rapid-sequence intubation in these patients will almost always fail and is a bad decision that should be avoided. A sedated awake intubation allows the patient to continue breath spontaneously and will provide extra time if the procedure does not go as planned. A sublgottic or surgical airway device will often be required. Transtracheal oxygenation or a jet insufflation device will provide oxygen to the patient but will not allow exhalation, resulting in hypercarbia and respiratory acidosis. If you have a patient with stridor, it is important to give the receiving facility early notification of your arrival and allow them time to alert and gather the necessary personnel and equipment.

In conclusion, identifying the specific cause of stridor in adults is not as important as identifying the seriousness of the situation. The common pitfalls to avoid are failure to recognize stridor, and more importantly, failing to identify the impending failure of the airway. Avoid the feeling of having to control the airway early, and remember that patients don't die from the lack of intubation, they die from the lack of ventilation. Some of the most important care provided in the prehospital environment is rapid and safe transport to the hospital.

SUGGESTED READINGS

Isakson M, Hugosson. Acute epiglottis: Epidemiology and streptococcal pneumoniae serotype distribution in adults. *J Laryngol Otol.* 2010;125(4):390–393.

Kuan WS, Quek LS. Stridor in an adult: not just a child's disease. *Eur J Emerg Med.* 2009;16(2):109–110.

Murphy P, Colwell C. Prehospital management of epiglottitis. *Emerg Med Serv.* 2000;29(1):41–49.

Wurtele P. Acute epiglottis in children and adults: a large-scale incidence study. *Otolaryngol Head Neck Surg.* 1990;103(6):902–908. Review.

34

PEARLS AND PITFALLS FOR TREATING STATUS ASTHMATICUS

JOHN P. FREESE, MD

Asthma is a complex disease process. In addition to the bronchospasm that we all associate with this disease, asthmatics experience increased airway secretions (which can lead to mucous plugging) and airway inflammation that narrows the smaller airways. The combination of these three elements leads to airflow obstruction and retention of air in the alveoli and smaller airways (so called "air trapping") and prevents effective exhalation.

To overcome these things, patients must increase their respiratory effort and use accessory muscles in order to generate sufficient pressure to overcome that resistance. In doing so, they increase their utilization of oxygen and production of carbon dioxide (CO_2) in the setting of a disease state that limits their ability to effectively oxygenate and ventilate. In addition, as the work of breathing increases, the increasing intrathoracic pressure reduces venous return and lowers preload, causing a reduction in cardiac output and systolic blood pressure.

If left untreated, this combination of hypoxia, elevated CO_2 levels (termed hypercarbia or hypercapnia), increased intrathoracic pressure, and cardiovascular compromise will lead to altered mental status, worsening respiratory depression, and even death.

And now, for the most severe of these patients, you are going to try to intubate them, a procedure that stimulates further bronchospasm and after which you will deliver ventilation with even more positive pressure. Almost seems counterintuitive, doesn't it? Well, with a few little tricks, you can avoid the potential perils of the intubated asthmatic.

1) *Before you reach for the laryngoscope, give epinephrine*
   The severe bronchospasm and airflow obstruction that lead to respiratory failure among asthmatics is typically refractory to inhaled beta-agonists because those drugs are unable to be effectively delivered to the small airways. Epinephrine given via the intramuscular route is a rapid and effective alternative for beta-agonist delivery. (And, in this age of epinephrine auto-injectors is a potentially life-saving therapy for asthmatics that both BLS and ALS providers can provide if allowed by their protocols or medical control.) The standard dose of epinephrine in adults is 0.3 mg IM (one adult auto-injector or 0.3 cc of a 1:1,000 solution).

Whenever bronchospasm is so severe that intubation may ultimately be required, and knowing that additional bronchospasm will
likely result from the intubation itself, administration of intramuscular
epinephrine prior to intubation should be considered standard therapy.

2) *While you're at it, add a little intravenous lidocaine*

Although the studies to date are mixed, there is evidence that intravenous lidocaine may attenuate bronchospasm that results from intubation. In one study, its administration not only reduced the degree of
bronchospasm that resulted from the intubation but it actually low-
ered airway resistance to a level below that which was present before
the intubation. When weighed in the context of a risk–benefit analysis,
improved airflow seems to argue for the administration of lidocaine. So
if the intubation is going to require a call to medical control anyway
(i.e., for sedation orders), throw 100 mg of intravenous lidocaine into
the mix.

3) *Don't stack the breaths*

Significantly elevated airway pressures can lead to decreased venous
return and cardiovascular compromise, and they can also lead to hyperinflation of the lung, progressive inability to ventilate, alveolar rupture,
accumulation of subcutaneous air, and pneumothorax. Such rises in
airway pressures result from "breath stacking"—ventilation provided
without allowing sufficient time for prior ventilations to be passively
exhaled, also referred to as "auto–PEEP (positive end-expiratory pressure)." To avoid this problem, you must allow for complete exhalation. This may require significant amounts of time (5 to 8 seconds) and
therefore requires the patient to be purposefully hypoventilated to allow
for a prolonged expiratory phase. If unable to effectively oxygenate the
patient in this setting, applying gentle manual pressure to the lower lateral chest wall during exhalation can assist with exhalation and reduce
airway pressures, allowing for improved ventilation and oxygenation.

4) *Treat the patient, not the numbers*

Following intubation, waveform capnography values for the asthma
patient will be elevated, but wrongly attempting to correct them
through hyperventilation will result in the "breath stacking" described
above. Remember that the patient may require hypoventilation in order
to minimize airway pressures and allow for effective oxygenation. Intentional hypoventilation and thereby purposefully allowing for this rise
in CO_2 values, the so–called "permissive hypercarbia" or "permissive
hypercapnia," may improve airway pressures and oxygenation, and this
technique has been shown to reduce the mortality among this patient
population.

5) *If they do arrest, reach for more epinephrine and consider tension pneumothorax*
The prognosis among asthmatics whose exacerbations progress to cardiac arrest is very poor. It is important to remember that these are asphyxial arrests, often presenting with bradyasystolic rhythms that were brought about by severe airway obstruction. The administration of intravenous epinephrine as part of pulseless electrical activity/asystole management may improve airway resistance, allow for effective oxygenation and ventilation, and achieve return of spontaneous circulation. Paramedics must also consider acidosis and pneumothorax (including the possibility of a tension pneumothorax) as likely and reversible causes, given the patient's hypercarbia and increased airway pressures, respectively. If a tension pneumothorax is at all a possibility, and the patient has not responded to the epinephrine, immediate needle decompression is indicated.

The goal in managing any critically ill asthmatic should be to avoid intubation. But if it is necessary, the early administration of epinephrine, considering the administration of lidocaine, avoidance of breath stacking, practicing permissive hypercarbia, and anticipating the reversible causes should the patient continue to deteriorate can help you to avoid the perils in this population.

SELECTED READINGS

Adamzik M, Groeben H, Farahani R, et al. Intravenous lidocaine after tracheal intubation mitigates bronchoconstriction in patients with asthma. *Anesth Analg.* 2007;104(1):168–172.

Brenner B, Corbridge T, Kazzi A. Intubation and mechanical ventilation of the asthmatic patient in respiratory failure. *J Allergy Clin Immunol.* 2009;124(2):S19–S28.

Darioli R, Perret C. Mechanical controlled hypoventilation in status asthmaticus. *Am Rev Respir Dis.* 1985;129:385–387.

Van der Touw T, Tully A, Amis TC, et al. Cardiorespiratory consequences of expiratory chest wall compression during mechanical ventilation and severe hyperinflation. *Crit Care Med.* 1993;21:1908–1914.

35

Toxic inhalation pitfalls

J. Brent Myers, MD

EMS providers are confronted with an array of potential toxic inhalation situations, ranging from the seemingly obvious cases such as a carbon monoxide suicide attempt with a running car in the garage to the far from obvious cases with multiple patients complaining of vague respiratory irritation after an unknown exposure. A standardized approach will both protect the EMS responder and provide the best possible outcomes for patients. Here are the pitfalls to be avoided:

1) *Don't omit the basics while confirming the agent(s) responsible for the inhalational injury*

   As with all responses, scene safety is the primary concern. Utilization of respiratory protection, establishment of staging upwind from an incident, and early involvement of special teams to help determine the agent or agents responsible will serve all responders well. Likewise, it is not possible for first arriving EMS providers to have immediate recall of the treatments unique to the myriad of agents capable of inhalation injury. Fortunately, standard treatment that includes management of airway, treatment for bronchospasm, correction of hypoxia, and supportive care is the preferred initial treatment for nearly all inhalational injuries. Thus, the provider can utilize familiar patient care practices while the agent is identified.

2) *Avoid overconfidence in scene safety and initial impression*

   A common mistake in response to toxic inhalation is the assumption that the toxin is known because of a provider's previous experience in the same or similar circumstance. This is best illustrated by two examples. First, during the Moscow hostage crisis, EMS providers assumed that when law enforcement and military personnel released "gas" into the building that it was nerve gas. Despite clinical presentations not consistent with nerve agent inhalation, the treatment provided was atropine and 2-PAM (protopam sulfate). In fact, aerosolized fentanyl had been utilized, and the patients were suffering from narcotic overdose that was imminently remediable with basic airway management and naloxone. It appears many lives were lost due to a rush to judgment. Likewise, "in-vehicle" suicides that historically have been due to carbon monoxide now may be due to hydrogen sulfide poisoning, requiring additional precautions and treatment modalities.

3) *Avoid treating the presumed exposure only—treat the patient*
   Obviously, it is prudent to treat for known and suspected exposures, such as consideration of treatment for carbon monoxide and cyanide exposure for an unconscious smoke inhalation victim. In this example, it is tempting to focus on the unusual and exciting treatment for presumed cyanide exposure and neglect thorough assessment of the patient for airway edema, traumatic injuries, and/or medical conditions such as myocardial ischemia that may have been triggered by the inhalation.

4) *Avoid over-reliance on medical monitoring with devices*
   When findings of hypoxia and/or elevated carboxyhemoglobin levels are consistent with the patient's history and presentation, such medical monitoring can be useful. In some cases, however, these devices can offer inaccurate findings. For example, the hypoxic patient may demonstrate falsely elevated carboxyhemoglobin readings. The provider who attributed the patient's respiratory distress to carbon monoxide exposure may not determine the actual cause of the respiratory distress and potentially provide suboptimal care.

The management of the patient with acute inhalational injury can be daunting. The provider who recalls the basics of scene safety and patient management does not rush to judgment regarding the agent or agents involved, and treats not only the inhalational injury but also associated traumatic and/or medical conditions, will offer the optimal care for their patient.

SELECTED READINGS

Cone DC, MacMillan D, Parwani V, et al. Threats to life in residential structure fires. *Prehosp Emerg Care.* 2008;12(3):297–301.

Feiner JR, Bickler PE, Mannheimmer PD. Accuracy of methemoglobin detection by pulse CO-oximetry during hypoxia. *Anesth Analg.* 2010;111:143–148.

Hall AH, Dart R, Bogdon G. Sodium thiosulfate or hydroxycobalamin for treatment of presumed cyanide poisoning? *Ann Emerg Med.* 2007;49:806–813.

http://scienceblogs.com/terrasig/2010/02/suicide_h2s_cary_warning.php [accessed May 19, 2011]

Wax PM, Becker CE, Curry SC. Unexpected "gas" casualties in Moscow: a medical toxicology perspective. *Ann Emerg Med.* 2003;41:700–705.

36

DON'T ADMINISTER TOO MUCH OR TOO LITTLE OXYGEN TO THE COPD PATIENT

TERENCE VALENZUELA, MD, MPH
JARROD MOSIER, MD

The method to provide oxygen to the acutely dyspneic patient with chronic obstructive pulmonary disease (COPD) in the field is a common and controversial challenge in EMS. Historically, EMS providers and physicians have been taught that breathing in severe COPD patients is driven by the amount of O_2 in the blood (hypoxic drive). In contrast, normal patients change breathing in response to the amount of carbon dioxide (CO_2) in the blood (hypercarbic drive). Unfortunately, in severe lung disease patients, the hypoxic drive to breathe is not strong until the amount of oxygen in the blood is at the border between adequate and inadequate; thus the regulation of breathing is neither sensitive nor precise in these patients. In contrast, normal patients using the hypercarbic drive use very small changes in blood CO_2 content to tightly regulate and control their breathing. Thus, because severe lung disease patients use the hypoxic drive, high-flow oxygen (facemask at 15 L/minute) can dramatically improve oxygenation to the point of extinguishing their hypoxic drive and causing the COPD patient to stop breathing.

Because of the risk of too much oxygen, in the past the prudent practice was to limit the O_2 administered even to the exhausted-appearing, confused COPD patient who grew less responsive by the minute. The disadvantage to that strategy was that inadequate oxygen support was provided allowing the patient to remain hypoxemic. This practice permitted the COPD patient to stay without sufficient oxygen in the blood to support the function and survival of critically important cells of the body, particularly in the brain and heart. Current EMS practice now recommends administration of high-flow O_2 to all patients with severe dyspnea, including the known COPD patient. Although high-flow oxygen might be dangerous long term, it was felt by most that a short course of maximum oxygenation posed little risk.

However, recent studies suggest that COPD and myocardial infarction patients may experience increased mortality and greater morbidity when treated with high-flow oxygen therapy, even if just during EMS transport. Possible mechanisms include decreasing coronary blood flow and increased pressure in the pulmonary circulation. These studies have methodological limitations; but, they generate the possibility that prehospital care should consider the possibility one may "overdose" the COPD by a mechanism(s) other than the "hypoxic drive" response previously taught. There is ongoing research in this area, but at the present time it appears that maximal oxygenation may increase the likelihood of your patient being intubated and having a higher mortality rate once at the hospital.

A feasible approach for prehospital providers is to assess the severity of the COPD patient's acute exacerbation. Those exhibiting signs and symptoms such as anxiety, insistence on sitting up (tripod position), use of accessory muscles of respiration, and diaphoresis are at greater danger of respiratory failure. If available, these patients will benefit from immediate CPAP use along with bronchodilators. Confusion and lethargy indicate that BVM or endotracheal intubation may be imminently needed to support ventilation.

Fortunately, the widespread use of the pulse oximeter in the field gives one a tool to assist in making decisions about how much oxygen to provide the patient. The oximeter measures the percentage of the hemoglobin molecules in the blood that are carrying oxygen. As most of the oxygen present in blood consists of oxygen bound to hemoglobin, the pulse oximeter is a reasonable approximation of the blood's oxygen content.

When the oximeter reading is 90%, blood contains enough oxygen to support cells in the body.

Additional oxygen may be dissolved in the blood plasma when 100% of hemoglobin molecules are saturated. If there is harm caused by high-flow oxygen, it will occur after the 95% threshold is passed.

The "dose" of oxygen given to a patient is represented by the fraction of air breathed that consists of the oxygen (FIO2). There is a rough correlation between the flow rate and FIO_2 with the various options for oxygen administration:

Non-rebreather mask at 16 L/min	FIO_2 70%
Face mask at 8 L/min	FIO_2 50%
Nasal prongs at 4 L/min	FIO_2 40%
Nasal prongs at 2 L/min	FIO_2 30%

Too little oxygen is worse than too much oxygen. Carefully titrate the amount of oxygen you provide. In severely ill patients, start with the highest FIO_2 available and, if transport time and circumstances permit, rapidly reduce the amount of oxygen administered to keep the pulse oximeter indicating the patient's hemoglobin is 90% to 94% saturated with oxygen. Be prepared with a BVM to support the patient's ventilation if he or she develops apnea at any time.

The task of EMS is to make critical decisions based on limited information in a short time. There follows an equally important responsibility: constantly monitoring the effects of one's decisions on the patient and readjusting when necessary. Nowhere are these principles more important than in providing oxygen therapy to the COPD patient.

SELECTED READINGS

Agusti AGN. Systemic effects of chronic obstructive pulmonary disease. *Proc Am Thorac Soc.* 2005;2:367–370.

Austin MA, Wills KE, Blizzard L, et al. Effect of high flow oxygen on mortality in chronic obstructive pulmonary disease patients in prehospital setting: randomized controlled trial. *BMJ.* 2010;341:c5462–c5470.

Farquhar H, Weatherall M, Wijesinghe M, et al. Systematic review of studies of the effects of hyperoxia on coronary blood flow. *Am Heart J.* 2009;158:371–377.

Wang CS. Does this dyspneic patient in the emergency department have congestive heart failure? *JAMA.* 2005;294:1944–1956.

37

Don't give up when it comes to interpreting tachycardias

Sean Covant, DO
Ray Fowler, MD

ECG interpretation can be challenging when the patient presents with a tachycardia. Instead of becoming dismayed, the astute field clinician must take a systematic approach to the evaluation of the rhythm.

In considering the evaluation of the patient with tachycardia, the EMS provider must first perform a physical assessment. For example, not all tachycardias that have a narrow complex and have a rate greater than 150 bpm are considered paroxysmal supraventricular tachycardias (we'll use the term "SVT" here for PSVT, meaning a narrow complex tachyarrhythmia). If the provider will use the formula 220 minus the patient's age, the patient's maximum possible rate of sinus tachycardia will be given. For example a 40-year-old patient would have a maximum sinus tachycardia rate of $220 - 40 = 180$ bpm. That's pretty fast! The maximum output sinus tachycardia in women is a little slower than in men, with a rate of 206 minus 88 percent of age. For example a 40-year-old female would have a maximum output sinus tachycardia of $206 - (40 \times .88) = 171$ bpm. For practical purposes, though, the 220 – age formula works fine for both sexes.

A very important point to be stressed here is that the EMS provider must understand that a patient with a heart rate at or close to their maximum sinus tachycardia output is likely critically ill if this rhythm is due purely to a physiological response, such as in sepsis or hemorrhagic shock. A 20-year-old female could muster a sinus tachycardia approaching 200 bpm. Yet, the medic may think that a narrow complex tachycardia in this female at a rate of 180 would likely be SVT rather than sinus tachycardia and might even think about giving adenosine to her. Yet, a 20-year-old woman bleeding internally from a ruptured ectopic pregnancy with a sinus tachycardia at 180 may be near death. The EMS provider must not confuse this point.

A general rule of thumb is that if the patient's heart rate significantly exceeds the maximum sinus tachycardia output, then a tachyarrhythmia is most likely present. The presence of a tachyarrhythmia must warrant a detailed search for the cause and can usually be placed into several identifiable patterns such as atrial fibrillation, atrial flutter, SVT, and multifocal atrial tachycardia (MAT). There are a few others, but they are relatively rare and will not be discussed here.

One very common presenting atrial tachycardia is atrial fibrillation. Atrial fibrillation is defined as an "irregularly irregular" rhythm that has a chaotic baseline with no reliably discernible P waves. In atrial fibrillation with a rapid ventricular response (AFRVR), the atria are "fibrillating" in a chaotic manner that is not coordinated with the ventricular contraction. This lack of coordination can lead to poor cardiac output. The AV node slows down somewhat the conduction of these many hundreds of chaotic atrial impulses per minute, commonly resulting in a ventricular response of usually between 100 – 180 bpm. The pitfall here for the provider is to miss the irregular irregularity, keeping in mind that AFRVR may be so fast that it is hard to see the irregularity in the rhythm.

Another common tachyarrhythmia is atrial flutter. In atrial flutter the atria contract in an organized rapid rate, usually between 250 and 350 bpm but with a very regular pattern. The classic appearance of atrial flutter on ECG is one showing a saw-tooth pattern in the baseline, especially seen in the limb leads, with oftentimes, but not always, a regular ventricular response. Typically, an atrial flutter pattern will present in a 2:1 or 3:1 atrial to ventricular ratio. For example, one can often see two to three sawtooth patterns for every one QRS that is conducted. The thorough clinician will consider a diagnosis of atrial flutter with a 2:1 ratio if the supraventricular rate is 140 to 150 bpm and regular. One clue to atrial flutter is when the rhythm is regular and the rate is solidly at 140, slightly slower than the slowest SVT. This suggests that an atrial flutter with 2:1 ratio is the source of the rhythm.

A paroxysmal SVT must always be considered when the heart rate is at or exceeds 150 bpm. In an SVT, the QRS complexes are typically "clock regular" and narrow. This rhythm is caused when an atrioventricular nodal reentry circuit forms, sending the impulses coming down from the atria to the AV node back up into the atrium. This is called a "circus movement." The nodal reentry circuit quickly sends another impulse down the conduction system at a rate of 150 to 250 bpm. The pitfall here is to call a regular narrow complex tachycardia at a rate above 150 "SVT" without determining if this rhythm COULD be sinus tachycardia (see discussion above). It is a pitfall to assume that perfectly regular narrow complex tachycardias at a rate of 150 or more are always SVT. Sinus tachycardia—implying a serious physiological response to some sort of stress—must be eliminated as the cause, if possible.

If a narrow complex tachycardia presents with three or more different types of P waves, then this may be MAT. MAT presents with a heart rate above 100 bpm with a PR interval that may vary. The P waves have different morphologies due to the origination of the atrial signal from sites other than the SA node. These alternate sites are "ectopic atrial pacemakers." The ventricular response, to the myriad of multiple ectopic signals, is an irregularly irregular rhythm. The provider may be likely to call this rhythm atrial fibrillation because it is irregularly irregular. Suspect MAT with the above features in the setting of a patient with known pulmonary disease and an ECG with the above features.

The few brief rules mentioned above, especially the rule about 220 – age, when applied carefully and regularly will help the EMS provider make rapid evaluation of tachyarrhythmias as well as giving further insight into the appropriate care of the patients suffering from these conditions.

SELECTED READINGS

AHA Atrial Fibrillation Summit. A Conference Report from the American Heart Association. *Circulation*. 2011;124:363–372, Published online before print June 27, 2011. doi: 10.1161/?CIR.0b013e318224b037.

Gulati M, Shaw LJ, Thisted RA. Heart rate response to exercise stress testing in asymptomatic women: the St. James women take heart project. *Circulation*. 2010;122(2):130–137. Epub 2010 Jun 28.

Multifocal Atrial Tachycardia, found at http://www.ncbi.nlm.nih.gov/pubmedhealth/PMH0001238/, last accessed 12/29/11.

38

DON'T GIVE UP WHEN IT COMES TO INTERPRETING BRADYCARDIAS

SEAN COVANT, DO
RAY FOWLER, MD

ECG interpretation can be challenging when the patient presents with a bradycardia. It is extremely important that the EMS provider understand the potentially lethal implications of certain bradycardias as evidenced by the interpretation of the ECG. This discussion will present several types of bradycardia of which the EMS provider must be aware. As with other rhythms, a systematic approach to the evaluation of the rhythm is essential.

The EMS provider must be aware of the potentially dangerous clinical scenarios evidenced by bradyarrhythmias. Many clinical conditions produce slow heart rates, and it is absolutely vital that the provider carefully assess the patient to determine if certain serious conditions are present. "Bradycardia" is generally defined as a heart rate—in an adult—of less than 60 beats per minute (bpm). The most common reason that a heart rate will be slow is that the patient has a "sinus bradycardia" that is normal for that person. A really fit athlete—a marathon runner for example—might have a resting heart rate in the 40s bpm. That's really slow! But, since the patient is in such great physical condition, the brain tells the heart that it doesn't need to beat so fast. The brain "turns up the vagal tone, increasing the parasympathetic response, and slowing down the firing of the sinus node." Most of our EMS patients are NOT marathon runners, however! So, we have to look for other causes of bradycardias in these patients.

The most common cause of a bradycardia in a patient who is not in great physical condition is a medication effect, most commonly a beta blocker medication such as atenolol or metoprolol. These medications slow down the firing of the SA node, slowing down the heart rate. Since blood pressure = cardiac output × peripheral resistance − and cardiac output is made up of pulse rate × stroke volume − then slowing the pulse rate naturally lowers the blood pressure. So, we commonly see beta blockers being used in the setting of hypertension.

The problem comes with beta blockers when the patient becomes toxic on them. If a provider sees a patient who looks ill and has a very slow pulse rate that is a sinus bradycardia—especially if it is a VERY slow rate such as in the 20s or 30s—then the provider should suspect beta blocker toxicity. Someone who has intentionally overdosed on a beta blocker, such as in a suicide attempt, may be desperately ill and may rapidly deteriorate. The beta blocker prevents the brain from being able to raise the pulse rate due to blocking the sympathetic receptors on the heart tissue. Fortunately there is at least one other path to stimulating the response of the sympathetic receptors and raising the pulse rate: The "glucagon receptor." In the setting of beta blocker toxicity to the point of profound bradycardia and shock, the provider must remember that glucagon given intravenously or intraosseously (possibly even intranasally) may be lifesaving. The problem is it may take a lot of glucagon for the treatment to work.

Finally, in evaluating a bradycardic rhythm, the EMS provider must always be on the lookout for the possibility of a third-degree atrioventricular (AV) heart block being present. In evaluating any ECG—but ESPECIALLY bradycardias—it is paramount that the PR interval on the ECG be assessed as part of a standard routine of interpretation. In a third-degree AV heart block, the electrical impulse generated from the SA node fails to make it through to the ventricles. The ventricles—with no electrical signal coming from the atria—then contract at the intrinsic rate of ventricular pacemakers, which is from 30 to 50 bpm, depending upon where the block is. Typically what is seen on the ECG is the presence of P waves and the presence of QRS complexes but with no regular relationship between the two complexes. The watchword is that the PR interval is "completely variable," and the P waves can often be seen "marching through" the QRS complexes. The prudent clinician must always suspect third-degree AV heart block if a bradycardia is present, the PR interval is completely variable, and there is no apparent relationship between the P wave and the QRS complex especially in the setting of bradycardia.

One pitfall for providers in evaluating third-degree AV block is that the actual site of the block might occur higher in the conduction system, such as at the AV node. When that happens, a junctional pacing site may take over, in the bundle of His. This means that the two bundle branches will be stimulated simultaneously, and the QRS complex will be narrow. This gives an ECG with a bradycardia, a completely variable PR interval, and a narrow QRS complex. If the block is in the bundle branches—where both bundles are blocked—then the site of the pacing stimulation comes from the ventricles, and the QRS complex will be wide and even slower.

It may be said in closing that bradycardias found in the field are both common as well as often indicative of something serious going on. The EMS provider must always carefully interpret the ECG, especially in light of the history and the clinical findings, to offer the most accurate evaluation and targeted management.

SELECTED READINGS

Arrhythmias. Found at http://www.ncbi.nlm.nih.gov/pubmedhealth/PMH0002091/, last accessed 12/29/11.

Brown L, Gough JE, Hawley CR. Accuracy of rural EMS provider interpretation of three-lead ECG rhythm strips. *Prehosp Emerg Med.* 1997;1(4):259–262.

Sherbino J, Verbeek PR, MacDonald RD, et al. Prehospital transcutaneous cardiac pacing for symptomatic bradycardia or bradyasystolic cardiac arrest: a systematic review. *Resuscitation.* 2006;70(2):193–200.

39

Don't be fooled by these ECG mimics

SEAN COVANT, DO

Mimics of ECG ischemia are commonplace and can easily mislead the unwary medic. One must consider many causes of ECG abnormalities such as early repolarization, pericarditis, electrolyte disorders, various toxins, and cardiac pacemakers as potential confounders in determining the presence of an ischemic event.

Astute field providers should always be vigilant in identifying an ST elevation myocardial infarction (STEMI). There are other conditions of the heart, besides infarction, that can cause the ST segments to become abnormal. One such condition to consider is "early repolarization" (ERP) which can be defined as an elevation of the QRS–ST junction of at least 0.1 mV from baseline with prominent T waves and manifested as QRS slurring or notching in at least two contiguous leads. In ERP, the heart repolarization occurs earlier than usual. This causes the ST segment to appear elevated but unlike in a STEMI due to myocardial ischemia there will not be reciprocal ST depressions noted in other ECG leads. Typically, ERP occurs in young people, athletes, and African-Americans and may be a benign finding. Recent work, however, suggests that there may be a very slightly higher long-term mortality (cardiac and arrhythmic) in the general population. The ST segments in ERP tend to be "concave upwards" as opposed to the "convex upwards" ST segments of STEMI. The pitfall here is that either the medic might assume that the ST segments on a patient with chest pain actually looked like ERP when, in fact, the patient was having a STEMI, or the medic might assume that the ST segments of ERP were actually a STEMI. Telling the difference takes training, practice, and good medical oversight.

Another cause of ST elevation is acute pericarditis. In pericarditis, there is generalized inflammation of the pericardium, the membranous sac that surrounds the myocardium. This diffuse inflammation causes widespread irritation of the surface of the heart which results in elevation of the ST segments. The typical pattern will be one of diffuse ST elevations across several leads to include noncontiguous leads. The ST segments due to a myocardial infarction are typically localized to the corresponding coronary vascular area and are not see diffusely. Additionally, in pericarditis, there may be depression of the PR interval in certain leads, such as Lead II, with the absence of pathologic Q waves. A pitfall here is that patients with pericarditis commonly have chest pain and with the elevated ST segments may be confused for having a STEMI.

The ECG can not only be used to determine the electrical status of the myocardium, but also one can gather a quick generalized idea of the state of the body's electrolytes. Cardiac myocytes are sensitive to electrolyte disorders. In particular, elevated or low potassium levels can have an adverse effect on cardiac function. Severe hyperkalemia can cause peaked T waves, and, if worsening, then cause the QRS to become widened and eventually devolve the QRS into a sinusoidal pattern that ultimately leads to ventricular fibrillation or asystole. Conversely, in hypokalemia, the T waves become flattened and then inverted, a U wave may also be present, and the PR interval becomes lengthened.

Although there are non-ischemic causes of peaked T waves such as an electrolyte disorder, the presence of peaked T waves must warrant a high suspicion for cardiac ischemia. Often when there is damage to the cardiac myocytes, the normal electrical flow is altered, and in some cases stopped entirely. This alteration of the normal electrical flow can cause ventricular repolarization to occur in a abnormal fashion resulting in abnormal T waves. Hyperacute T waves are often seen in the early stages of a STEMI, preceding the appearance of ST elevation and the formation of Q waves.

The ECG can also be a tool to help identify potentially life-threatening drug overdoses. In one instance, such as in a tricyclic antidepressant overdose, one can see widened QRS (greater than 120 msec) and a large terminal R wave in lead aVR. This may be the only clue to help identify the nature of the overdose in a patient with altered mental status. Another drug of abuse to consider is cocaine. Diffuse ST elevations secondary to cocaine-induced coronary vasospasms may be prominent. Most ECG changes will present within 3 hours of the use of cocaine, although signs and symptoms have been attributed to cocaine for up to 4 days after use. Additionally, there have been instances where the drug GHB has caused peaked T waves on the ECG. This effect was not due to the GHB itself but due to the potassium salts that are used to synthesize the GHB.

One must also consider the patient's additional comorbid conditions. If a patient has a cardiac pacemaker, then oftentimes a left bundle branch (LBBB) pattern is seen on the ECG, immediately preceded by a pacing spike. The typical LBBB pattern that can be seen is a QRS that is greater than 0.12 sec (120 ms), broad monophasic R waves in Lead I and V6, and broad monophasic S waves in V1. These changes can make it difficult to determine the presence of a STEMI in a patient who has a pacemaker. The Sgarbossa criteria are a validated clinical decision-making tool to help identify the presence of an acute myocardial infarction in the presence of a LBBB. The Sgarbossa criteria are:

- ST elevation greater than 1 mm in leads with a positive QRS complex such as lead V6.
- There may be ST depression greater than 1 mm in leads V1 to V3. The ST depression is in the same direction as the QRS complex in those leads.
- There may be ST elevation greater than 5 mm in leads V1 to V3. This ST elevation is in the opposite direction as the QRS complex in those leads.

Learning the conditions that mimic STEMI is a challenge for every clinician that interprets ECGs. Only through great training, continuous application of ECG evaluations, and good feedback from knowledgeable mentors can the ECG become a partner in the evaluation of the many different conditions that cause ECG abnormalities.

SELECTED READINGS

Derval N, Shah A, Jais P. Definition of early repolarization: A tug of war. *Circulation.* 2011;124:2185–2186.

Haïssaguerre M, Derval N, Sacher F. Sudden cardiac arrest associated with early repolarization. *N Engl J Med.* 2008;358:2016–2023.

Sgarbossa EB, Pinski SL, Barbagelata A. Electrocardiographic diagnosis of evolving acute myocardial infarction in the presence of left bundle-branch block. GUSTO-1 (Global Utilization of Streptokinase and Tissue Plasminogen Activator for Occluded Coronary Arteries) Investigators. *N Engl J Med.* 1996;334(8):481.

40

Don't forget that there are many causes of chest pain

David Lehrfeld, MD

Traditional risk factors for cardiac disease come from the large Framingham cohort and include diabetes, hypertension, hyperlipidemia, and smoking. More recently, conditions such as chronic kidney disease, lupus, and the immunocompromised have been found to be strongly associated with acute coronary syndrome (ACS). The connection between the traditional and emerging risk factors is that they all cause damage to the coronary arteries and other organs as well. Although risk factors are predictive of lifelong risk for cardiac disease, they are less helpful in evaluating whether the current complaints are related to ACS.

The history of present illness (HPI) that is consistent with angina is more predictive than risk factors in identifying ACS. Angina is a poorly localized discomfort of the chest that may radiate to the arm. Angina is generally defined as discomfort in the above areas that is aggravated by exertion and relieved by rest or nitroglycerin. When evaluating a patient for ACS, it is important to keep in mind that not everyone will have a chief complaint of angina.

Atypical symptoms are common presentations among the old and those with multiple cardiovascular risk factors. Atypical ACS complaints can include pain in the arm, neck, and back as well as complaints other than pain such as dyspnea, nausea, or fatigue. More alarmingly, in a recent review, patients who did not complain of typical symptoms were treated less aggressively and suffered higher mortality.

Any patient complaining of typical symptoms should have a 12-lead ECG performed promptly to determine the presence of ST elevation myocardial infarction (STEMI) as this will affect the choice of destinations for these patients. Communicating the results of the 12-lead ECG (and/or transmitting the ECG to the receiving hospital) will allow the early alerting of their cardiology team, activating a plan of action before patient arrival. The performing of the early 12-lead ECG will also affect the therapies given. For instance, inferior STEMIs that affect the right ventricle can make the cardiac output "preload dependent." In this case, the typical practice of giving nitrates could precipitate severe hypotension. Anterior septal infarcts may give rise to cardiogenic shock and might be an indication to withhold IV B-blockers early on. The 12-lead ECG can also be helpful in the diagnosis of atypical pain. Syncope, altered mental status, and dyspnea might be the only signs of acute myocardial infarction (AMI) in the elderly.

In the contexts of the patient presenting with chest pain in the pre-hospital arena—whether with typical or atypical symptoms—it is best to recognize that if a patient lacks ischemic risk factors, and the HPI and ECG are not consistent with ischemia or STEMI, then an alternate diagnosis must be considered in addition. 12-lead ECGs may help in the consideration of the differential diagnosis of chest pain. Deadly arrhythmias, pulmonary embolism (PE), and aortic dissection (AD) should always be considered in patients presenting with syncope, dyspnea, or chest pain.

The classic risk factors for PE are known as "Virchow's triad," which consists of stasis, hypercoagulability, and vascular injury. Many conditions may cause stasis, such as paralysis from strokes or immobility from surgery, splinting, or casting. Hypercoagulability can be caused by conditions such as pregnancy, cancer, and sickle cell disease. There are scoring systems available for evaluating the risk of PE in a given patient, and the provider must remember that no single ECG finding can make the diagnosis of PE. In patients with PEs, ECG findings are often either nonexistent or transient.

The most common ECG finding in PE is sinus tachycardia, although this is a very nonspecific sign of illness in general. However, in the face of no ischemic changes on the ECG, the presence of sinus tachycardia in a patient with chest pain should prompt an alternate explanation for the patient's symptoms. Classically, right-axis deviation is associated with PE (due to right heart strain, which shifts the axis of the hears to the right side), although left-axis deviation is actually more common. The classic S1-Q3-T3 pattern (S wave in I, Q wave in III, T wave inversion in III) is an indication of right-ventricular strain. Only PEs large enough to sustainably reduce blood flow out of the right ventricle might cause this finding, and it occurs in less than a quarter of PEs that are diagnosed. Right bundle branch blocks can also occur, but their association with PE is highly variable (the provider should keep in mind that all bundle branch blocks may cause ST and T wave changes that can mimic ischemia). Both ST and T wave changes have been found in patients with PE, with T wave inversions being much more common, especially in the precordial V1 to V3 leads. Although there are no definitive findings in the ECG for PE, when combined with a good HPI, a 12-lead ECG can be helpful in differentiating ischemic from non-ischemic chest pain.

It is said of AD: "The difficulty in diagnosis, delayed diagnosis, or failure to diagnose, is so common as to approach the norm for this disease, even in the best of hands, rather than the exception." Risk factors include hypertension, collagen vascular disease, age, male sex, and family history. The HPI is highly variable. Acute AD can often present with symptoms typical of ACS, with chest pain, dyspnea, and diaphoresis, but on the other hand, some cases don't even present with pain. Because dissection can extend to the descending aorta, symptoms above and below the diaphragm—chest AND abdominal pain—should prompt thoughts of AD. Unequal pulses or cold limbs are present in about 15% of dissections. Disruptions in the aortic root can produce new aortic murmurs in one-third of these patients. Dissections into the coronary and carotid arteries can cause AMIs and strokes. Because of this constellation of findings, any patient with a combination of acute cardiac and neurological symptoms should be suspected to have an AD. This is important for the prehospital provider to remember.

The ECG is not a specific test for dissection. It may be normal, show nonspecific signs such as T-wave inversion, or present with STEMI should the coronary arteries be affected by the AD. Even when the ECG confirms the finding of AMI, in the presence of neurologic deficits—such as syncope, paralysis, or paresthesias—AD should be considered as well as occlusive coronary disease. The implications for this can be profound, as giving antiplatelet agents or heparinizing a patient with AD could prove fatal. Lastly, the provider should be suspicious of multiple complaints that seem to have no common cause in patients with HPI findings such as syncope, leg pain, dyspnea, and nausea. This could be the initial presentation of AD, with syncope and leg pain being the neurological symptoms while dyspnea and nausea being atypical findings suspicious for STEMI or non-STEMI but in fact being associated with the dissection.

SELECTED READINGS

Canto JG, Goldberg RJ, Hand MM, et al. Symptom presentation of women with acute coronary syndromes: myth vs. reality. *Arch Intern Med.* 2007;167:2405–2413.

El-Menyar A, Zubaid M, Sulaiman K, et al. Atypical presentation of acute coronary syndrome: A significant independent predictor of in-hospital mortality. *J Cardiol.* 2011;57(2): 165–171.

Esdaile J, Abrahamowicz M, Grodzicky T, et al. Traditional Framingham risk factors fail to fully account for accelerated atherosclerosis in systemic lupus erythematosus. *Arthritis Rheum.* 2001;44(10):2331–2337.

Hsue PY, Giri K, Erickson S, et al. Clinical features of acute coronary syndromes in patients with human immunodeficiency virus infection. *Circulation.* 2004;109:316–319.

41

DON'T FORGET TO ANALYZE WIDE COMPLEX TACHYCARDIAS

DAVID LEHRFELD, MD

Wide complex tachycardias (WCTs) encompass a variety of rhythms that can be difficult to distinguish. The main differentiation that needs to be made is between ventricular tachycardia (VT), supraventricular tachycardia (SVT) with aberrancy due to bundle branch block (BBB), and SVT with aberrancy due to Wolf–Parkinson–White syndrome (WPW). It is important to make this determination as it will affect the subsequent treatment.

VTs are more likely with elderly people who have known heart disease such as myocardial infarction, congestive heart failure, or a family history of sudden cardiac death. In addition to eliciting this in the history, the provider should look for signs of previous medical interventions such as the presence of sternotomy scars or automated internal cardiodefibrillators (AICDs). The provider should consider VTs when the WCT is sustained for more than 30 seconds and especially if the patient becomes unstable. VT is typically often monomorphic, that is, a regular rhythm with the QRS complexes on a consistent axis.

The main exception to the rule is in the setting torsades de pointes (TDP, or "twisting of the points"), a WCT in which the QRS axis changes direction, called "polymorphic tachycardia." This WCT is associated with long QT syndrome. With torsades the QRS complex changes direction, appearing to alternatively go above and then below the ECG baseline. It is a lethal rhythm that often degenerates to ventricular fibrillation (VF) if not treated immediately.

Other helpful signs in determining if the rhythm is VT are if all the QRS complexes from V_1 to V_6 are in the same direction, either all up (R waves) or all down (known as the "QS complex") without any RS complexes. Also, if the QRS has the same morphology as previous premature ventricular contractions, this is a good indicator that the rhythm is of ventricular origin, especially if the rhythm lacks typical bundle branch patterns across the precordial leads. Also, very wide QRS complexes (of 160 ms or greater) and ECGs that show a WCT with an extreme right axis deviation are suggestive of ventricular origin.

If there is AV disassociation with a WCT—where the P waves are not related to the QRS complexes—then the rhythm is almost certainly VT. This can be hard to see at ventricular rates greater than 150 bpm, but actually sometimes P waves can be seen within the QRS complex, either spontaneously generated, or from retrograde conduction of a ventricular beat. The presence of fusion beats—which are supraventricular impulses that are transmitted to the ventricle and triggered a complex on top of an ectopic beat activation—is a useful sign of VT.

SVTs such as AV nodal reentrant tachycardia (formally known as paroxysmal SVT, but now generally called SVT) can also cause WCT in the presence of a BBB or in the preexcitation syndrome WPW. This is referred to as "SVT with aberrancy." SVT is a regular rhythm that is more likely to be found in younger patients, though can be seen at virtually any age. Patients often have a history of palpations that were resolved with adenosine. This history is not necessarily diagnostic as adenosine can terminate VT. If the ECG was taken before the tachycardia began, it might show a BBB with the same morphology as the WCT—indicating that this rhythm is most likely SVT with aberrancy—or shows sign of WPW such as a PR interval of less than 120 ms and the presence of delta waves. If the QRS follows a normal progression for a left bundle branch block or right bundle branch block across V_1 to V_6, the rhythm is likely SVT with aberrancy. At slower rates, P waves might be seen in the QRS complex indicating a supraventricular origin of the rhythm.

Irregularly irregular WCT rhythms suggest atrial fibrillation with aberrancy. Atrial flutter with BBB will be regular if the conduction is fixed (such as the common 2:1 conduction ratio with an atrial rate of 300 bpm and a ventricular response of 150 bpm), though flutter may be irregular if the AV conduction is variable, which often happens if the patient is on an anti-arrhythmic medication.

It's rare that the prehospital provider can be 100% certain that a rhythm is SVT with aberrancy, so if in doubt and the patient is unstable, then treatment for VT should be begun. Non-sustained VT terminates spontaneously, usually without hemodynamic compromise. Sustained VT lasts >30 seconds, and it usually requires an intervention for termination. Sustained VT may produce severe hemodynamic compromise and/or syncope, and it may degenerate into VF.

Recognition of the type of tachycardia has a profound implication on therapy. If the wrong therapy is applied, it might not only fail to terminate the tachycardia but could prove fatal for the patient. Patients with unstable WCT need fast effective treatment in the form of cardioversion.

SELECTED READINGS

Mattu A, Brady W. The "cardiac" literature in 2006: an annotated review for the emergency physician. *Am J Emerg Med.* 2007;25:960–976.

Page R. *Multi-Lead Medics.* Available at www.multileadmedics.com

Wagner G, Marriott H, Lim T. *Marriott's Practical Electrocardiography.* 11th ed. Philadelphia, PA: Lippincott Williams & Wilkins, 2008.

42

DON'T MISS THE SUBTLE ECG FINDINGS OF STEMI

A.J. KIRK

Paramedics should be expert in interpreting electrocardiographic tracings for ST segment elevation myocardial infarctions (STEMIs). Not all myocardial infarctions (MIs) produce a classic ST segment injury pattern appearance; however, paramedics must not be falsely reassured by the lack of a classic injury pattern in a patient having chest pain. Furthermore, not all ST segment elevations are consistent with injury and acute coronary syndrome. It is important for prehospital providers to understand both of these concepts and to correctly interpret ECGs to assist them in correctly caring for patients.

First and foremost, a paramedic must remember to treat the patient rather than relying on any one single test. While the so-called "silent MI" is an important consideration, most patients having a STEMI have some signs and symptoms that should be worrisome to the paramedic. It is always important to remember why a patient is having an ECG performed in the first place, whether it is a routine part of a protocol or whether the paramedic is suspicious of a possible cardiac event. Also, it is really important to remember that some symptoms and signs might be "anginal equivalents," such as altered mental status (AMS) in an elderly person being the only presenting sign of a STEMI.

Some basic rules of ECG interpretation are critical. For example, the paramedic in the prehospital setting should be cautious about deciding whether an elevated ST segment is a STEMI or is "early repolarization." They look very much alike, and "ruling out" a STEMI because the paramedic decides that the tracing is early repolarization and not a STEMI would be a clinical error. Instead, the provider must care for the chest pain patient (or anginal equivalent) according to a STEMI protocol (or other appropriate protocol, including a stroke protocol in a patient with AMS). Conversely, should a 50-year-old male with crushing chest pain and a strong family history of coronary artery disease be ashen gray, diaphoretic, short of breath, and clutching his chest but yet have a normal 12-lead ECG, the paramedic must still suspect myocardial ischemia and treat the patient accordingly.

Many medical therapies—including those for STEMI—have some degree of risk, such as the irreversible aspirin-induced platelet inhibition as a risk for bleeding in aortic dissection or nitroglycerin-induced refractory hypotension in cardiogenic shock. Thus, the prompt transport of the patient with chest pain to the closest appropriate emergency department (ED) is one of the most important parts of the care of these patients, appropriately conveying the patient's condition to the receiving team, including therapies given and changes in condition. Sadly, a common pitfall during further evaluation of these patients is in the underestimation of the patient's condition after successful prehospital treatment. Patients who receive supplemental oxygen, aspirin, nitroglycerin, analgesia, reassurance, and rest may often have improvement of their ECG findings upon arrival to the hospital. It is essential for the paramedic to provide the prehospital ECG tracing(s) to the ED as well as a meaningful and intelligent report on the change in condition. Providers should remember to write the patient's name on the prehospital ECG if it is not already on the tracing! An ECG without a name on it doesn't belong to anybody!

It would be uncommon for deteriorating conditions to be missed by emergency medical services and ED personnel. Improved conditions, however, can give false reassurance to all providers that the patient is not suffering from a serious condition. This may lead to under-triage in the setting of a patient actually suffering from a dangerous problem, and it could delay definitive care such as percutaneous coronary intervention in a patient suffering from a STEMI.

Sometimes prehospital ECGs look a bit different from the in-hospital ECG. Twelve leads produced in the field have comparable quality to in-hospital ECG machines. Placement of the ECG electrodes and the position of the patient may produce differences in the tracings. It can be difficult for paramedics to position patients appropriately during ECG acquisition in the back of an ambulance, for example. ECG limb leads are often placed on the torso near the extremities rather than on the limbs where they should be placed. Placement of the limb leads on the torso may produce "pseudo-Q waves" and "pseudo-ST segment elevations." Should leads be placed adjacent to or partially on top of other electrodes, including defibrillation pads, this may also lead to a "pseudo-ST segment elevation" tracing. Performing an ECG with the patient sitting in a 90-degree upright position may decrease the inferior lead amplitude, making an inferior STEMI more difficult to recognize *(Figs. 42.1, 42.2, and 42.3)*.

Paramedics are often very comfortable interpreting inferior, anterior, and lateral STEMI on ECGs. Avoiding the pitfall of missing the less obvious posterior MI or inadequately recognizing the perils of ST elevation in

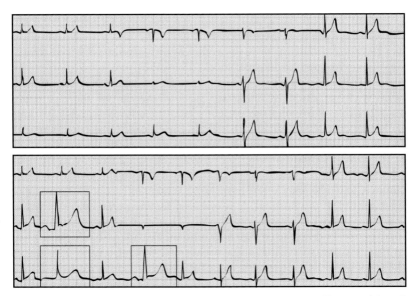

FIGURE 42.1. **Top:** Correct placement of electrodes. **Bottom:** Torso position of electrodes causing pseudo–ST segment elevation.

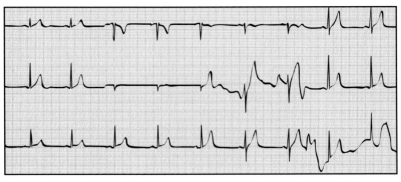

FIGURE 42.2. Pseudo–ST segment elevation from telemetry electrodes being placed on top of ECG electrodes.

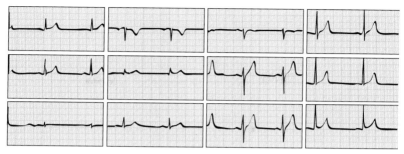

FIGURE 42.3 Decreased inferior amplitudes in ECG performed on a patient sitting upright at 90 degrees.

aVR are also essential. aVR is often neglected during ECG evaluation but, should it contain ST elevation, especially with ST elevation in aVL, it may be associated with left main coronary artery disease. Thus, aVR ST elevation should be recognized in the prehospital and ED setting with suspicion being generated for STEMI *(Fig. 42.4)*.

Acute posterior MI may be difficult both clinically and electrocardiographically to appreciate. Providers may both be less familiar with the criteria for diagnosis and less comfortable making the diagnosis on ECG. Posterior MIs are manifested on ECG with prominent, fully evolved with prominent R waves with ST segment depression in a mirror image of acute injury in leads V_1 through V_3. Placing right-sided chest leads (V_4R, for example) and/or posterior chest leads (V_7, V_8, V_9) may be helpful in making the diagnosis of posterior MI. It is essential that medics not miss a posterior STEMI for lack of an actual ST segment elevation on a 12-lead ECG. Finally, the combination of inferior ST elevation with ST depression in V_1, V_2, or V_3 is consistent with an "inferoposterior" MI. In that setting, the ST depression in the V leads is not reciprocal depression but indicative of a posterior infarction as well *(Fig. 42.5)*.

In summary, it is vital to prehospital patients that paramedics continuously study the technique of 12-lead ECG interpretation. Only through a lifetime of continued practice and improvement can the spectrum of electrocardiography be confidently mastered by the prehospital provider.

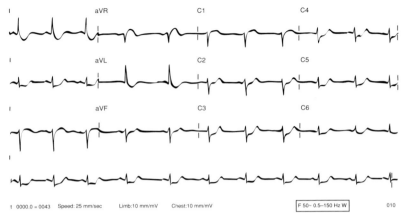

t 0000.0 = 0043   Speed: 25 mm/sec   Limb:10 mm/mV   Chest:10 mm/mV   F 50~ 0.5–150 Hz W   010

FIGURE 42.4. ST elevation in lead aVR consistent with a STEMI.

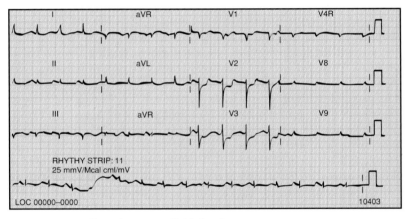

FIGURE 42.5. Posterior myocardial infarction.

SELECTED READINGS

Baranchuk A, Shaw C, Alanazi H, et al. Electrocardiography pitfalls and artifacts: the 10 commandments. *Crit Care Nurse.* 2009;29:67–73.

Chase C, Brady WJ. Artifactual electrocardiographic change mimicking clinical abnormality on the ECG. *Am J Emerg Med.* 2000;18(3):312–316.

Cone D, O'Connor R, Fowler R, et al. *Clinical Aspects of Prehospital Medicine.* Dubuque, IA: Kendall Hunt, 2009.

Hori T, Kurosawa T, Yoshida M, et al. Factors predicting mortality in patients after myocardial infarction caused by left main stem coronary artery occlusion. Significance of ST segment elevation in both aVR and aVL leads. *Jpn Heart J.* 2000;41:571–581.

Mozid AM, Sritharan K, Clesham GJ. Acute total left main stem occlusion treated with emergency percutaneous coronary intervention. *BMJ Case Rep.* 2010; doi:10.1136/bcr.05.2010.3036.

Rudiger A, Hellermann JP, Mukherjee R, et al. Electrocardiographic artifacts due to electrode misplacement and their frequency in different clinical settings. *Am J Emerg Med.* 2007;25(2):174–178.

Thompson J. Country cardiograms case 4: acute posterior myocardial infarction. *Can J Rural Med.* 1997;2(2):76.

43

DON'T OVERLOOK THE ROLE OF HANDS-ONLY CPR IN COMMUNITY-BASED STRATEGIES FOR SURVIVAL

JENNIFER TRIACA, RN, NREMT-P

Compress *and* ventilate, or just compress? That is the question being examined with renewed interest and enthusiasm. The American Heart Association's (AHA) 2010 guidelines for cardiopulmonary resuscitation (CPR) and emergency cardiac care devote an entire section to the discussion of this particular topic. Current recommendations for trained rescuers call for administration of both compressions and ventilations. However, there is some evidence to suggest a role for compression-only, or "hands-only," CPR.

Resuscitation, simply put, means to revive. CPR, as defined by the Merriam-Webster dictionary, "is a procedure that is used to restore normal breathing after cardiac arrest. This involves clearing air passages, artificial respiration, and heart massage by exerting pressure onto the chest from an exterior source." In most cases, CPR is performed with manual chest compressions and artificial respiration via mouth to mouth or mask to mouth.

Educating the public in the chain of survival and the importance of performing immediate and high-quality CPR is paramount. Most laypeople believe that their most important and only role in out-of-hospital cardiac arrest is to activate emergency medical services via 911. Kern et al. conducted a study to evaluate the effectiveness of compression-only CPR. It is commonly accepted that lay rescuers are reluctant to perform mouth-to-mouth resuscitation due to the fear of contracting an illness from the victim. Kern used animal models to study the efficacy of compression-only CPR. He reported that 24–hour survivability was similar between the compression-only and compression–ventilation group. Experimental studies were also performed to simulate worst-case scenarios involving completely occluded airways. One group received 6 minutes of compression–ventilation CPR while another group received 6 minutes of compression-only CPR. There was no difference in 24–hour survival rates between the two groups. Researchers concluded that compression-only CPR is as efficacious as traditional CPR for the first few minutes of cardiac arrest. The AHA guidelines cite several "observational studies" which show similar outcomes for victims of cardiac arrest who receive hands-only CPR versus conventional CPR. Furthermore, bystanders may be likely to perform the compression-only method since there is no risk of disease transmission.

Since initiation of bystander CPR is a key to survival, AHA encourages laypersons to provide chest compressions "(either Hands–Only or conventional CPR…) for anyone with a presumed cardiac arrest."

Emergency medical dispatch (EMD) protocols may function as another avenue for the examination of compression-only CPR. A recent study published in *the New England Journal of Medicine* examined the utility of providing CPR instructions via telephone to callers requesting help for victims of presumed cardiac arrest. Standard protocols, including chest compressions and ventilations, were compared to instructions that incorporated only chest compressions. Emergency medical dispatchers randomly gave standard CPR instructions versus compression-only instructions for witnessed out-of-hospital cardiac arrest. A total of 1,276 patients were included in the study—620 patients received compression-only instructions, and 656 patients were assigned to "standard" CPR. The 30-day survival rate was 8.7% (54 of 620 patients) for patients who received compression-only CPR and 7.0% (46 of 656 patients) who received standard CPR. No statistically significant difference in survival was found at 30 days in compression-only versus standard CPR. The study examined other factors crucial to the initiation of bystander CPR. Compression-only CPR instructions resulted in the delivery of more compressions per minute. In addition, compressions were started in a more timely manner. It is commonly held that survival from cardiac arrest correlates with the delivery of uninterrupted and high-quality compressions. Interruptions in chest compression occurred more frequently in the "standard CPR" study arm. Laypersons took on average 16 seconds to ventilate as opposed to the 1.5 to 2 seconds recommended for healthcare providers.

The debate over standard versus compression-only CPR will continue. To date, there is no research or evidence to conclude that one method is superior with respect to increased survival. From a public health perspective, it seems reasonable that a "hands–only CPR" protocol would encourage bystanders to provide CPR. Improved bystander CPR will increase community-wide survival from out-of-hospital cardiac arrest. EMS systems should take a long, hard look at the possibility of incorporating a "hands-only" strategy into EMD protocols. Compression-only CPR should not be overlooked as a valuable link in the chain of cardiac arrest survival.

SELECTED READINGS

American Heart Association's "Hands-Only CPR" website http://handsonlycpr.org. Videos and mobile smartphone applications are available free of charge for download.

Berg RA, Hemphill R, Abella BS, et al. Part 5: Adult basic life support: 2010 American Heart Association guidelines for cardiopulmonary resuscitation and emergency cardiovascular care. *Circulation.* 2010;122:S685–S705.

Cone DC. Compression-only CPR. *J Am Med Assoc.* 2010;304(13):1493–1495. doi: 10.1001/jama.2010.1420.

Kern KB, Helwig RW, Berg RA, et al. Efficacy of chest compression-only BLS CPR in the presence of an occluded airway. *Resuscitation.* 1998;39(3):179–188.

Svensson L, Bohm K, Castren M, et al. Compression-only CPR or standard CPR in out-of-hospital cardiac arrest. *N Engl J Med.* 2010;363:434–442.

44

DON'T OVERLOOK THE USES OF CAPNOGRAPHY IN CARDIAC ARREST

MAX PATTERSON, EMT-P
JONATHAN C. WENDELL, MD

The use of capnography, otherwise known as continuous monitoring of partial pressure of end-tidal carbon dioxide ($PEtCO_2$), has become widely accepted for prehospital emergency care. Detection of $PEtCO_2$ is already the gold standard for endotracheal tube placement confirmation and is being used increasingly for suspected asthma patients and patients with undifferentiated respiratory distress. With respect to cardiac arrest, however, many providers use only a fraction of capnography's true potential. In this chapter, we will review how $PEtCO_2$ benefits both provider and patient in cases of cardiac arrest.

Numerous studies have demonstrated a correlation between $PEtCO_2$ measurements and the relative success rate of resuscitation. We know that $PEtCO_2$ directly correlates with the partial pressure of arterial CO_2 ($PaCO_2$), which is related to metabolism and cardiac output. With cardiac arrest there is cessation of cardiac output, thus diminishing $PEtCO_2$ return. Cardiac output is augmented through the delivery of high-quality and uninterrupted chest compressions. The increased cardiac output reestablished gas exchange and transport of carbon dioxide. However, $PEtCO_2$ returns to only a fraction of the normal level due to the anaerobic state that accompanies cardiac arrest.

USE OF CAPNOGRAPHY TO MONITOR OUR CPR EFFICACY

Even with optimal compressions, cardiac output only reaches 25% to 33% of normal values. It logically follows that both the uptake of oxygen from the lungs and the delivery of carbon dioxide to the lungs are reduced. Initial levels of $PEtCO_2$ are increased due to the elimination of accumulated byproducts of cellular distress. However, the $PEtCO_2$ typically diminishes over time if return of spontaneous circulation (ROSC) is not established. Maintaining continuous capnography during cardiac arrest can provide real-time feedback of the quality of compressions. In the majority of cases, the slower the $PEtCO_2$ decreases, the more effective the compressions. Optimal cardiopulmonary resuscitation (CPR) will produce greater CO_2 exchange. Conversely, a rapid decline in levels of $PEtCO_2$ should prompt providers to reconsider the quality of chest compressions. With less effective CPR, a comparably lower amount of CO_2 is exchanged. In cases of cardiac arrest, you should continuously monitor for a slowly descending $PEtCO_2$ value as an indicator of efficient resuscitative efforts.

PROGNOSTIC VALUE OF CAPNOGRAPHY IN CARDIAC ARREST

In an early study, a $PEtCO_2$ of 10 mm Hg following 20 minutes of advanced cardiac life support (ACLS) was 100% specific in determining death in patients. Subsequent studies have linked a low $PEtCO_2$ reading to a grim prognosis. Studies in Europe also support the prognostic role of capnography, though their observed futility threshold is a $PEtCO_2$ value of 16 mm Hg. However, these studies only included individuals who were declared deceased in the emergency department (ED). A 2008 study of 737 out-of-hospital cardiac arrests showed that after 20 minutes of advanced life support, a $PEtCO_2$ of 11.3 mm Hg in patients with a shockable rhythm accurately predicted death. For patients with a non-shockable rhythm, a value of 14.3 mm Hg was a reliable predictor of death. Although the exact $PEtCO_2$ levels vary, the literature is clear that persistently diminished $PEtCO_2$ is prognostic of cardiac arrest mortality. It is reasonable to consider integrating end-tidal CO_2 values into termination of resuscitation protocols.

USE CAPNOGRAPHY TO DETERMINE RETURN OF SPONTANEOUS CIRCULATION

Perhaps even more useful than being able to determine futility of resuscitation is the ability of $PEtCO_2$ to detect ROSC. An increase in cardiac output and return of aerobic metabolism follows ROSC. This results in a measurable increase in the patient's $PEtCO_2$. Multiple studies have shown a sharp and sudden increase of >10 mm Hg can be observed at the moment that ROSC begins. This finding carries such profound implications that the American Heart Association included a Class IIa recommendation for $PEtCO_2$ monitoring during ACLS. The savvy clinician can utilize this finding (or lack thereof) to avoid frequent pulse checks during cardiac arrest. Ultimately, the literature is clear that limiting interruptions in chest compressions is key to improved patient outcomes. Continuous capnography can limit these interruptions and should be implemented during the resuscitation effort.

Improving survival from out-of-hospital cardiac arrest is a goal for every prehospital provider. To achieve this goal, we must realize the full potential of the equipment at our disposal. PEtCO2 is a valuable diagnostic and quality improvement tool. Capnography can be used to monitor our CPR efficacy, provide prognostic value, and help determine ROSC. Effective utilization of $PEtCO_2$ and capnography directly improves patient care, particularly in situations of cardiac arrest.

SELECTED READINGS

Kolar M, Krizmaric M, Klemen P, et al. Partial pressure of end-tidal carbon dioxide success-fully predicts cardiopulmonary resuscitation in the field: a prospective observational study. *Critical Care.* 2008;12:R115.

Kupnik D, Skok P. Capnometry in the prehospital setting: are we using its potential? *Emerg Med J.* 2007;24:614–617.

Neumar RW, Otto CW, Link MS, et al. Guidelines for Cardiopulmonary Resuscitation and Emergency Part 8: Adult Advanced Cardiovascular Life Support: 2010 American Heart Circulation. *J Am Heart Assoc.* 2010;122(183):S729.

Pokorná M, Necas E, Kratochvíl J, et al. A sudden increase in partial pressure end-tidal carbon dioxide ($PEtCO_2$) at the moment of return of spontaneous circulation. *J Emerg Med.* 2010;38(5):614–621.

Sanders AB, Kern KB, Otto CW, et al. End-tidal carbon dioxide monitoring during cardiopulmonary resuscitation: a prognostic indicator for survival. *J Am Med Assoc.* 1989; 262(10):1347–1351.

45

DO NOT INTERRUPT CPR FOR MORE THAN 10 SECONDS: IT CAN BE THE DIFFERENCE BETWEEN STAYING ALIVE AND BITING THE DUST

JONATHAN WENK, MD

In a landmark study published in the February 2002 edition of the journal *Circulation*, researchers determined that neurologic outcomes of cardiac arrest survivors were improved with continuous chest compressions. It has since been demonstrated that interruptions in chest compressions negatively impact overall mortality and the neurologic outcomes of cardiac arrest survivors. These findings prompted the American Heart Association (AHA) to change its official guidelines in 2010 so that laypeople would provide compression-only cardiopulmonary resuscitation (CPR). Similarly, it is critical for prehospital providers to administer continuous chest compressions for cardiac arrest victims. This is a huge shift from emergency medical services tradition where the importance has always been placed on tracheal intubation, intravenous access, rhythm analysis, and other advanced life support interventions.

The goal behind performing chest compressions is to perfuse end organs with oxygenated blood. The brain is the organ most susceptible to damage from hypoxic events. Therefore, cerebral perfusion pressure must be maintained during cardiac arrest to ensure improved neurologic outcomes. Timerman et al. concluded that uninterrupted chest compressions promoted higher cerebral and coronary perfusion pressures, leading to an overall decrease in mortality and poor neurologic outcomes.

The most common cause of interrupted chest compressions is multiple or prolonged attempts at securing the airway. While ventilating and oxygenating the lungs is important, it is also important to note that cells are able to extract oxygen from any available circulating hemoglobin. This exchange can take place even when partial pressures of oxygen (PaO_2) in arterial blood are extremely low. This finding highlights the importance of providing continuous chest compressions to circulate oxygenated hemoglobin to the cells.

It is now known how frequently CPR is disrupted during the resuscitative sequence. In a landmark paper published in the journal *Circulation* in 2005, Valenzuela et al. determined that frequent and prolonged stops in chest compressions occur in 57% of out-of-hospital nontraumatic cardiac arrests. The authors cite this fact as chiefly responsible for the dismal 7% survival rate for out-of-hospital arrest victims.

If intubation attempts are unsuccessful while chest compressions continue, alternative airway management techniques should be employed. The use of oropharyngeal/nasopharyngeal airway adjuncts, in conjunction with two-person bag-valve-mask ventilation, or the insertion of an extraglottic device (i.e., laryngeal mask airway), or a dual-lumen airway (i.e., easy tube), are all excellent alternatives to tracheal intubation. The bottom line—don't interrupt chest compressions to attempt intubation!

Chest compressions are also sometimes temporarily halted during placement of intravenous catheters. If movement from continuous chest compressions genuinely prevents the prehospital provider from obtaining intravenous access, resuscitation drugs should be administered via the intraosseous route.

Two other common causes of disrupted chest compressions involve the use of defibrillators. Practitioners often stop chest compressions to apply ECG electrodes, defibrillation pads, while charging the defibrillator, and during pulse checks after delivering a shock. Chest compressions should be interrupted only during actual delivery of an electrical shock, and resumed immediately thereafter, for a full 2 minutes.

Rhythm analysis is another common cause of interrupted chest compressions. The cardiac rhythm should be quickly analyzed prior to delivering an electrical shock, or at the end of every 2-minute compression cycle. A prolonged interruption in chest compressions to analyze the cardiac rhythm is an absolute mistake. It is also best practice for prehospital providers to analyze the ECG rhythm while assessing the pulse.

If prehospital personnel become fatigued while performing chest compressions, a replacement provider should take over in a coordinated and choreographed manner to minimize the interruption. In addition, consideration should be given to the use of automated CPR devices. Similarly, physical transfer of cardiac arrest patients from bed to bed should be coordinated and performed as quickly as possible to allow for minimal interruption of chest compressions.

Finally, it is worth mentioning that compressions should be performed at a rate of at least 100 beats/minute. This has been demonstrated to be the ideal rate to circulate oxygenated blood. A slower compression rate will introduce built-in interruptions that should be avoided. Performing chest compressions to the beat of the popular Bee Gees song, "Stayin' Alive," ensures a rate of 100 compressions per minute. Less optimistic providers can listen to Queen's, "Another One Bites the Dust," for the same time signature.

In summary, uninterrupted chest compressions performed at a rate of at least 100 beats/minute has been shown to decrease mortality and improve

neurologic outcomes in survivors of cardiac arrest. Many prehospital defibrillators have a metronome feature to assist providers in determining the
ideal chest compression rate. If available, mechanical chest compression
devices provide uninterrupted chest compressions at the proper rate and
depth. Whether these devices are superior to human chest compressions,
however, is controversial.

SELECTED READINGS

Kern KB, Hilwig RW, Berg RA, et al. Importance of continuous chest compressions during
    cardiopulmonary resuscitation: improved outcome during a simulated single lay-rescuer
    scenario. *Circulation.* 2002;105:645–649.

Matlock JW, Hafner EG, Bockewitz LT, et al. "Stayin' Alive": a pilot study to test the effec-
    tiveness of a novel mental metronome in maintaining appropriate compression rates in
    simulated cardiac arrest. *Ann Emerg Med.* 2008;52(4):S67–S68.

Rea T, Fahrenbruch C, Culley L. CPR with chest compression alone or with rescue breathing.
    New Engl J Med. 2010;363:423–433.

Timerman S. Improved hemodynamic performance with a novel chest compression device
    during treatment of in-hospital cardiac arrest. *Resuscitation.* 2004;61:273–280.

Valenzuela T, Kern K, Clark L, et al. Interruptions of chest compressions during emergency
    medical systems resuscitations. *Circulation.* 2005;112:1259–1265.

46

PAY CLOSE ATTENTION TO BLS INTERVENTION!

JOEL HIGUCHI, I/C, ACLS I/C

You are dispatched to a cardiac arrest. Your partner runs for the intubation gear, and the firefighter medics are setting up an intravenous line (IV). With all the paramedic help at the patient's side, there can be no doubt about survival, right? WRONG!

ACLS is thought of as the "gold standard" when rendering treatment to victims of cardiac arrest. Recent literature suggests that basic life support is equally, if not more, important and paramedics often overlook this component. In 2005, <6% of out-of-hospital cardiac arrest patients survived to hospital discharge. In that same year, the American Heart Association published two studies that documented poor quality of cardiopulmonary resuscitation (CPR) performed during in-hospital and out-of-hospital resuscitations. Prehospital cardiac arrest has poor survivability; there is no doubt. To increase the survivability, renew your emphasis on good BLS care, specifically CPR.

There are many procedures for patients in cardiac arrest: Chest compressions, endotracheal intubation, venipuncture, medication administration, etc. Of these, compressions may have the highest therapeutic value. Studies have repeatedly shown an increase survival of ventricular fibrillation (VF) patients with early CPR and defibrillation. When CPR is performed properly, you can maintain a cardiac output of 25% to 30% of normal values. This is a vital amount of blood flow necessary to perfuse core organs such as the heart, brain, and lungs. During VF, the patient's heart is depleted of oxygen and energy. Compressions can deliver the oxygen and energy to the heart, increasing the likelihood that a shock will both eliminate VF and be followed by return of spontaneous circulation (ROSC). The current standards reflect a compression rate of at least 100 per minute, a depth of at least 2 in., allowing for adequate recoil, minimizing interruptions, and avoiding excess ventilations. This can be difficult to maintain consistently throughout an entire call. Making an effort to periodically step back and assess the overall quality and focus of patient care can significantly change patient outcome.

Pay special attention to your ventilatory rate. One of the most common pitfalls in BLS care is unintentional hyperventilation. When a patient breathes in normally, the diaphragm flattens and lowers, causing a negative intrathoracic pressure. This pulls air into the lungs and enhances blood return to the heart. When a patient is ventilated, the diaphragm does not react physiologically and air is forced into the lungs creating a positive pressure. Positive pressure ventilation inhibits blood return to the heart. When hyperventilating our patients, we are actually decreasing cardiac preload and therefore cardiac output.

All too often we take unnecessary or longer than necessary breaks in CPR for intubation, patient movement, or IV's. To maintain cardiac output and optimize patient outcome it is also important to ensure quality compressions throughout the patient encounter, especially while moving the patient into the hospital. It is very difficult to get the proper compression depth, rate, and recoil with the stretcher at its highest height setting. Often, this can be easily accomplished by lowering the stretcher to allow for proper technique. Minimize interruptions in compressions by becoming more efficient. Perform CPR during attempts at intubation and intravenous or intraosseous access. If you must stop, only stop for the bare minimum amount of time to perform the skill. Early defibrillation has shown to be the most significant intervention when treating your patients in VF and pulseless ventricular tachycardia and should be performed as efficiently as possible. Do not stop CPR to place defibrillation electrodes on the patient or charging the defibrillator. Good BLS care continues to be the backbone of cardiac arrest treatment even during the ACLS interventions. Treatments should be performed around consistent and quality CPR to provide the best chance of survival. Cardiac arrest medications will not yield their maximum effect if they are not properly circulated. To allow medications, the best chance at performing, it is best to administer these medications as soon as possible during the 2-minute cycles of CPR. Properly performed CPR will give medications more time to circulate and reach their site of action.

The goal in every resuscitation event is ROSC and discharge from the hospital with intact cardiocerebral function. All too often we overlook and underemphasize the BLS components of cardiac arrest care. Remember to periodically step back and assess quality and focus of patient care. Maintain proper compressions, minimize interruptions, and become a more efficient practitioner when performing interventions. Hyperventilation will reduce cardiac preload and output, so be sure to maintain the proper rate of ventilation throughout patient care. The better BLS care is instituted, the more impact ALS interventions can have.

SELECTED READINGS

Berg RA, Hemphill R, Abella BS, et al. Adult basic life support: 2010 American Heart Association guidelines for cardiopulmonary resuscitation and emergency cardiovascular care. *Circulation.* 2010;122:S685–S705.

Ewy G, Kellum M, Bobrow B. Cardiocerebral resuscitation. *EMS World Magazine.* 2008; 38(6):41–49.

Field JM, Hazinski MF, Sayre MR, et al. Executive Summary: 2010 American Heart Association guidelines for cardiopulmonary resuscitation and emergency cardiovascular care. *Circulation.* 2010;122:S640–S656.

Ramsay PT, Maxwell RA. Advancements in cardiopulmonary resuscitation: increasing circulation and improving survival. *Am Surg.* 2009;75(5):359–362.

47

REFER YOUR PATIENTS WITH ROSC TO THE MOST APPROPRIATE FACILITY

BRUCE G. VANHOY, NREMT-P

As prehospital providers, we work diligently to resuscitate our patients who have suffered out-of-hospital cardiac arrest (OOHCA). When the patient has a return of spontaneous circulation (ROSC), our job remains far from complete. It is our responsibility to transport patients to the closest appropriate facility. With respect to cardiac arrest, the closest hospital may not always be the most suitable receiving facility.

Prehospital patient care is only one component of a larger, regionalized system that needs to be in place for the proper care of a patient who has suffered OOHCA with ROSC. As emergency medical services (EMS) systems have adopted newer, evidenced-based cardiopulmonary resuscitation guidelines, there has been improvement in both survival and neurologic outcomes. Regional systems for survival and the designation of "cardiac resuscitation centers (CRCs)" have their roots in an improved understanding of cardiac arrest physiology and interventions associated with survival. CRCs are committed to collaboration with local EMS systems, the initiation of therapeutic hypothermia, and percutaneous coronary intervention (PCI). Though there is not currently a nationwide standard for the CRC designation, potential elements of a specialized cardiac arrest receiving center include:

- Ability to perform PCI
- Ability to initiate and maintain therapeutic hypothermia
- Coordinated, multidisciplinary care plan for post-arrest patient care
- Provides cardiopulmonary resuscitation (CPR) and advanced cardiac life support training for patients, community, and staff
- Maintains data registry for the purpose of tracking, improving, and monitoring outcomes

Understanding the components of a regionalized, post-resuscitation transport algorithm allows the prehospital provider to be a functional component of positive outcome driven care. Key prehospital interventions and benchmarks include:

- Early hemodynamic stabilization
  - Treatment of reversible causes of the cardiac arrest
  - Initiation of vasopressors for patients with low blood pressures
- Initiation of therapeutic hypothermia

- Being prepared to react to re-arrest
- Early notification of the receiving CRC
- Transport the patient to a CRC

The last two items illustrate the importance of the "closest appropriate" facility for patients in cardiac arrest. CRCs that offer hypothermic therapy and possibly post-arrest PCI may significantly contribute to improved outcomes. These hospitals represent state-of-the-art, evidence-based care for the patient with ROSC from cardiac arrest. Though several jurisdictions have embraced the idea of resuscitation centers, other EMS simply encourage providers to transport patients with ROSC to the closest hospital. Just as trauma patients benefit from the specialized care and resources of credentialed trauma centers, patients resuscitated from cardiac arrest may fare better when taken to hospitals capable of providing coordinated, post-arrest care. The "system of survival" represents a unique opportunity for collaboration between local hospitals, medical directors, and system administrators. Drs. Bobrow and Kern, two pioneers of cardiocerebral CPR, state that the goal of directed patient transport is to get "the right patients to the right place in the right time."

Tracking and reporting data on patients suffering from OOHCA is another important component of a regionalized system. Prehospital interventions need to be reviewed by a continuous quality improvement (CQI) process. This allows for feedback and highlights both strength and weakness in the prehospital phase of care. Data collection is also integrated into the CQI process. Analysis of data permits a thorough evaluation of system efficiency. The Arizona Department of Health began designating cardiac arrest centers (CACs) in 2007; data from their system of survival is collected in order to "shed light on key resuscitation questions such as how to optimize cooling, emergent PCI, and other interventions." The Arizona consortium of CACs, as of 2008, includes 19 hospitals and key stakeholders such as community leaders and specialists from emergency medicine, cardiology, and critical care. Data are collected and shared on an ongoing basis in order to ensure the delivery of up-to-date, evidence-based cardiac arrest care.

EMS providers play an important role in optimizing outcomes from cardiac arrest. It is no longer just about the ROSC. Cardiac arrest is a complex medical condition that requires specialized resources and expertise. The local EMS system is uniquely positioned to "refer" patients to hospitals best suited to the delivery of post-arrest care.

SELECTED READINGS

Bobrow BJ, Kern KB. Regionalization of postcardiac arrest care. *Curr Opin Crit Care.* 2009; 15:221–227.

Graham N. Regional cardiac resuscitation systems of care. *Signa Vitae.* 2010;5(suppl 1):50–54.

Jacobs I, Nadkarni V, Bahr J, et al. Cardiac arrest and cardiopulmonary resuscitation outcome reports. *Circulation.* 2004;110:3385–3397.

Nichol G, Aufderheide T, Eigel B, et al. Regional systems of care for out-of-hospital cardiac arrest. *Circulation.* 2010;121:709–729.

Rittenberger J. Therapeutic hypothermia: a potent therapy. *EMS1.com,* July 27, 2010. http://www.ems1.com/medical-clinical/articles/854210-Therapeutic-hypothermia-A-potent-therapy/

48

IT'S A COLD DAY ON THE HORIZON: CHILL YOUR ROSC PATIENTS OUT!

RICK LEONARD, AAS, NREMT-P
KEVIN G. SEAMAN, MD, FACEP

Have you ever needed a patient to just "chill out" to make the situation better? Here's an intervention that does exactly that!

The concept of therapeutic hypothermia was born from observed clinical cases of accidental hypothermia where patients were found in states of moderate or severe hypothermia, clinically deceased, and were able to not only be revived and re-warmed but found to be completely (or nearly completely) neurologically intact. This led to two large studies utilizing methods that included cold IV fluids and ice packs, respectively, to cool comatose survivors of cardiac arrest. These landmark studies, published in 2002, demonstrated improved neurologically intact survival in those patients who had been cooled. An additional benefit is that only six to seven patients would need to be cooled to produce one neurologically intact survivor. The data from these studies were strong enough to be included in the 2005 AHA guidelines; subsequent studies have revealed that only a minority of hospitals and emergency medical services (EMS) have instituted cooling. For this reason, the American Heart Association has recognized and recommended the therapy for prehospital care as part of coordinated patient care efforts with receiving facilities. It is anticipated that therapeutic hypothermia (TH) will be as commonplace for the post-arrest patient as cardiopulmonary resuscitation is to the cardiac arrest victim.

As TH is relatively new for EMS implementation, the goal of this section is to anticipate the possibility of pitfalls and mitigate them. The objective is to establish best practices for EMS system implementation including initial training for providers and quality controls. These best practices should clearly identify the therapeutic window for the initiation of cooling and the complications that occur outside of those boundaries. An ongoing quality assurance program will ensure that the latest, evidence-based practice is incorporated into any prehospital protocol for TH.

COMMON PITFALLS
- Failure to initiate protective hypothermia immediately after return of spontaneous circulation (ROSC), resulting in delays in core temperature reduction and diminished protection against free radical formation.

- Failure to monitor core temperature to maintain therapeutic core temperatures between 32° and 34°C.
- Relying on pulse-oximetry to determine oxygen perfusion when peripheral circulation is minimal during post-arrest states and compounded by induced hypothermia. Tissue respiration is better monitored by measured end-tidal carbon dioxide.
- Initiation of therapeutic hypothermia prior to ROSC. This reduces the bio-availability of resuscitative medications and may hinder efforts to regain ROSC.
- Failure to coordinate with local emergency departments and ensure that patients with ROSC are transported to a facility capable of TH and post-cardiac arrest critical care.

WHO GETS THE COLD SHOULDER (TREATMENT)?

The 2010 AHA guidelines recommend therapeutic hypothermia solely for those patients who are comatose, post-resuscitation with ROSC. Therapeutic hypothermia should be induced as quickly as possible, but only after successful resuscitation. Use of a cooling device or cold IV fluids during resuscitative efforts will hinder the bio-availability of medications and could instigate lethal arrhythmias rather than alleviate them. One small study indicated that rapid infusion of 2 L of 4°C Ringer's lactate or normal saline is sufficient for lowering the core to the desired temperature. Further research is needed to detail what other patient populations may benefit from this strategy. Some studies have even explored the concept of intra-arrest cooling.

HOW LOW CAN YOU GO?

Multiple studies cite the best outcomes from patients maintained between 32° and 34°C. This temperature range is classified as mild hypothermia and translates to a core body temperature of roughly 90° to 93°F. Temperatures above 34°C are not effective for preventing cardiac instability or the release of toxic radicals thought to be responsible for destruction of neural tissue and instigating multisystem organ failure. Temperatures below 32°C are known to allow crystallization of tissues and certain blood components and decreases circulation to clinically detrimental levels. Getting there is only half the battle, though; the pitfalls to avoid are over-cooling and passive re-warming. Caregivers must continuously monitor the patient's core temperature to assure maintenance of this therapeutic range.

SO, WE'VE CHILLED OUT.... NOW WHAT?

It is critical to understand that therapeutic hypothermia is a single facet of post-arrest care. In addition to TH, providers must continue to support cardiac output and monitor $PEtCO_2$ for adequate tissue perfusion.

In addition to the intervention, pre-planning is a critical factor in the total management of care. EMS systems are encouraged to collaborate with hospitals and even state and regional care systems to

1) standardize equipment and methodologies
2) develop standardized protocols and procedures
3) identify facilities with hypothermia and cardiac intervention capabilities
4) allow for transport to these specialty centers, which may involve bypass of the closest hospital

This system-wide approach integrates resuscitation science, prehospital care, and emergency department care. A coordinated approach to TH affords cardiac arrest survivors the best chance for a meaningful neurologic outcome. EMS providers are in a unique position to advocate for their patients and participate in the development of regionalized protocols. TH is a low-cost and potentially high-impact treatment strategy that is rapidly becoming the standard of care for patients with ROSC. Put your system on ice!

SELECTED READINGS

Arrich J. Clinical application of mild hypothermia after cardiac arrest. *Crit Care Med.* 2007; 35:1041–1047.

Bernard SA, Gray TW, Buist MD, et al. Treatment of comatose survivors of out-of-hospital cardiac arrest with induced hypothermia. *N Engl J Med.* 2002;346:557–563.

Field JM, Hazinski MF, Sayre MR, et al. Executive Summary: 2010 American Heart Association guidelines for cardiopulmonary resuscitation and emergency cardiovascular care, *Circulation.* 2010;122:S640–S656.

Gaieski DF, Band RA, Abella BS, et al. Early goal-directed hemodynamic optimization combined with therapeutic hypothermia to improve the neurologic outcome after cardiac arrest. *Resuscitation.* 2009;80:418–424.

Hypothermia After Cardiac Arrest Study Group. Mild therapeutic hypothermia to improve neurological outcome after cardiac arrest. *N Engl J Med.* 2002;346:549–556.

Kim F, Olsufka M, Longstreth WT Jr, et al. Pilot randomized clinical trial of prehospital induction of mild hypothermia in out-of-hospital cardiac arrest patients with a rapid infusion of 4°C normal saline. *Circulation.* 2007;115:3064–3070.

49

Chest compressions are your most "advanced" BLS technique

Gregory R. Valcourt, AAS, NREMT-P
Kevin G. Seaman, MD, FACEP

Survival from cardiac arrest is dependent on many factors. One of the most important factors is the production and continuance of blood flow by rescuers with cardiac compression until normal or physiologic cardiac flow is restored. The quality of cardiac flow is determined by the quality of cardiac compressions. The goal of high-quality team resuscitation is to provide the highest possible coronary and cerebral blood pressure during cardiac arrest (no-flow) states. Coronary blood pressure is determined by subtracting right arterial "diastolic" pressure from the aortic "diastolic" pressure ($CPP = Ao_d - Ra_d$). The most important determinant of cerebral perfusion is the arterial pressure generated during external chest compressions. The quality of cardiac compressions is determined by several factors: Compression surface, compression rate, compression depth, compression recoil, compression interruption, compression feedback, and compressor fatigue. Let's look at each one of these factors individually and how we can maximize the quality of our compressions.

Compression Surface
A common sense rule, of course, is to place the patient in a supine position on a firm surface. Performing cardiac compression in a bed or on the stretcher may allow for ineffective compression as the mattress or stretcher pad allows for downward displacement of the patient instead of the patient's sternum against their spine. If necessary, a board can be placed between the patient and the bed or the patient can be quickly and safely placed on the floor for effective cardiac compressions. Also, performing manual cardiac compression on a moving stretcher will affect compression performance and probably produce less blood flow than when the patient is stationary. Resuscitation should generally be conducted where the patient is found.

Compression Rate
According to the 2010 American Heart Association guidelines for cardiopulmonary resuscitation (CPR) and emergency cardiovascular care (2010 AHA), chest compressions should be performed at a rate of at least 100 per minute. The rate refers to the speed of compressions, not the actual number of compressions delivered per minute. The number of chest compressions

delivered per minute is an important determinant of return of spontaneous circulation (ROSC) and neurologically intact survival. Extrapolation of data from out-of-hospital observational study showed improved survival to hospital discharge when at least 68 to 89 chest compressions per minute were delivered; the study also demonstrated that improved survival occurred with chest compression rates as high as 120 per minute.

COMPRESSION DEPTH
Compressing the sternum creates flow or cardiac systole. A depth of at least 2 in. (5 cm) is the current adult compression depth according to 2010 AHA. An earlier study found that deeper compressions (greater than 50 mm or 2 in.) resulted in conversion to an organized cardiac rhythm in 100% of the cases.

COMPRESSION RECOIL
With complete chest recoil, you create cardiac diastole or refill. Many studies reveal that incomplete chest wall recoil was common, particularly when rescuers were fatigued. Incomplete recoil during cardiac compression is associated with higher intrathoracic pressures and significantly decreased hemodynamics, including decreased coronary perfusion, cardiac index, myocardial blood flow, and cerebral perfusion.

Good cardiac compressions require equal downstroke and upstroke for CPR to produce maximum flow in the cardiac arrest patient.

COMPRESSION INTERRUPTION
Once cardiac flow is established, it is important to maintain it. Interrupting compression for unnecessary reasons only decrease the patient's chance of survival. Currently, interruptions should be for less than 10 seconds. With good team training and practice, rescuers can switch compressors, perform a pulse check, defibrillate, and resume compression within 10 seconds or less. Maintaining continuous cardiac flow is the key to surviving cardiac arrest.

COMPRESSION FEEDBACK
There are numerous feedback devices on the market that can assist with rescuers improving the quality of compressions. One study evaluated CPR quality with auto feedback and it found that it improved short-term outcomes, and there was trend toward improved survival (2.9% control versus 4.3% with feedback).

Some of these devices provide both visual and audio prompts as to the quality of compressions, whereas others are incorporated into automated external defibrillators or cardiac monitors. When real-time feedback was combined with debriefing, compression rate guideline compliance significantly improved, from 45% to 84%. In addition, the study found that both rate and depth of compression improved from 29% to 64%, nearly doubling the measured quality of CPR.

COMPRESSOR FATIGUE

As with any manual repetitive skill, the longer it is performed continuously, there will obviously be a decrease in performance of that skill. The same holds true for cardiac compressions. Significant fatigue and shallow compressions are common after 1 minute of CPR, although rescuers may not recognize that fatigue is present for greater than 5 minutes. The CPR Improvement Working Group formed to help improve CPR skill performance reported in November 2009 at an AHA conference in Orlando, Florida, that 75% of healthcare professional perceived their skill at performing CPR as being quite high. However, only 26% stated perceived performance of rate, depth, and ratio in compliance with the AHA/ILCOR 2005 CPR guidelines. In addition, 55% of healthcare professionals surveyed believe that studies report CPR quality is good, very good, or excellent. This survey showed the gaps that exist in perception versus reality of CPR performance by healthcare professionals.

With so many factors affecting the quality of compressions, the imperative of ongoing research is clear. Research, training, feedback, and critique are central to maximizing resuscitation techniques and improving survival from cardiac arrest.

SELECTED READINGS

Berg RA, Hemphill R, Abella BS, et al. Part 5: Adult basic life support: 2010 American Heart Association guidelines for cardiopulmonary resuscitation and emergency cardiovascular care. *Circulation.* 2010;122(suppl 3):S685–S705.

Edelson DP, Litzinger B, Arora V, et al. Improving in-hospital cardiac arrest process and outcomes with performance debriefing. *Arch Intern Med.* 2008;168(10):1063–1069.

Edelson DP, Abella BS, Kramer-Joansen J, et al. Effects of compression depth and pre-shock pauses predict defibrillation failure during cardiac arrest. *Resuscitation.* 2006;71(2):137–145.

Kim JA, Vogel D, Guimond G, et al. A randomized, controlled comparison of cardiopulmonary resuscitation performed on the floor and on a moving ambulance stretcher. *Prehospital Emergency Care.* 2006;10(1):68–70.

Kramer-Johansen J, Myklebust H, Wik L, et al. Quality of out-of-hospital cardiopulmonary resuscitation with real time automated feedback: a prospective interventional study. *Resuscitation.* 2006;71:283–292.

50

CPR DEVICES: DON'T BELIEVE EVERYTHING YOU HEAR

SAM MATTA, RN, CEN, CCRN, NREMT-P

Over the last few years it seems like every conference you go to or every journal you open, there are new devices that claim to help you resuscitate a patient more effectively. Such advertisements and representatives make claims such as

- "Twice as many patients achieved return of spontaneous circulation (ROSC),"
- "Doubles blood flow to the heart, and can increase blood flow by 75%."

Are these claims true? In this chapter we will examine the effectiveness of current CPR devices and come up with the ones you should convince your medical directors/EMS captains are worth the money. The two types of mechanical compression devices and currently available airway adjunct devices will be discussed.

One example of a mechanical compression device is a piston style device manufactured by Jolife, a division of Medtronic. Although piston style devices have been on the market for some time, the LUCAS device offers the advantage of active decompression technology. The LUCAS uses a suction cup at the end of the piston. The concept for this design was reportedly initiated after an EMS crew witnessed a man performing CPR on his elderly father using a bathroom plunger. It is proposed that with this technology, the chest is actively decompressed and the suction creates more negative intrathoracic pressure than the intrathoracic pressure created with standard CPR. In theory, this concept appears to be sound; however, the majority of literature addressing this type of technology provides little to no advantage over manual CPR.

The second design type of mechanical compression device that is available is the belt or cuff design. These types of devices use a load distributing band or cuff to constrict the entire chest cavity from front to back during the compression process. Presently, the Zoll AutoPulse® is the most commonly used device of this type. In a major metropolitan prehospital study, the belt or cuff style device revealed a 15% increase in ROSC using this type of device than what was obtained using manual CPR. The results of this study have not been supported or duplicated by any additional research. Other research indicates that belt or cuff devices provide similar or inferior outcomes than the outcomes that result using manual CPR.

A more promising resuscitation device is the impedance threshold device (ITD). The ITD is a small device that is placed between the BVM/resuscitator device and the mask/airway device (ETT/LMA/Combitube) and functions as an adjunct to airway management. The ITD limits air entry into the lungs during recoil of the chest during CPR. The resulting decreased air entry into the lungs reduces intrathoracic pressure and ultimately enhances venous return. With increased venous return, the heart is filled more effectively, thereby greatly increasing the cardiac output with each compression. The increased cardiac output translates to improved coronary perfusion pressures and cerebral perfusion pressures. While there has been little evidence of increased long-term survival with the use of ITD, there is convincing evidence that the device improves hemodynamic parameters during resuscitation. Presently, the most commonly used ITD device is the ResQPOD® manufactured by Advanced Circulatory Systems. The ResQPOD® also incorporates a set of timing lights that blink 10 times a minute to help guide the provider to deliver appropriate ventilation cycles thus decreasing the risk of hypo- or hyperventilating the patient. The cost of ITDs is approximately $100 and the benefits provided may be well worth the cost of the product.

The mechanical compression devices were developed to address the problem of providing effective compressions while performing CPR in both inpatient and outpatient settings. Multiple studies have indicated that compressions failed to be delivered at the correct rate and/or depth more than 50% of the time whether performed by highly trained providers or those not highly trained. Research also indicates that the quality of compressions deteriorates significantly after only 1 minute of starting compressions. Although research does not indicate that any of these compression devices significantly improves CPR outcomes, one distinct advantage that does exist with any of these devices is they provide an increased margin of safety during transport. If these devices can be perfected, they will allow EMS providers to remain restrained during transport while still providing effective circulatory support. Although these mechanical compression devices appear to provide some benefits, they have not been proven to be superior to well-trained providers. Clearly, it is the well-trained EMS provider who represents the most effective CPR device on the market!

SELECTED READINGS

Halperin H, Carver D. Mechanical CPR devices. *Signa Vitae*. 2010;5:69–73.

Shuster M, Swee L, Deakin C, et al. CPR techniques and devices. *Circulation*. 2010;122: S338–S344.

Wik L, Kramer-Johansen J, Mykelbust H. Quality of cardiopulmonary resuscitation during out-of-hospital cardiac arrest. *JAMA*. 2005;293:363–365.

51

CONFIRMATION IS ABOUT MORE THAN DIRECT VISUALIZATION, ESPECIALLY IN CARDIAC ARREST

SCOTT H. WHEATLEY, BS, NREMT-P
ELIZABETH MOYE, BA, NREMT-P

As prehospital care providers, we do not get constant and continuous practice with endotracheal intubation as we do with the insertion of intravenous lines or the application of oxygen masks. However, the one thing that has to be a constant in our management of the intubated patient is confirmation and security of the endotracheal tube after it is placed. During resuscitation from cardiac arrest, the chance of tube dislodgement becomes even higher due to patient movement from external forces of compression, either human or mechanical. Similarly, the chaotic and high-pressure environment of the resuscitation may contribute to mistakes and oversight. Current studies indicate that endotracheal tube dislodgement may occur with much more frequency than previously believed. Securing the tube is an absolute imperative, and commercial tube holders provide additional insurance against tube migration.

Throughout resuscitation efforts, your natural adrenaline is flowing high as you cope with challenges of securing and maintaining the airway. Direct visualization of the endotracheal tube as it goes through the cords is a useful tool and can be constituted as firm evidence of a correctly placed endotracheal tube. However, multiple additional techniques should be utilized to confirm the placement. Do not rely solely on your eyes! After visualization occurs, ventilate the patient and auscultate the abdomen and chest. Even though you visualized the passage of the tube, movement or improper anatomy recognition may give the provider a false sense of security. Make sure you start at the abdomen. By starting in the abdomen, you may be able to recognize an improperly placed endotracheal tube much quicker than starting over the lung fields. Once you assure that there are no sounds in the abdominal area, move to the lungs. Lung sounds provide an additional but incomplete measure of security. Patients who have excessive air in their stomach or who have aspirated gastric contents can have lung sounds that are "falsely positive." In other words, the lung sounds may not indicate that the tube is squarely in the trachea. The utilization of capnography is the next and final piece of the confirmation puzzle. In one study, 23% of misplaced endotracheal intubations were associated with failure to utilize continuous $EtCO_2$ monitoring. A multimodal strategy of tube confirmation meets current American Heart Association recommendations of the verification of endotracheal tube placement. Remember that a misplaced endotracheal tube is not an immediate life-threatening problem. The failure to recognize misplacement, however, is something for which providers should have zero tolerance. An unrecognized esophageal intubation has disastrous consequences for your patient.

Once the endotracheal tube has been confirmed to be in the correct place, maintaining the security of the endotracheal tube is your next challenge. In the early years of prehospital intubation, one method and one method only was utilized for endotracheal tube securing and that was tape. Tape was useful and served a purpose unless it became contaminated with blood, vomit, or other bodily fluids or substances. In some instances there were records of skin tears or other adverse effects while removing the "taped" endotracheal tubes. Now as time has progressed we have moved forward with innovation and invention. We now have many different commercial endotracheal tube holders available that will make your job easier in the field. The goal is to find one that works with you, for you, and is within the budget restraints of your particular department.

As you secure the endotracheal tube think about what could dislodge it. Think about all the outside forces that may play against you with normal patient movement, road movement, and/or a spontaneous return of circulation with alertness and consciousness. If utilizing tape, remember that simple things such as water, vomit, blood, and/or sputum can dislodge the tape and keep it from sticking and securing the endotracheal tube to the patient. If utilizing a commercial device, assure that the device remains attached to the patient. Sometimes when moving the patient, a commercial device may become detached and permit migration of the endotracheal tube.

When moving the patient down steps and from the back of the ambulance, disconnect the endotracheal tube from the bag valve mask. This assures that with normal movement and/or a change in elevation that the tube remains in place and not changed due to human height or lack of attention to pulling or pushing the bag valve mask. Remember to constantly check both clinical assessment factors of endotracheal tube confirmation and visual confirmation of teeth marks and line of depth recording. During cardiac arrest situations, this will have to be continuously monitored due to constant movement of the patient not only from the residence but lifting and moving the patient to the transport vehicle, road bumps, and of course movement to the receiving facility's stretcher. Providing emergency department personnel with a visual record in the form of a carbon dioxide waveform is indisputable proof that you have done your job in inserting, maintaining, and securing the endotracheal tube.

During resuscitations, it is extremely challenging to simultaneously address the issues of endotracheal tube confirmation and security. The goal is to make a plan, execute it, and confirm that your intervention was successful. Utilizing the systematic approach, confirming your intervention, and continuously reassessing your interventions will prevent, if not eliminate, misplaced prehospital endotracheal intubations.

SELECTED READINGS

AHA. *Guidelines 2000.* Dallas: AHA; 2000.

Grmec S. Comparison of three different methods to confirm tracheal tube placement in emergency intubation. *Intensive Care Med.* 2002;28(6):701–704.

Owen R, Castle N, Hann H, et al. Extubation force: a comparison of adhesive tape, non-adhesive tape and a commercial endotracheal tube holder. *Resuscitation.* 2009;80(11):1296–1300.

Silvestri S, Ralls GA, Krauss B, et al. The effectiveness of out-of-hospital use of continuous end-tidal carbon dioxide monitoring on the rate of unrecognized misplaced intubation within a regional emergency medical services system. *Ann Emerg Med.* 2005;45(5):497–503.

Verification of endotracheal tube placement. *Ann Emerg Med.* 2009;54(1):141–142.

Yilmaz B, Colakoglu K, Gurunluoglu R. Skin avulsion injury during endotracheal tube extubation—case report of an unusual complication. *Patient Saf Surg.* 2008;2:12.

52

KNOW WHEN TO SAY, "WHEN!" TERMINATION OF RESUSCITATION EFFORTS IN CARDIAC ARREST

THOMAS G. CHICCONE, MD, FACEP

Prehospital providers will be well served to remember who benefits most from resuscitation. The 2010 AHA Guidelines for cardiopulmonary resuscitation (CPR) and ECC address this issue early in their document.

The vast majority of cardiac arrests occur in adults, and the highest survival rates from cardiac arrest are reported among patients of all ages who have a witnessed arrest and an initial rhythm of ventricular fibrillation (VF) or pulseless ventricular tachycardia (VT).

Consider this: United States paramedics respond to 300,000 victims of cardiac arrest every year. Fewer than 8% will survive. What then are the barriers to suspension of prehospital resuscitative efforts? Focus groups of emergency physicians and EMS medical directors at the 2008 National Association of Emergency Medical Physicians meeting reached consensus on this issue. Some states mandate that arrest victims get transported to a hospital. This may be based on the public misperception that more will happen for arrest victims in the hospital, or that more will survive. In addition, reimbursement issues drive policy decisions about transport versus no transport. This creates potent disincentive to terminate efforts on scene when transports pay more. Spending more healthcare dollars, however, is a feeble strategy and ultimately will not raise the dead. Then comes the thorny issue of how to manage the acute grief of loved ones in this emotionally charged setting. Finally, providers voice frustration that evidence-based medicine continues to erode their spectrum of care activities, and that CPR is the pinnacle of prehospital interventions.

The AHA has recently offered two-tiered advice for termination of resuscitative efforts for adults who experience out-of-hospital cardiac arrest. Tier 1 deals with suspending efforts by withdrawing BLS support (before the arrival of ALS) provided the following conditions are met.

- Arrest not witnessed by EMS provider(s) or first responder
- No return of spontaneous circulation (ROSC) after three complete rounds of CPR and automated external defibrillator (AED) analyses
- No AED shocks delivered

Tier 2 deals with ALS termination of resuscitation in the out-of-hospital arrest before transport. Again, all of the following conditions must be met.

- Arrest unwitnessed by anyone
- No bystander CPR
- No ROSC after complete ALS care in the field
- No shocks delivered

In both instances, online medical control is included.

Other groups have wrestled with the problem of when to say, "when." Suggestions include (for normothermic patients)

- Duration of efforts exceeding 30 minutes without ROSC
- Initial rhythm asystole
- Interval delay between arrest onset and resuscitation
- Patient age and comorbidities
- Absent brainstem activity

In the setting of traumatic prehospital arrest, certain mechanisms are felt to simply be incompatible with life. These include, but are not limited to, subjects burned beyond recognition, victims of blunt trauma to the chest and/or abdomen without vital signs. Once resuscitative efforts proceed, clinical circumstances such as blunt versus penetrating trauma may play a role in the decision to withdraw support.

Any protocols empowering prehospital providers to withhold or terminate care should be legally enlightened and cautiously developed. The unique features of any given EMS system require active physician oversight. In a timely position statement approved by its Board of Directors, the National Association of Emergency Medicine Physicians advocated that, as a first step, EMS systems have written protocols that allow for termination of resuscitation by EMS providers in nontraumatic cardiac arrest. Perhaps this powerful endorsement will stimulate collaboration between jurisdictional (local) medical direction and providers to implement these urgently needed changes.

Interested readers are directed to the National Association of EMS Physicians (NAEMSP) resource document published in the fall of 2011. The authors are quick to point out that just as the science of resuscitation is evolving, so is the science of termination of resuscitation. Adoption of termination protocols is in the interest of public health. In nontraumatic cardiac arrest, evidence-guided protocols include arrests not witnessed by EMS providers, absence of shockable rhythms, and no ROSC before transport. Perhaps their conclusion says it best: "In general, resuscitation for nontraumatic cardiac arrest should occur on scene rather than during transport."

SELECTED READINGS

Bailey ED, Wydro GC, Cone DC. Termination of resuscitation in the prehospital setting for adult patients suffering nontraumatic cardiac arrest. National Association of EMS Physicians Standards and Clinical Practice Committee. *Prehosp Emerg Care.* 2000;4:190.

de Vos R, Oosterom L, Koster RW, et al. Decisions to terminate resuscitation. Resuscitation Committee. *Resuscitation.* 1998;39:7.

Haller JS Jr. The beginnings of urban ambulance service in the United States and England. *J Emerg Med.* 1990;8:743.

Hampton OP Jr. Transportation of the injured, a report. *Bull Am Coll Surg.* 1960;45:55.

Hazinski MF, ed. *Highlights of the 2010 American Heart Association Guidelines for CPR and ECC.* Dallas, TX: American Heart Association, 2010; 2, 24.

Horsted TI, Rasmussen LS, Lippert FK, et al. Outcome of out-of-hospital cardiac arrest—why do physicians withhold resuscitation attempts? *Resuscitation.* 2004;63:287.

Marco CA, Bessman ES, Schoenfeld CN, et al. Ethical issues of cardiopulmonary resuscitation: current practice among emergency physicians. *Acad Emerg Med.* 1997;4:898.

Millin MG, Khandker SR, Malki A. Termination of resuscitation of nontraumatic cardiopulmonary arrest: resource document for the National Association of EMS Physicians Position Statement. *Prehosp Emerg Care.* 2011;15:547–554.

Mohr M, Bahr J, Schmid J, et al. The decision to terminate resuscitative efforts: results of a questionnaire. *Resuscitation.* 1997;34:51.

Morrison LJ, Visentin LM, Kiss A, et al. Validation of a rule for termination of resuscitation in out-of-hospital cardiac arrest. *N Engl J Med.* 2006;355:478.

National Association of EMS Physicians Position Statement. Termination of resuscitation of non-traumatic cardiopulmonary arrest. 2/18/2011.

53

NONINVASIVE AIRWAY MANAGEMENT IN CARDIAC ARREST: THINK BEYOND INTUBATION

ALEXANDER J. PERRICONE, BS, NREMT-P

"I cannot wait to tube somebody!" Does this phrase sound familiar to you? Every new paramedic eagerly awaits their first opportunity to intubate a patient in the field. Dropping an endotracheal tube has long been regarded as a benchmark of competency and experience in the EMS arena. Prehospital endotracheal intubation (ETI) has long been regarded as the golden standard of airway management for the patient in cardiac arrest. Recent studies, however, indicate that paramedics may not have enough training and continuing practice with the skill to maintain proficiency. Furthermore, prehospital intubation has not been linked to improved outcomes or survival. The airway can be safely, effectively, and efficiently managed by noninvasive means. The American Heart Association has even down played the use of invasive airway management in its 2010 cardiac arrest resuscitation recommendation. The focus of this chapter is to present the prehospital provider with an alternative to invasive airway management in cardiac arrest.

Emergency medical technicians (EMTs) are taught the importance of airway maintenance as well as noninvasive methods of ensuring airway patency. A significant amount of classroom time is spent learning about noninvasive airway management. Skill practice sessions and practical testing ensure that EMTs can reliably demonstrate these techniques on actual patients. Topics such as patient positioning, airway adjuncts, suction, and bag-valve-mask (BVM) techniques are all introduced during initial EMT training. What happens to these skills as we transition to a higher level of care? It's very clear that paramedics still rely on the endotracheal tube despite numerous academic studies, guideline changes, and recommendations in favor of noninvasive airways in the prehospital setting.

It is well established that prehospital providers must maintain a high level of proficiency in airway assessment and noninvasive airway management techniques. Providers must perform a thorough assessment of the patient's airway and make rapid decisions on how to manage the airway during cardiac arrest. Failure to act quickly results in airway/respiratory compromise and can lead to further deterioration of the patient. Providers must assess the impact of invasive airway management on patient outcome.

If chest compressions are interrupted, even for only a few seconds, the invasive airway techniques place the patient at greater risk for poor neurologic outcomes. This can simply be avoided by using noninvasive airways instead of intubation. The proper use of noninvasive airway adjuncts such as the oropharyngeal, nasopharyngeal, and BVM device will allow for constant and consistent CPR, a key goal for successful out-of-hospital ROSC.

Training programs place a huge emphasis on the importance of ETI. Noninvasive skills need to be treated with the same importance. Field supervisors, senior medics, and Quality Assurance Officers should ensure that providers working under their care are appropriately trained and possess the ability to assess the airway and properly use noninvasive airway adjuncts.

Airway management in cardiac arrest involves selecting the most appropriate tools and employing effective techniques to ensure that the patient is adequately ventilated and oxygenated. Providers should focus on airway management while ensuring uninterrupted chest compressions. One method of ensuring sharp focus during cardiac arrest management is to follow the "Ten Commandments of Airway Management." In 1999, Dr. Corey Slovis expertly articulated the priorities of prehospital airway control:

1) Oxygenation and ventilation are the top priorities.
2) Airway management does not mean intubation.
3) Be an expert at BVM ventilation.
4) Know your equipment.
5) Know at least one rescue ventilation technique.
6) Develop a personal airway algorithm.
7) Don't let your ego get in the way.
8) Invest time in learning airway skills.
9) Use an end-tidal CO_2 ($EtCO_2$) detector and/or esophageal detector device to confirm every intubation.
10) When seconds count, don't count on seconds.

Simple noninvasive maneuvers and airway adjuncts are the most beneficial to our patients. This concept is emphasized by the first five commandments. Commandment 2 expressly deemphasizes ETI. Providers must evaluate the risks and rewards of using invasive airways during cardiac arrest.

ETI is not the only choice for securing an airway. It is an option reserved for patients with a failed or dislodged tracheostomy catheter and those that can't be adequately ventilated with BVM. Airway maintenance should be accomplished simultaneously while treating the causes of cardiac arrest. Prehospital providers should carefully evaluate the need for

ETI during cardiac arrest and be comfortable with the use of noninvasive, "BLS" airway adjuncts.

Selected Readings

Benumor J. *Airway Management: Principles and Practice.* Mosby: St. Louis: Mosby, 1996.

Clawson JJ, Dernocoeur KB, Rose B. *Principles of Emergency Medical Dispatch.* 4th ed. Salt Lake City: Priority Press, 2008.

Kovacs G, Bullock G, Ackroyd-Stolarz S, et al. A randomized controlled trial on the effect of educational interventions in promoting airway management skill maintenance. *Ann Emerg Med.* 2000;36:301–309.

Neumar RW, Otto CW, Link MS, et al. Advanced cardiovascular life support: 2010 American Heart Association guidelines for cardiopulmonary resuscitation and emergency cardiovascular care. *Circulation.* 2010;122:S729–S767.

Slovis C. Ten commandments of airway management. *JEMS.* 1999;34(1):31.

54

DO NOT FAIL TO ENSURE QUALITY CHEST COMPRESSIONS!

CERISA C. SPEIGHT, NREMT-P
DALE E. BECKER, NREMT-P

Press hard, press fast—why are we telling you this? You know the components of quality CPR; you must compress at an adequate rate and depth, allowing full recoil and minimizing interruptions. We know what to do, so what's the problem? The problem is that studies are showing, time and time again, that we don't administer quality CPR without practice and feedback.

Feedback, for our purposes, will be defined as any way of measuring the efficacy of our interventions before, during, or after the event. Feedback is important. You wouldn't administer a nebulizer treatment to an asthma patient and then fail to auscultate lung sounds, or give a fluid bolus to a hypotensive patient and then never take another blood pressure, would you? So why are we administering chest compressions and just assuming that what we are doing is having the desired effect?

The fact is that we aren't nearly as good at CPR as we think. Even though our average rate of compression is above 100 per minute, when we factor in interruptions, we are actually compressing closer to 65 per minute. Studies have shown that we may deliver compressions of adequate depth less than 25% of the time. Now consider that there is a direct correlation between the depth of compressions and the success of defibrillation. Compression depth also determines coronary perfusion pressure (CPP) and CPP has been found to be the best single predictor of return of spontaneous circulation (ROSC). The use of feedback during chest compressions has been shown to increase the amount of effective compressions by nearly 50% and the conclusion is clear: Feedback ensures quality and ensuring quality saves lives.

The first part of CPR quality assurance starts before the call. In paramedic school, we learn that the response starts with dispatch. We will take it a step further: When it comes to a skill as vital as CPR, the response starts with attitude. We must change the culture of EMS, such that cardiac arrests are no longer regarded as skill drills or "Hollywood codes." With a national survival disparity as vast as 5% to 50%, we have to believe that if we change the way we approach out-of-hospital cardiac arrests, our outcomes will change. For things to get better, we must try something different, and the first change will have to be our expectations.

Now that we have the proper attitude, we need to train with an emphasis on quality compressions. This should be a team approach. Like all things that involve the participation of numerous people, it will require a lot of practice and communication. Commercially available feedback devices such as metronomes and accelerometers can help ensure that we are compressing at the appropriate rate and depth, but only practice can ensure that we are limiting hands-off time and increasing compression fraction by coordinating interventions. We should also have a "game plan" before the call. Consider assigning duties to members of your team so that everyone knows their responsibility.

For the next part of our QA program, we need to ensure the effectiveness of CPR in real time. One way to provide real-time QA is to assign someone whose sole job is to ensure that compressors switch out every 2 minutes and that CPR is performed as effectively as possible. It's very easy to allow compressions to become secondary to more advanced interventions (intubation, IV/IO access, medication administration, etc.) All of these interventions take time and have their own quality assurance processes. It's important to work around those providing CPR and limit interruptions at all times. Data suggest that every 5-second reduction in the pause preceding defibrillation nearly doubles the odds of a successful shock. Make no mistake; next to rescuer safety, effective chest compressions are the most important part of running a code!

Another way to provide QA is the aforementioned feedback devices. While these items haven't been proven to be effective in improving patient outcomes, they have been proven to improve the quality of CPR. A standard "musical" metronome will help ensure that compressions are at the appropriate speed. Some cardiac monitor/defibrillators have this feature built in. Compression quality feedback devices can be as simple as an accelerometer that measures the distance that the device moves downward (and then provides a visual or audible indicator of depth) or part of a more complex system that integrates with the cardiac monitor defibrillator (such as Philips' QCPR.) There are even CPR "apps" that work with smart phones using built-in accelerometers for training purposes.

Assessing end-tidal carbon dioxide ($EtCO_2$) levels through the use of waveform capnography is another way to evaluate the efficacy of resuscitative efforts. $EtCO_2$ levels may correlate with CPR quality by providing a visual indicator of effectiveness. For example, the rescuer at the monitor may begin to see a decreasing size in waveform height, as the compressor's quality declines. A spike in $EtCO_2$ levels has been shown to provide one of the earliest indicators of ROSC.

One final method of ensuring quality in compressions occurs after the code is over. Regardless of the result, debriefing helps providers improve their skills by acknowledging what was done well and what could be improved on the next call. Software, such as Physio-Control's Code Stat, can provide information for analysis after the incident allowing hard data to guide the debriefing process.

Quality assurance is essential to improving patient care. The organizations that are leading the way in resuscitative care are arguably the most introspective. Through vigilance in training, re-training, education, and data analysis, it is possible to improve the outcome for victims of sudden cardiac arrest.

PEARLS

- Train with other rescuers to minimize interruptions in compressions
- Practice compressions with feedback devices to improve your skills
- Approach every working code as a viable patient until proven otherwise
- Coordinate ALS interventions so that compressions remain paramount
- Limit pulse checks to less than 10 seconds
- Always switch compressors after 2 minutes
- Use waveform capnography to assess effectiveness
- Debrief every code

SELECTED READINGS

Berg RA, Hemhill R, Abella BS, et al. Part 5: Adult basic life support: 2010 American Heart Association guidelines for cardiopulmonary resuscitation and emergency cardiovascular care. *Circulation.* 2010;122(suppl 3): S685–S705.

Bhanji F, Mancini ME., Sinz E, et al. Part 16: Education, implementation, and teams: 2010 American Heart Association guidelines for cardiopulmonary resuscitation and emergency cardiovascular care. *Circulation.* 2010;122(suppl 3):S9200–S9933.

"Code-Stat 7.0." *Lifenet Systems.* Available at: http://www.physio-control.com/uploadedFiles/products/data–management/product_data/CODE-STAT_Spec_3206829-001.pdf

Edelson DP, Abella BS, Kramer-Johansen, et al. Effects of compression depth and pre-shock pauses predict defibrillation failure during cardiac arrest. *Resuscitation.* 2006;71(2):137–145.

Heightman AJ. The ultimate trend setter. *Measuring life and breath: the benefits of capnography in EMS. J Emer Med Services.* 2010;7. http://www.jems.com/special/measuring-life-breath

Kramer-Johansen J, Myklebust H, Wik L, et al. Quality of out-of-hospital cardiopulmonary resuscitation with real time automated feedback: a prospective interventional study. *Resuscitation.* 2006;71(3):283–292.

Leonard S. Accelerometer provides real-time feedback for handheld CPR device. *Medical Product Manufacturing News.* January/February 2011. Available at: http://www.qmed.com/mpmn/article/28425/accelerometer-provides-real-time-feedback-handheld-cpr-device

Paradis NA, Martin GB, Rivers EP, et al. Coronary perfusion pressure and the return of spontaneous circulation in human cardiopulmonary resuscitation. *JAMA.* 1990;263(8):1106–1113.

"Pocket CPR." Zoll Medical Corporation. Available at: http://www.pocketcpr.com/iphone.html

Wik L, Kramer-Johansen J, Myklebust H, et al. Quality of cardiopulmonary resuscitation during out-of-hospital cardiac arrest. *JAMA.* 2005;293(3):299–304.

55

INVOLVE YOUR COMMUNITY IN CARDIAC ARREST: TOGETHER YOU CAN MAKE A DIFFERENCE

CASSANDRA MARIA CHIRAS GODAR, BS, NREMT-P

KEVIN G. SEAMAN, MD, FACEP

INTRODUCTION

EMS providers are met with many challenges while resuscitating a patient in cardiac arrest. Providers at all levels participate in these resource-intensive cardiac arrest calls. Did you know there is another team member that can improve survival and not cost a dime in salary? Other than volunteer firefighters or well-intentioned bystanders, who could that be? The answer: The community. This chapter will explore the idea of using the community as the first "first-responder." People have their emergencies where they live, work, and play; it only makes sense to make use of the bystanders to deliver initial CPR and care.

- EMS response is a pivotal step in the chain of survival, but not the only one.
- Many arrests occur at home, in the presence of family members who are available to perform bystander CPR.

At times, cardiac arrest can seem overwhelming and providers feel that success or failure rests solely in their hands—don't make that mistake! Broaden your team to include your community to provide initial care. Since the early days of EMS, providers have recognized the value of bystander involvement to combat the time-dependent emergency of cardiac arrest. In 1972, Medic Two of Seattle, WA, was the first system in the world to incorporate citizens into the emergency response of cardiac arrests. They realized that even with the best response by emergency vehicles, patients would be without CPR for too long and they acted to train citizens to provide CPR until the EMS rescuers arrived.

SCIENCE BEHIND CARDIAC ARREST SURVIVAL

Patient survival seems to be a worthy enough resuscitation goal, but we have to remember that the patient must also be neurologically intact to be able to walk out of the hospital and maintain a good quality of life. Many patients do achieve a return of circulation during transport, only to die in the emergency room soon after arrival. This is a disappointing situation for everyone involved in the resuscitation, but we have to remember that many factors both in and out of our control can affect the survivability of an arrest. Studies have identified three essential factors that influence neurologically intact cardiac arrest survival.

- Time to CPR
- Time to defibrillation
- Provision of timely and proficient ALS care

Ideally, we'd like to keep these times as short as possible, and there are many ways to do this.

Similarly, resuscitation research demonstrates that some factors don't increase neurologically intact survival to hospital discharge as much as we previously thought (if at all).

- ACLS drugs
- Devices (i.e., automated CPR devices, impedance threshold devices)

IMPROVING SURVIVAL: WHAT STEPS CAN WE TAKE?

How can your community members help?

- They can learn compressions-only or "hands-only" bystander CPR. Community-oriented classes are available free of charge and over the internet.
- Increase aggressive telephone CPR instructions. Dispatchers trained in emergency medical dispatch (EMD) protocols can instruct the caller to provide CPR in real time.
- Increase awareness about public access defibrillation (PAD) and training in the lay population.

What can you do as an EMS provider?

- Individually:
  - Efficient turnout time from the station: Move as if you're responding to a fire in your first due area.
  - Bring all essential equipment with you upon arrival (don't backtrack!).
  - BLS: Don't be afraid to ask for help and upgrade to ALS.
- As a crew:
  - Assign provider roles prior to the response, or practice/review roles before you even get a call.
  - Continuing education—chest pain, SOB, syncope, and seizures can be arrest imposters, or they can deteriorate into an arrest situation. Be aware of this and respond with urgency to all of these calls.
  - Remember that basic life support interventions (such as high quality, uninterrupted compressions) should take priority.

- As a system:
  - Cardiac arrest is resource intensive. The presence of more providers permits a more coordinated approach to resuscitation and helps avoid the problem of rescuer fatigue.
  - Rapid dispatch of units is essential (because time saved is muscle saved!).
  - Attempt to evaluate CPR performance in real time throughout the call. (Read the chapter on real-time QA of CPR if you want to learn more!)

Taking It to the Next Level: Implementing QA Feedback and Formal Programs

What else can be done to improve cardiac arrest survival in your community?

- Implement a system to measure metrics and bystander CPR performance rates.
- Implement citizen CPR programs (which will decrease time to CPR).
- Give dispatchers feedback on telephone CPR instructions.

Evaluate discrepancies in PAD locations versus arrest locations and rethink placement if necessary. (Goal: Get AEDs where the arrests are happening.)

Conclusion

Improving cardiac arrest survival rates in your community seems like a monumental task, but it can be done.

- Involve your community and let them help you! (Make them the first "first-responders.")
- Do what you can do individually.
- Do what you can do as a crew/in your station.
- Educate your supervisors about system changes that can be made.

Selected Readings

Berg RA, Hemphill R, Abella BS, et al. Part 5: Adult basic life support: 2010 American Heart Association guidelines for cardiopulmonary resuscitation and emergency cardiac care. *Circulation.* 2010;122(suppl 3):S685–S705.

Bobrow BJ, Spaite DW, Berg RA, et al. Chest compression-only CPR by lay rescuers and survival from out-of-hospital cardiac arrest. *JAMA.* 2010;304(13):1447–1454.

Eisenberg MS. *Resuscitate! How Your Community Can Improve Survival from Sudden Cardiac Arrest.* Seattle, WA: University of Washington Press; 2009.

Travers AH, Rea TD, Bobrow BJ, et al. Part 4: CPR overview: 2010 American Heart Association guidelines for cardiopulmonary resuscitation and emergency cardiac care. *Circulation.* 2010;122(suppl 3):S676–S684.

56

Teamwork in cardiac arrest: no one codes alone

Elizabeth L. Seaman, NREMT
Kevin G. Seaman, MD, FACEP

Have you ever been involved in a cardiac arrest where the code seemed chaotic or poorly run? Conversely, have you been involved in a cardiac arrest that proceeded in an organized way and flowed well (like clockwork)? Are these differences occurring solely from chance alone? Or, is there a way to accomplish the "code like clockwork" more consistently? The answer is emphatically, "yes!" This chapter will provide you with good examples of team–oriented approaches to resuscitation.

Publication of the *2010 American Heart Association Basic and Advanced Life Support Guidelines* reemphasizes that the two most important factors affecting survival in cardiac arrest are time to effective CPR and time to first defibrillation. Adding to our knowledge are new articles which demonstrate that higher percentage of time spent doing chest compressions for each minute, termed chest compression fraction or CPR density, also improves survival.

Pearls (Errors to Avoid)

- Mistaking gasping, weak, ineffective respiratory efforts (agonal breathing) as adequate and not starting chest compressions
- Not timing the resuscitation/not monitoring the compression interval (less than 2-minute cycles of CPR)
- Not monitoring compression quality (depth of chest compressions, adequacy of chest recoil)
- Failure to minimize interruptions in CPR (most common pauses are to shock or ventilate)
- Failure to integrate basic life support (BLS) and advanced life support (ALS) roles during the resuscitation
- Failure to assign tasks for cardiac arrest resuscitation prior to the call
- Failure to efficiently rotate chest compressors leading to rescuer fatigue and ineffective compressions

Cardiac arrests in the field are chaotic enough; to improve survival, chest compression fraction must be maximized. Just as the Boy Scout motto is, "Be Prepared"; implementing this maxim to assign roles for the different tasks in cardiac arrest will make CPR more efficient. Just as fire suppression roles are defined prior to the first call at morning turnover, so can roles for cardiac arrest resuscitation be predefined. For a four-person crew, these assignments might look like this:

Officer—timekeeper and CPR conductor
Driver—AED operation
FF1—compressions
FF2—ventilations

In an EMS system with a tiered response, the BLS suppression crew is typically the first to arrive. Each team member begins in their assigned role. The officer keeps time and advises the team upon completion of the first 2-minute compression interval. The AED operator analyzes the rhythm as the compressor and ventilator switch roles. By switching roles, the members performing compressions stay fresh and maintain good quality CPR can be continued. The officer monitors the quality of CPR and provides real-time feedback about compression rate, quality, and depth. The officer also ensures that rescuers permit full chest recoil in between compressions.

Arriving ALS providers present new challenges for the continuity of care during resuscitation. ALS interventions such as intubation and switching from AED to a manual monitor-defibrillator can cause unacceptably long pauses in CPR. Here, as well, teamwork is the key to success. The officer can call out time remaining to switch and let the ALS crew know that they have that time to plan their interventions. If bag-valve-mask ventilation is adequate, intubation can be delayed. The ALS providers can focus on defibrillation, IV access, and medication administration. Intubation, when indicated, can be done with chest compressions ongoing or can be accomplished during a pause in CPR not longer than 10 seconds.

As crews get used to their new roles in cardiac arrest, opportunities for improvements in chest compression fraction (that fraction of time per minute spent compressing the chest) are many. Some of these process improvements take some faith—continuing chest compressions while the AED is charging requires confidence in the AED operator not pressing to shock until they truly confirm, "all clear!" That said, the risk of shock from biphasic defibrillators is extremely low. The compressor can improve efficiency by hovering their hands 6 to 10 in. over the chest while the countershock is delivered. CPR resumes immediately following the shock. The team should not pause for the traditional pulse check. Taken together, all of these efficiencies (role assignments, teamwork, minimizing pauses in CPR, and integration of ALS) have been termed "high-performance CPR."

(See Box.) You can learn more about these techniques of CPR and view a video of high-performance CPR by visiting the Resuscitation Academy's website: http://www.resuscitationacademy.org/index.htm

Time to first CPR, quality of CPR, and time to first defibrillation all contribute to neurologically intact survival following cardiac arrest. Believe that you can make a difference. Change what you can about the way you personally, and your team, deliver CPR. Make improvements in the CPR delivery and technique. Provide feedback to crews on their performance and continually reassess benchmarks like compression fraction, compression depth, and compression rate. Newer technologies permit feedback delivery to take place in real time. Before you know it, you too will be seeing results from treating CPR as a team sport!

Roles in Cardiac Arrest Based Upon Team Size

- Two-person response team
  - First BLS responder: Defibrillator, timekeeper, and chest compressions
  - Second BLS responder: Ventilator, sets rate ≥ 100 and counts compressions
  Rotate positions every 2 minutes.
  Upon ALS arrival the first BLS responder assumes the role of the timekeeper.
  For all response teams with > two responders, the defibrillator operator does not change position until ALS is on the scene.

- Three-person response team
  - First BLS responder: Defibrillator and timekeeper
  - Second BLS responder: Ventilator, sets rate and counts compressions
  - Third BLS responder: Chest compressions
  Rotate second and third persons every 2 minutes.
  Upon ALS arrival the first responder rotates into the timekeeper position.
- Four-person response team
  - First BLS responder: Defibrillator
  - Second BLS responder: Ventilator, sets rate and counts compressions
  - Third BLS responder: Chest compressions
  - Fourth BLS responder: Timekeeper and radio
  Rotate second and third persons every 2 minutes.
  Upon ALS arrival the fourth person remains the timekeeper.
- Five-person response team
  - First through fourth responder same as four-person team
  - Fifth BLS responder: ready to assume CPR compressions in rotation
  Rotate second, third, and fifth persons every 2 minutes.
  Upon ALS arrival the fourth person remains the timekeeper.

Adapted from the Resuscitation Dance, Thurston County Medic One

SELECTED READINGS

Berg RA, Hemphill R, Abella BS, et al. Part 5: Adult basic life support: 2010 American Heart Association guidelines for cardiopulmonary resuscitation and emergency cardiovascular care. *Circulation.* 2010;122(suppl 3):S685–S705.

Christenson J, Andrusiek D, Everson-Stewart S, et al. Chest compression fraction determines survival in patients with out-of-hospital ventricular fibrillation. *Circulation.* 2009; 120:1241–1247.

Eisenberg MS. *Resuscitate! How Your Community Can Improve Survival from Sudden Cardiac Arrest.* Seattle, WA: University of Washington Press; 2009.

Field JM, Hazinski MF, Sayre MR, et al. Part 1: Executive summary: 2010 American Heart Association guidelines for cardiopulmonary resuscitation and emergency cardiovascular care. *Circulation.* 2010;122(suppl 3):S640–S656.

Lecture Handout, Cynthia Hambly, Thurston County Medic One, presented at the Resuscitation Academy, Seattle, WA, October 2010.

Resuscitation Academy website: www.resuscitationacademy.org

57

THINK ABOUT WHERE TO BEGIN YOUR RESUSCITATION

GREGORY R. VALCOURT, AAS, NREMT-P
KEVIN G. SEAMAN, MD, FACEP

In the global picture of cardiac arrest management, providers may often overlook the simple question of where to begin a resuscitation. The obvious answer might be the following: Treat the patient where you find him! And like me, you probably have responded to a cardiac arrest where the initial responders have begun treatments in an inappropriate and inadequate location, for example, on the bed, on the small bathroom floor, or even in a car. In one such case, I was dispatched to a call for an unconscious person. Upon my arrival, I located the EMTs who were attempting to take blood pressure on the "unconscious patient" who was slumped over on the toilet with his pants down by his ankles. When I asked the EMTs if the patient was breathing or had a pulse, they responded that they hadn't checked them yet. And, you guessed it: The patient was in cardiac arrest. With their assistance, we removed the patient from the bathroom, down the narrow hall, and out to the living room. I made this movement decision first because there was far more room to begin our assessment and care of the patient on the living room floor than in the small bathroom where care was initially started. Sometimes, small spaces prevent the treatment team from functioning effectively. Something as simple as adequate working room can make the difference between successful and stressful resuscitations. Just as with any other emergency call, it is important to perform a scene size-up. Resuscitation team leaders must consider physical obstacles and hazards to ongoing resuscitation. Without the information gathered in the size-up, often the wrong decision is made in regards to what attack method is used and oftentimes the initial wrong decision is followed, sometimes to a disastrous result. I have heard this described as "backing a loser (bad decision)."

Ample space is required for the performance of high-quality, team-based cardiac resuscitation. Well, just how large does the space need to be to allow an adequate working space? I like to think of the space needed to perform effective resuscitation as the "CPR action circle." This action circle allows the team to have rescuers on both sides of the victim's chest so that continuous cardiac compression can be maintained and to allow for quick switching of compressors at 2-minute intervals. There also need to be room on both sides of the patient for the cardiac monitor and for the initiation of intravenous or intraosseous lines. In addition, there needs to be ample room at the patient's head for airway personnel to perform necessary basic and advanced airway skills. Furthermore, adequate space is required to transfer the patient to a backboard, a stretcher, and a waiting ambulance. There have been times when we have turned the patient's bed up against the wall to allow for ample space to work in the patient's bedroom.

Another simple rule to follow is to "look as you walk." As you walk through the house or incident location, look for a large area to "hold the resuscitation" as you eventually reach your patient. By looking for the space before you reach the patient, you can quickly move them to the spot you "discovered" during your scene survey and entry. Another factor to consider is the amount of light in the resuscitation area. As you "go through the house" turn on the lights. By lighting the way, this also allows you to spot any potential scene dangers. If the patient's room does not supply enough light, move to a room that has adequate lighting to make the resuscitation more effective.

During paramedic classes, I simulate a cardiac arrest in my small office with the lights off. Almost every time, the students will work the simulated cardiac arrest in the dark office where they found the patient. Yet just 10 ft away is the well-lit, large hallway they just walked down to reach the simulated patient! Often prehospital providers prefer to move the patient from the location where they are found to the back of our ambulance or "office" to run the code. In dangerous situations or bad weather, this strategy might have merit. But after the patient is secured in the back of the ambulance, the amount of room ("CPR action circle") available for the performance of effective cardiac resuscitation is greatly decreased. In conclusion, the decision of "where to resuscitate" is the most important step in the total care of the cardiac arrest patient. Take the time to think of the answer of "where to resuscitate" before you actually begin to resuscitate!

SELECTED READINGS

Havel C, Schreiber W, Riedmuller E, et al. Quality of closed chest compression in ambulance vehicles, flying helicopters and at the scene. *Resuscitation.* 2007;73(2):264–270.

Stone CK, Thomas SH. Can correct closed-chest compressions be performed during prehospital transport? *Prehosp Disaster Med.* 1995;10(2):121–123.

Vadeboncoeur T, Bobrow BJ, Clark L, et al. The Save Hearts in Arizona Registry and Education (SHARE) program: who is performing CPR and where are they doing it? *Resuscitation.* 2007;75(1):68–75.

58

REMEMBER TO TAKE A THOROUGH PATIENT HISTORY!

PATRICK BRADY

Neglecting to take a thorough patient history is a commonly committed EMS pitfall that is really classified as a "subset" of the larger failure of the provider to perform a thorough and complete assessment of the patient. Acquiring the medical history of our patients is a critical element of the care of EMS providers. Unfortunately, providers can often be found not to have acquired important information related to the history of the patient, and this omission can dramatically impact the patient's care in a negative manner.

The failure of providers to take a thorough patient history is common, especially in the heat of the moment associated with fast-moving events such as a major trauma case. One element of their medical history, which *can* be a key answer to the patient at hand, should be asked for all trauma patients: *How and why did this trauma happen in the first place?* Knowing, for example, that a patient is on a beta-blocker for hypertension could explain why, in the setting of hemorrhagic shock due to trauma, a tachycardia response was not exhibited by the patient. Do prehospital providers have to be so excessively detail-oriented? Noticing the little things can more often than not make a big difference indeed. EMS providers who fail to discover important information readily available to them might be lulled into complacency due to, for example in this trauma case of a patient on a beta-blocker, the absence of tachycardia when in fact the patient is critically ill.

Providers must always include the basic "SAMPLE" history: Signs and symptoms, Allergies, Medications, Pertinent past history, Last oral intake, and Events leading up to the injury or illness. Other more specific and situational questions must be asked as well. It is a good idea to ask important yet detail-oriented questions, to which the answers are not always readily apparent. For example, can you think of situations in which the following questions might be very revealing?

- Did the patient become unconscious before the auto accident or as a result of it?
- Did the elderly patient become unconscious before or after the fall that they were witnessed taking?
- Was this assault victim actually the *perpetrator*, but they are changing their story in front of you? Answers to such a question would guide the need to have a public safety officer present on scene.

- Does this victim have a history of any underlying psychological issues or alcohol and drug use?

Paramedic training stresses the value of a good patient assessment, but the academic environment and the field environment are drastically different. In the "real world," providers are frequently extremely busy, answering multiple calls per day, and have difficulty finding the time—and mental energy—to dedicate to a comprehensive approach to each and every patient encounter. To be sure, providers must focus on "the basics," such as the general impression of how sick patients seem to be, the primary and secondary surveys, and then getting on with the business of getting them to where they need to go. It's tempting for prehospital personnel to say, "*they are just going to do all of this assessing again once the patient is delivered to the Emergency Department, so why perform history and physical tasks that don't seem to change anything?*" Such an attitude is directly contradictory to the current-day concept of the team approach to EMS: Assessment and care begins in the field and seamlessly transitions into the emergency department. All members of the team are critical to improve the patient's outcome.

There are a few important things that field personnel can do in order to save time while providing the best quality patient assessment possible. First, it is tempting for medics to bury their heads in the paperwork—either electronic or written records—minimizing the examination and observation of the patient for whom they are providing care. This early completing of the paperwork seems to speed up the call, enhances the patient transfer effort at the emergency department, and gets the ambulance back in service quicker. Time spent completing the medical record should not prevent the provider from continuing evaluation of the patient's condition. Patient care reports may be completed following the patient encounter so that the provider can maintain vigilant observation of the patient. The patient-centered focus will dramatically help the quality of provider assessments.

Second, many patients have with them a long list of medications, many of which the provider may not be aware of the intended use or the side effects. A pocket drug guide, or in this age of Smart Phones, a downloaded application can also help the provider reference this material. The field crew members will be regularly surprised by the sheer amount of medical disorders that many patients—regardless of their overall education level—simply don't know they have or don't view as important enough to tell you about.

Simply stated, the taking of a good (and thorough) health history is of extreme importance. In the thick of the effort to care for a critically ill patient—even when it seems like the patient's chief complaint is readily apparent—the answers to these important questions must not be overlooked, lest the absence of important historical information lead to the patient's detriment.

SELECTED READINGS

Chapleau W, Burba A, Pons P, Page D. *The Paramedic*. 2nd ed. Columbus, OH: McGraw-Hill Publishing; 2011.

Elling B, Elling KM. *Principles of Patient Assessment in EMS*. Florence, KY: Delmar Cengage Learning; 2002.

The patient assessment: don't fail to do it right every time

Patrick Brady

The failure of a provider to perform a complete physical assessment on a patient may happen for several reasons. We can all pick out the obvious problems when we first assess the patient who has the bone sticking out of somewhere that we really do not want to think about. What about the more subtle, yet equally dangerous warning signs?

When faced with a major (or sometimes not-so-major) trauma, we, as first-line medical crews, are often startled by how serious a noticeable and severe injury appears, and also how remarkable the mechanism of injury might look. Many times when faced with such cases the first instinct is to focus on the obvious and plainly apparent injuries. While this is a natural response, especially for younger providers, we must still force ourselves out of this dangerous mental habit.

The problem comes when we assume, without thinking, that *this is the only injury that the patient has,* and as a result we fail to complete a thorough assessment on our patients. Everybody who has spent any amount of time in emergency medicine can relate to this and probably has stories from the past that pertain to missing a critical detail on a patient. Examples might possibly include the discovery and treatment of a bullet entry wound but missing the exit wound, or not palpating or inspecting the back when a major trauma victim is found lying face up on the ground.

Another assessment error that is commonly made includes not check-ing for the presence of pulses, motor, and sensation in all extremities. Why is this always necessary? It's simple: Because we can never know that some-thing is wrong unless we thoroughly check for ourselves! While this is a straightforward point, one would be surprised how often it is overlooked. For example, when assessments are conducted while patients are lying flat or sitting up (or in any body position other than standing or ambulating), the fact that their legs are not working properly simply is not noticed. Another set of circumstances that sometimes throws medical crew members off is when the patient is unusually calm for the circumstances. Thus the medical practitioner often just simply assumes that the patient is "fine" and has no other complaints other than the obvious. They are conscious, so if they had a major problem, they would let us know, right?

Another common error is not taking the time to thoroughly palpate all areas of the body. This especially includes the extremities—which can occasionally have deformities or other injuries—and also pulse, motor, and sensory deficits that can escape our attention. In cases involving thoracic trauma, for example, which requires thorough examinations and definitive interventions, it can be easy to miss some extremity wounds that in the absence of other injuries would seem blatantly obvious. It can be remarkable how sometimes our attention span can be reduced to one or two obvious injuries to the exclusion of all else, especially while responding to a major accident, when our own adrenaline levels are high.

The provider must not fail to continually reassess the patient's level of consciousness while en route to the receiving facility. A patient's level of consciousness can change quickly, particularly in the setting of major trauma. Furthermore, in the setting of a trauma victim with an altered level of consciousness, the provider must also consider when the altered mental status actually occurred: Did this change of consciousness take place before or after the main traumatic event? Is this loss of consciousness just a one-time thing or will it come or go with the passage of time and with changes of the body's condition, such as a shock state that improves with treatment or worsens in spite of treatment? Most important of all: Is the patient fully conscious at the moment? The sheer complexity of the patient's brain can make assessment difficult at times. Further questioning can reveal that the patient may have memory loss, either for the events leading up to the event or ongoing memory loss for subsequent events. The provider should give the patients his or her first name and ask them to remember it. Failure of the patient to be able to remember the name is indicative of altered mental status for any of a number of reasons including traumatic brain injury. A useful tip to know, with the patient who is suspected to have altered mental status (such as memory loss) is for the provider to state, "My name is _____, and I'm going to be taking care of you. I want you to remember my name." Then, the provider should wait a few minutes while otherwise taking care of the patient and, a few minutes later, ask if the patient remembers the provider's name. Failure of the patient to remember the name is indicative of altered mental status, perhaps due to concussion, substance intoxication, or dementia. Had the provider not asked the question, though, then the situation might not be obvious.

There are many examples of the assessment pitfalls that the EMS provider should guard against making. A thorough and complete assessment, such that no area of the body is left unexamined and no injury is overlooked, is of utmost importance and cannot be overstated.

The principal point of this discussion is that a full patient assessment must be done correctly and thoroughly every time. To fail to do so is to gain experience, and as the old adage goes, "experience is the costliest tutor."

Selected Readings

Campbell JE. Trauma Assessment and Management. In: *International Trauma Life Support.* 7th ed. Upper Saddle River, NJ: Prentice Hall; 2011.

Elling B, Elling KM. *Principles of Patient Assessment in EMS.* Florence, KY: Delmar Cengage Learning; 2002.

60

BE SURE TO AVOID THESE PITFALLS
IN CONFIRMING DEATH AT SCENE

PATRICK BRADY

Stories such as the following continue to surface from time to time. By those of us who provide emergency medicine as a profession, they are not quickly forgotten.

An EMS crew evaluates a horrific car accident late one rainy night, finding all the victims to be "obviously dead." Public safety secures the scene, the coroner comes, and the crew returns to the station. After their shift ends, they are shocked to be called back to EMS Administration. To their horror, they are told that one of the victims was still alive during the coroner's examination hours later, and the crew is now placed on administrative leave pending further investigation.

Such a scenario could happen to any EMS provider unless some basic rules of determining death at scene are followed.

First, due diligence should be undertaken with each victim. One can only imagine both the pain that the victim's family members feel from the event itself and the anger that they would understandably feel toward the emergency medical crew that could have done something on scene for the patient but did not do so. There is simply no excuse for lack of attention to detail and lack of the most basic step in the patient assessment—the ABCs.

Even if the patient appears obviously dead, unless decapitation or incineration have occurred, the provider should check each patient's heart rhythm in two leads using the monitor/defibrillator, even when it seems intuitive or obvious that the patient is dead. Thus, it should not be assumed that a patient is dead unless proven so. Remember, *it never hurts to look.* Providers must conduct a thorough patient assessment. Absence of respirations, for example, may be secondary to the patient's positioning.

Checking the patient's heart rhythm on a monitor when the patient seems apparently dead may seem unnecessary. Many times the field medical crew might be advised or otherwise influenced explicitly *not* to check a rhythm because even if the rhythm is found to be asystole (confirmed in two different leads), then even checking an ECG rhythm requires the team to work the patient as a full cardiac arrest. This pitfall could appear to be a "Catch 22" of sorts—if they are dead (no cardiac activity) then they must be worked anyway. The apparent signs of death of the patient would seem to some providers to eliminate the need for hooking the patient to the monitor.

It is true that every medic has a protocol for cardiac arrest with the patient in asystole. A "determination of death at scene protocol" allows for situational and clinical judgment. Thus, providers should never hesitate to check a cardiac rhythm on a patient to confirm whether or not death at scene can be confirmed. The EMS provider has an obligation to check for any signs of life, and due diligence should always be exercised. Providers should care for their patients as they would want another crew to care for their loved ones. If there is *any possibility of life at all*, then medics should do absolutely everything they possibly can to salvage it. Carefully thought out protocols that address current concepts of field determination of death should be prospectively crafted by the EMS Medical Director together with the medical community.

As far as where to take the patient, local protocols should be deferred to and followed with regard to the transport/no transport decision or the choice of destination. The type of trauma the patient suffers from (such as blunt versus penetrating or complications to the trauma such as shock) can and should many times be the deciding factor on the transport destination, based on the capabilities of the hospital.

SELECTED READINGS

Pepe PE, Swor RA, Ornato JP, et al. Resuscitation in the out-of-hospital setting: medical futility criteria for on-scene pronouncement of death. *Prehosp Emerg Care.* 2001;5(1):79–87.
The University of Texas Southwestern EMS Clinical Operating Guidelines, Version 2011. Available at www.biotel.ws, last accessed December 22, 2011. http://www.biotel.ws/TreatmentGuidelines2010/BioTel%20Guidelines%20February%202012%20to%20December%202013.pdf

61

IT'S NOT OVER UNTIL YOU DOCUMENT, AND YOU HAVE TO DO IT RIGHT!

PATRICK BRADY

Let's face it: Paperwork is *boring*! Paperwork is *time-consuming*. Paperwork is a *pain in the neck*. Johnny and Roy never had to be too concerned with documentation on "*Emergency!*," so why should we?

Besides, the chances of this particular call going to court are slim, anyway. Right? Well, this is all true, but no matter what: The documentation must be done, and done *thoroughly*, after each and every call. If not, then you, the medical provider, may have just compromised tragically your patient's health, your department, and yourself as a provider.

First, should somebody decide to litigate, incomplete or flawed documentation will increase the chances of you being brought to court to defend your actions. Think about it from the perspective of the plaintiff's attorney whose job is ultimately to get money for their clients. Which is the easier target to lay blame upon: The medic who has clearly and at the outset exhibited a lack of thoroughness and attention to detail, or the other medical providers who have at the very minimum properly documented their actions and findings? The answer is obvious.

Second, but no less important, with incomplete documentation you have also made the job of defending yourself and your actions more difficult once you get on the stand, should the situation escalate to that level. You, the medical crew member, might have done nothing at all that caused any adverse effects on the patient, but through incomplete documentation, it is not so obvious to a third party who unfortunately knows nothing other than what you wrote down: Or rather, failed to record. Doubts might be raised about the quality of care that was rendered should be medical record be found lacking in documentation. While this may not seem fair, it is indeed reality.

By properly documenting your work in the care of your patients, you not only demonstrate your competence but can refer to it while under oath. Often, trials take place years after the accident itself has occurred. Proper documentation allows you to refer back to the incident and review your actions. It is there for your benefit and memory.

While it is true that your chances of getting to the point of having to defend yourself in court are slim as an EMS provider, if you use this logic to justify not doing a thorough job on documentation, then you have very unwisely just increased your own chances of going through this unpleasant experience. Remember that legal action likely could be directed toward your partner, your fellow crewmembers, and employer! Thus, incomplete documentation of a call can put the entire team—even the EMS agency and the Medical Director—at increased liability risk. This is guaranteed to be very unpopular. And it is possible that it could also cost you your job.

Third, but certainly not the least important, is the impact that an accurate and thorough initial patient report has when used as reference later on in the patient's care. Often the hospital emergency staff members or other medical team member will need to access this information for consideration in their clinical judgment. It can act, in effect, as both the "eyes and ears" of the physician as well as a proxy of your initial assessment of the patient. This is particularly relevant when it comes to medical cases, for example, in which transitory episodes of altered level of consciousness are exhibited, or of pain that comes and goes or moves around to different regions of the body, such as in cardiac chest pain or an aortic dissection.

A complete report to the hospital can provide important details about the patient's initial compliant. Hospital providers will usually refer to your patient care report if details about the patient history are unobtainable. The value of the prehospital provider's assessment of the scene and of the care provided augment's the emergency department staff to accurately deal with the patient's problems.

Finally, it is critical for the provider to remember that appropriate documentation is also a legal requirement, the failure to perform which could result in action by the state EMS agency. Regulations in the state of Texas, for example, provide for potential revocation of EMS provider licenses in the event of failure to meet appropriate documentation standards.

By far, however, the most important thing we must remember is the old adage that has been pounded into all of our heads since almost the very first day we started training: *If it wasn't documented, then it wasn't done!*

Selected Readings

Harkins S. Documentation: Why is it so important? *Emerg Med Serv.* 2002;31(10):89–90, 93–94.

Laudermilch DJ, Schiff MA, Nathens AB, et al. Lack of emergency medical services documentation is associated with poor patient outcomes: A validation of audit filters for prehospital trauma care. *J Am Coll Surg.* 2010;210(2):220–227.

Texas Administrative Code Title 25, Part 1, Chapter 157, Subchapter C, Rule 157.36 on **Criteria for Denial and Disciplinary Actions for EMS Personnel and Voluntary Surrender of a Certificate or License** states in Part B *Nonemergency suspension, decertification and revocation of a certificant or paramedic licensee: "The department may suspend* *or decertify an EMS certificant or suspend or revoke a licensed paramedic for, but not limited to, the following reasons:*

(3) failing to make accurate, complete and/or clearly written patient care reports documenting a patient's condition upon arrival at the scene, the prehospital care provided, and patient's status during transport, including signs, symptoms, and responses during duration of transport;

(4) falsifying any EMS record; patient record or report; or making false or misleading statements in a oral report; or destroying a patient care report." (Retrieved May 2, 2012, from http://info.sos.state.tx.us/pls/pub/readtac$ext.TacPage?sl=R&app=9&p_dir=&p_rloc=&p_tloc=&p_ploc=&pg=1&p_tac=&ti=25&pt=1&ch=157&rl=36)

62

DON'T TRANSPORT A PATIENT TO AN INAPPROPRIATE FACILITY

PATRICK BRADY

The capabilities of hospitals across the spectrum of patient care may differ significantly. Important to remember is that standards for hospitals have been established in various medical and traumatic conditions based principally on what types of cases can be managed at those *hospitals*, and not only upon the capabilities of the emergency departments at those hospitals. In this era of specialization of hospital facilities, it is clear that certain types of patients benefit from care at certain types of facilities. For example, evidence strongly suggests that a victim of penetrating trauma who appears to be in critical condition should be taken to the closest *appropriate* hospital for those injuries, in this case a trauma center, if one is readily available.

Moment of stress during the care of a critically ill patient can cause pressure among EMS crews to simply "hand the patient off" to the closest hospital. Part of the stress can come from the fact that the medics feel that they have done everything in the field that can be done, and any hospital can always do more than they can in the ambulance. Acting on this pressure might have serious adverse (and even potentially fatal) consequences for the patient, such as in the setting of transporting a patient with an ST-elevation myocardial infarction (STEMI) to a hospital without capabilities of performing timely percutaneous coronary intervention. As the saying goes "Time is Muscle" and in those cases the medical crews have wasted both.

Difficulty clinical situations in the field naturally produce uncertainty at times about which protocols to follow and where to take the patient. Clinical suspicious must often be scaled up or down as the patient's assessment and response to treatment unfolds. Providers should maintain a low threshold for transporting patients to a trauma center in certain clinical situations, for example, and when in doubt online medical direction could be consulted, if available, to discuss the transport the patient to the most appropriate facility.

A patient should be transported to a destination facility that provides prompt, optimized care for the clinical condition. It is always better to "over triage"—that is, take the patient to a higher level of care than may be necessary for the condition. Factors to consider in this decision-making process include:

— Critically ill trauma patients need a trauma team and a dedicated facility, not just an ER staff!

— Often the *only* achievement gained by taking an EMS patient to an inappropriate hospital destination is *lost time for the patient.*

— Initial transport to a higher level of care may prevent a secondary transport later, which could be adverse to time-sensitive conditions such as major trauma, STEMI, or stroke.

— Pre-existing familiarity by the EMS agencies with area air ambulance capabilities may facilitate transports.

— EMS agencies and their medical directors should delineate the specialty referral centers for their locales under community agreement and protocol.

— EMS crews should optimize the use of air ambulance resources, including the perimeters and conditions in which air transport is or is not indicated.

— It must also be remembered that it is not *always* faster to use air transport for a critical patient than using ground transport.

In summary, responding medical crews must be diligent to transport their patients to the proper facility for the presenting clinical condition. The principal concern must always be to transport the patient to the proper facility and by the route that best serves the patient's time-sensitive condition.

Selected Readings

Billittier AJ, Lerner EB, Moscati RM, et al. Triage, transportation, and destination decisions by out-of-hospital emergency care providers. *Prehosp Disaster Med.* 1998;13(2–4): 22–27.

Lerner EB, Shah MN, Swor RA, et al. Comparison of the 1999 and 2006 trauma triage guidelines: Where do patients go? *Prehosp Emerg Care.* 2011;15(1):12–17.

Stewart KE, Cowan LD, Thompson DM, et al. Factors at the scene of injury associated with air versus ground transport to definitive care in a state with a large rural population. *Prehosp Emerg Care.* 2011;15(2):193–202.

63

AVOID PITFALLS IN SPINAL IMMOBILIZATION

Patrick Brady

Applying cervical collars and long backboards for critical trauma patients is a common part of EMS care. When it is late at night and an ambulance crew is responding to a wreck on the highway that involves major vehicle damage and requires a prolonged extrication time, it is obvious to even the least experienced EMS providers that immobilization is essential. Everybody in the prehospital business also knows to apply backboards and C-collars to patients who might seem unharmed, yet have been involved in major events in which other patients were critically injured. These behaviors are instinctive, and are the "low-hanging fruit"—so to speak—of EMS judgment calls.

Where we as professionals seem to frequently go wrong is when it comes to the less obvious cases. The need for spinal immobilization of a patient who has been involved in a *minor* traumatic event may be overlooked, perhaps to potentially disastrous consequences. How many times have you, or a medical crew with whom you are familiar, responded to a senior citizen's fall from a standing position down to lying on the floor? This is, as we all know, a very routine call, given the aging of our populations. It is tempting to simply help such patients onto the EMS stretcher, placing them in a position of comfort. They have no obvious injuries other than a little pain, and this care may seem appropriate under the circumstances. They do not take into account that many times the elderly patient already has a difficult time ambulating, and any new pain from the fall may be difficult to distinguish from chronic pain. Add into the mix the prevalence of osteoporosis in the geriatric community, which causes the bones to be brittle and easily broken, and it makes it even more probable that your patient might be suffering from a more serious source of pain. Moreover, while the reduction of pain is well intended, caution must be used in making the decision to withhold application of spinal immobilization. Spinal immobilization is often not the most comfortable position for the patient, but providers should remember that there are ways to reduce discomfort, such as by padding the backboard at certain key points of contact.

The process of padding the backboard is straightforward. It is virtually always best to accomplish this after the patient is positioned on the board, and it is often surprising to see just how small the amount of padding is that is required to get the job done. Typically, all that is needed is to pad the small of the back, the hips' points of contact, or where the shoulders and the backboard touch. One or two small pillows are ordinarily all that is needed for the job, but any number of everyday objects can be improvised for the task on short notice. A paper towel roll, elasticized bandage rolls, or a stack of soft cot sheets have been known to be a great relief indeed for the uncomfortably immobilized patient.

In short, the discomfort of immobilization must be properly prioritized against the possibly compromised patient's need for immobilization, especially to ensure against any possible spinal insult. It does not take that much extra time to both do the job right and also ensure patient comfort.

Another frequently encountered prehospital miscalculation could be in the setting of rear-impact auto accidents, which produce "whiplash-like" (extension–flexion) neck trauma. These patients are commonly out of the vehicle and ambulatory on-scene. It may not be evident at a chaotic EMS scene that such a patient requires cervical immobilization. Providers must avoid any temptation to minimize any patient's report of pain, possibly to the detriment of our patients.

Providers must not take an incorrect message away from the rapid clearing of a cervical spine by the attending emergency department (ED) staff upon arrival to the hospital, often without even an exploratory X-ray taken. Emergency physicians staffs are trained in how to determine whether significant spinal injury is suspected, often from the history of the event supplied by EMS providers from the scene. Indeed, it may be annoying to EMS providers to see such rapid spinal clearance, perhaps sending an incorrect message that all of the prehospital spinal precautions were unnecessary. Nothing could be further from the truth, and EMS crews must continue to weigh the benefit of spinal immobilization against the discomfort of being held still until safely cleared by ED staff members. The logic is always in doing the "right thing for every patient, every time." It only takes one time to wrongly guess the question of "is it necessary to immobilize this patient?" to potentially cause irreparable harm to a patient from failure to use spinal precautions.

The current concepts of which patients benefit most from spinal immobilization are being revisited, as will be discussed in the next paragraph. Patients that would seem most appropriate for spinal immobilization include:

- Trauma victims who have experienced loss of consciousness or are currently unconscious.
- Patients who seem to have suffered a concerning mechanism of injury, such as high speed impacts.
- Elderly patients.
- Patients with significant distracting injuries such as long bone fractures, and
- Patients who demonstrate an abnormal neurological examination after trauma, such as one-sided focal weakness.

Occasionally providers will be confronted with a patient requiring consideration for immobilization for spinal conditions not caused by injury, such as spinal infections and concerning presenting neurological signs and symptoms.

It is important to note that the routine use of spinal immobilization for victims of trauma is being re-studied at this time. An important "re-look" at the field was conducted by the Cochrane Collaboration in 2009, and they stated "the effect of spinal immobilization on mortality, neurological injury, spinal stability and adverse effects in trauma patients remains uncertain." The implication of this work is that further randomized testing needs to be conducted to determine if alternative strategies for spinal immobilization are acceptable. Providers should keep an open mind on this subject in coming years, as new strategies emerge.

What do providers do with this new information that seems to be changing the EMS landscape? What will likely come of this is that we will be more selective of the use of spinal immobilization to settings where real concern for serious spinal lesions is raised, as opposed to just routinely applying immobilization. After all, some risks are present by keeping patients on long spine boards for prolonged periods. These risks include pressure sores and diminished pulmonary function. Thus, routine, non-selective spinal immobilization might not benefit and indeed may perhaps harm some patients. EMS systems should select which patients may benefit from immobilization and weigh the risks and benefits. Potential benefit, which in most clinical settings seems to be small, is also weighed against more than discomfort. What should providers do with this evolving area in EMS care? They should work carefully with their Medical Directors, agency leadership, and medical communities to determine the optimal treatment of the spectrum of patients confronted by EMS systems for whom spinal immobilization might be considered. Future research efforts in this arena will be very revealing.

SELECTED READINGS

Domeier RM. Indications for prehospital spinal immobilization. *Prehosp Emerg Care.* 1999; 3(3):251–253.

Kwan I, Bunn F, et al. Spinal immobilisation for trauma patients. *Cochrane Collaboration,* 2009.

Streger MR. Spinal immobilization. *Emerg Med Serv.* 2001;30(3):34.

Don't forget to look for a "cardiac cause" of an accident

Stephen Bock

Primary cardiac illness leading to a road accident has been shown to be a relatively rare cause of these events. Only about 0.1% of reportable road accidents are attributed to medical causes, with an even smaller percentage being specifically due to cardiac events. While these numbers may seem to be statistically insignificant, according to the National Highway Transportation Council, in 2008 there were 10.2 million traffic accidents in the United States with 39,000 reported deaths. This sheer volume of accidents places estimates of potentially thousands of road accidents per year that may have involved a patient having a cardiac cause, including primary arrhythmias having caused the event.

A field provider who fails to look for a possible cardiac cause of an accident may miss a number of medical events that could be lethal. A patient suffering an acute myocardial infarction, for example, may present with a dysrhythmia which could have caused the patient to momentarily lose consciousness. Since the patient may have lost consciousness, causing the accident, he or she may not even have recollection that any medical complaint preceded the accident.

Trauma from safety belts and air bag deployment may mask the symptoms of this event. It is common for a patient to complain of chest or shoulder pain after experiencing a motor vehicle collision. The first field provider might naturally assume that the chest discomfort was produced by contact with the seat belt or air bag, failing to consider the question of which came first, the chest pain or the obvious blunt trauma event.

Complicating assessment for potential cardiac causes of an accident includes patients who may have distracting injuries. A fractured femur may be causing such pain to a patient that chest discomfort may be overlooked. In addition, it is very natural for a provider to "go to the obvious injury" and possibly neglect to perform a head-to-toe assessment. This sort of tunnel vision—while understandable—must be resisted by the experienced provider. Initial training for trauma focuses on the rapid extrication and transport of the victim of trauma, especially major trauma. This appropriate limitation of field time can also be part of what might prevent a thorough patient assessment.

A trauma patient in shock and/or with significant bleeding presents even more difficult triage decisions. The options of "load and go" due to the trauma versus taking the time in the field for a more thorough assessment—including a 12-lead ECG—may seem inappropriate for this patient's condition. If the field treatment decision is expanded to treatment for a cardiac event, protocols commonly call for aspirin, nitroglycerin, and analgesics, treatments that could clearly worsen the condition of a patient in shock from trauma. Aspirin could possibly enhance bleeding in a patient suffering from uncontrolled hemorrhage. Nitroglycerin could increase hypotension in a patient suffering from acute hemorrhage. On the other hand, failure to provide rapid transport to an appropriate trauma center for a patient with chest pain but suffering from traumatic shock could potentially result in the transport of a major trauma victim to a non-trauma facility. These difficult decisions must be based on thoughtfully derived clinical protocols that provide clear guidance, including gaining input from both cardiology and trauma experts during the production of EMS clinical guidelines. In addition, online medical direction can help the field providers manage these challenging patients.

Difficulty in evaluating a major trauma victim for cardiac causes of the event can be presented in the patient with severe chest trauma. The severely diaphoretic patient, or the patient with rapid respirations presents difficulty in obtaining a 12-lead ECG. While the ECG monitor may give some indication of the potential for a cardiac cause of the accident—such as an obvious dysrhythmia on the monitor—nonetheless, using the monitor only to evaluate the patient, rather than performing a 12-lead ECG, may not reveal the complete clinical picture.

If the provider suspects both a traumatic as well as a cardiac event in the same patient, consultation with online medical control may be helpful due to the relative rarity of patients suffering a cardiac event that is the cause of a motor vehicle accident.

Field providers must ALWAYS complete a thorough initial assessment, secondary survey, and, when possible, a careful patient history. If the patient has chest discomfort of any sort after an accident, the provider should consider performing a 12-lead ECG to rule out a cardiac event that may have led to the accident, especially if the patient history is indicative of previous cardiovascular disease. As mentioned previously, caution should be exercised when administering medications such as aspirin and nitroglycerin in the setting of a patient with significant trauma.

Rapid transport of patients sustaining serious trauma is always important. The provider who has concern for a potential cardiac event as the cause of the accident will have to choose the appropriate time to perform the 12-lead ECG.

Thorough assessment of the victim of major trauma must include searching for the actual cause of the event. Finding the occasional victim whose acute cardiac event produced an accident will help both to determine the state of the patient's critical condition and to optimize care.

SELECTED READINGS

Campbell J, et al. *International Trauma Life Support Manual.* 7th ed. Downer's Grove, IL: ITLS, 2011.

US Census Bureau, Statistical Abstract of the United States. Retrieved from http://www.census.gov/compendia/statab/2011/tables/11s1102.pdf

US Department of Transportation, Federal Highway Administration. *Conference on Cardiac Disorders and Commercial Drivers.* Bethesda, MD: 1987. Publication No. FHWA–MC-88-040.

65

DON'T UNDERESTIMATE HEMORRHAGE FROM PELVIC AND LONG BONE FRACTURES

STEPHEN BOCK

According to the Centers for Disease Control in 2004 there were 320,000 hospital admissions for fractures of the pelvis. This number could be expected to rise with an aging population and rising incidence of osteoporosis. EMS providers are commonly dispatched to this type of "injured person call" involving falls with possible fractures of the pelvis or femur. Many if not most of these emergencies involve the elderly, with the majority of them being female.

Because of the size of the bones involved and the large vessels adjacent to them (including the femoral artery), a significant amount of blood loss may have occurred due to pelvic and femur fractures. Several arteries branch off in the thigh to bring oxygenated blood to the femoral head and neck. This blood supply is often described as tenuous because fractures of the femoral neck can disrupt the blood supply to the femoral head. In addition, on physical examination, swelling due to a fracture on the proximal thigh may not be as obvious as a fracture associated with a distal part of an extremity. If the patient doesn't look sick following a fall, that patient may be transported without a sense of urgency with a low priority transport status, a "no lights or sirens" transport. In addition, a change in vital signs might be attributed to the narcotic analgesic administered prior to transport. The fact that hemorrhagic shock due to a pelvic fracture may be the cause of a vital sign change may be missed. Thus, mortality can be as high as 30% with unstable pelvic ring injuries, with much of this excessive mortality risk being due to internal blood loss.

On first patient contact, the quick question during assessment is "did the person fall and injure the hip or did the hip appear to give and the patient then fell." An important distinction is this: If the hip is fractured, the foot on the affected side may appear to be rotated laterally, while a hip dislocation generally appears as the thigh and lower leg rotated medially.

Paramedics are trained to manage this type of patient by stabilization of the pelvis with either commercial splints or with the use of a simple tied bed-sheet splint. In the elderly, initially stable vital signs may not have real significance unless the patient had been down for a long period of time prior to arrival of EMS. If the patient does not visibly look sick, the paramedic might consider elevated vital signs as an indicator of pain or preexisting hypertension. While initial hypotension *MAY* be accurately attributed to the box of medications the patient is taking due to other preexisting medical conditions, these assumptions demand continued reassessment en route to the Emergency Department.

Remember that the initial assessment may not be indicative of the severity of the injury. Bleeding within the pelvis may be subtle at first, and the patient may have lost substantial blood volume due to internal hemorrhage before shock becomes readily apparent. Also, the fact that a patient may be elderly may be distracting to the provider due to other concurrent medical problems that might be present. Remember that a patient with pelvic or long bone injuries may have been injured due to a medical reason, such as falling after a stroke occurs.

Don't give excessive amounts of intravenous fluid to patients with shock due to uncontrolled hemorrhage. Current guidelines call for giving sufficient intravenous fluid to maintain the presence of a patient's radial pulse. Careful titration of narcotic analgesia is important in patients suffering potential pelvis and/or long bone fractures due to the potential for inducing hypotension.

Providers should use caution when palpating a patient's pelvis for potential fracture. Excessive force on an unstable pelvis could potentially induce increased internal bleeding. Also, extra care should be taken to appropriately stabilize an unstable pelvic fracture with either the use of commercial pelvic splints or simple bed sheets. Long bone fractures should be stabilized to prevent motion of the extremity.

EMS providers caring for victims of lower extremity and pelvic trauma must be ever watchful for the possibility that a patient may have substantial internal blood loss that may place the patient's life in danger. Complicating factors include medications (such as beta blockers) that may mask early signs of shock. Frequent, repeated assessments and the transport of patients to appropriate hospital facilities will help optimize outcomes.

SELECTED READINGS

Centers for Disease Control and Prevention National Center for Injury Prevention and Control. Falls and Hip Fractures Among Older Adults.

Cooper C, Campion G, Melton LJ 3rd. Hip fractures in the elderly: a world wide projection. *Osteoporos Int*. 1992;2(6):285–289.

Fowler R, et al. Shock evaluation and management. In *International Trauma Life Support Manual*. 7th ed. Downer's Grove, IL: ITLS, 2011.

Kobziff L, MS, BSN, BS, RN, C, ONC Orthopaedic Nursing.

Winkley G. Fractures, Hip. www.emedicine.com/emerg/topic198.htm.

66

AVOID THESE PITFALLS IN VASCULAR ACCESS IN THE TRAUMA PATIENT

STEPHEN BOCK

Patients in profound shock due to trauma require minimizing scene time, transport time, and delays in the emergency department. Operative care is often life-saving. Field providers have historically made great effort in gathering information to inform the receiving facility of the actual mechanism of injury, appropriately immobilizing the patient, administering oxygen, applying monitoring equipment, and providing intravenous access to administer crystalloid solutions. Growing evidence suggests that intravenous access in major trauma victims—especially for the purpose of administering large boluses of fluid to victims of uncontrolled hemorrhage—may worsen outcomes.

Establishing field intravascular access is still widely considered a part of an "advanced life support" protocol for trauma patients before arriving at a trauma center. While this treatment has not been shown to improve patient outcomes in the setting of hemorrhagic shock, paramedics are still often expected by the receiving physician and staff to obtain an IV (or IVs) before arriving at the ED. Since patients in profound shock have decreased peripheral circulation, the paramedic must become skilled in not only finding an appropriate vein in which to place a large-bore IV catheter but often to perform this skill in a moving ambulance.

It is generally accepted that delays in transport must be avoided with a significant trauma event, and delaying on-scene for many minutes while an IV attempt is made (or more than one attempt) may literally endanger the patient's welfare if active hemorrhage is occurring. This makes the need for starting the line in the back of the ambulance all the more necessary—AND challenging! This is not to say that paramedics are unable to provide this skill. The success rates for initiating IV therapy en route to the hospital is high—quoted as high as 92% for trauma patients. It has also been reported that if an appropriate vein is not available, the paramedic still feels compelled to place "something" prior to arrival at the ED. It is not uncommon for an 18 or 20 gauge IV to be established in an adult patient. This small-bore IV is of marginal value to the surgeon or emergency physician standing by to prepare the patient for the operating room. These patients may require large volumes of blood products to be administered both before the operating room and during surgery, and small-bore IV lines will be of little assistance in giving these products.

Once intravascular access has been obtained, it is not uncommon that providers will use this access to infuse large volumes of fluid, even inadvertently. It is now in most standard training protocols to minimize large fluid boluses during care of the trauma victim, and it is important to point out that no subset of trauma patients has demonstrated a survival advantage when prehospital IV fluid resuscitation has been performed in uncontrolled hemorrhagic shock. The paramedic must be vigilant to assure that only the minimum volume of fluid called for in protocol be administered en route to the ED.

Studies support this fact with the opinions of many trauma providers that the routine use of IV catheter placement and fluid administration for all trauma patients should be discouraged, to prevent the outcomes from being worse. Several mechanisms for these bad outcomes associated with IV fluid administration have been suggested, including dislodgement of clot formation within bleeding vessels, dilution of clotting factors, and acceleration of hemorrhage caused by elevated blood pressure. The only exceptions to this treatment modality would be in the cases of altered sensorium that is directly due to the shock state, if the radial pulse cannot be palpated, or if systolic blood pressure is below 80 mm Hg. Under these conditions small fluid boluses should be given to "maintain life until definitive care is possible." It is now a standard recommendation that in the setting of a patient with uncontrolled hemorrhage, the provider should not attempt to normalize blood pressure by administering large volumes of fluid. Rather, the amount of fluid administration should be limited to that needed to restore a peripheral pulse, which is approximately 80 mm Hg.

When routine IV access cannot be successfully obtained, the availability of an intraosseous (IO) needle may provide an option of a "non-collapsible" peripheral line prior to arrival at the emergency department. The rate of infusion varies with the size and site of the IO needles, though, and may be less optimal for volume resuscitation, especially during the administration of blood products.

The time expended achieving intravenous access in a victim of major trauma may actually be time wasted in the field. In addition, since this line may become a route for over-zealous volume administration and possibly worsening the outcome for patients with uncontrolled hemorrhage, serious consideration should be given to starting the line en route since the actual value of the line—in the setting of patients with uncontrolled hemorrhage—seems to be in question. Only in the cases of profound shock with highly defined parameters should IV administration of crystalloids be stressed, and only to administer enough fluids to help return a peripheral pulse.

It is important to point out that in the setting of hemorrhagic shock that can be controlled—such as in an extremity amputation—it is reasonable to consider giving sufficient fluid to normalize blood pressure. Ideally, giving sufficient fluids in a judicious manner to ensure a normal urinary output is the most optimal way to treat these patients. Some patients with controlled hemorrhage may already have Foley catheters in place, and prehospital personnel must understand "intake and output" in these patients, lest they give more or less fluid than the patient requires.

It is important to remember that the actual placing of an intravenous or intraosseous line itself may place the medic and other transporting personnel at risk during transport due to the possibility of infectious disease exposure. Thus, EMS clinical protocols calling for this procedure in the setting of trauma should be authorized by EMS medical directors in consideration of current concepts of trauma care in the field.

SELECTED READINGS

Fowler R, Gallagher JV, Isaacs SM, et al. The role of intraosseous vascular access in the out-of-hospital environment (resource document to NAEMSP position statement). *Prehosp Emerg Care.* 2007;11(1):63–66.

Seymour CW, Cooke CR, Hebert PL, et al. Intravenous access during out-of-hospital emergency care of noninjured patients: A population-based outcome study. *Ann Emerg Med.* 2011;253(2):371–377.

67

The patient's airway: manage it the right way!

A.J. Kirk

A provider's ability to manage a patient's airway is predicated upon assessing the patient's ability to protect the airway, adequately ventilate, and maintain ventilatory effort. Providers must be very familiar with the causes of respiratory distress and failure as well as the treatment modalities for these conditions. While proper advanced airway management requires technical proficiency involving both manual dexterity and hand/eye coordination, the provider's ability to form and execute contingency plans—should initial airway management techniques fail—is of the utmost importance.

Airway management begins with careful evaluation of airway patency, patient's mental status, patient's ability to protect the airway with gag and cough reflexes, and evaluation of adequate ventilation. Airway status is dynamic and must be continuously re-evaluated. Failure to appreciate impending respiratory failure or compromise will leave the provider without adequate time to intervene to prevent aspiration, hypoxia, hemodynamic instability, and possibly death.

When evaluating a patient's airway, the provider's level of training must always guide what airway management capabilities the provider possesses. An airway management algorithm is an important guide to the order of the airway management steps. Providers must also use available information to assist in airway management. The standard of care for airway evaluation includes the patient's level of consciousness, pulse oximetry, either capnometry or waveform capnography, and monitoring the heart rate. Where pulse oximetry provides a window into oxygenation, capnography may provide the first indications of loss of an adequately patent airway and/or abnormal ventilation.

Airway management starts in the classroom with the understanding of the axes of the head and neck. A provider should be familiar with the normal anatomy and physiology of the upper airway as well as techniques to align the axes and relieve obstructions. The oropharyngeal, hypopharyngeal, and tracheal axes may be better aligned with flexion of the neck and extension of the atlanto-axial joint. A simple jaw thrust is a highly effective and often underutilized technique for beginning to align these axes, as well as to project the base of the tongue anteriorly and out of the main line of the airway. The jaw thrust technique requires placement of the fingers behind

Airway axes alignment and exposure of the glottic opening

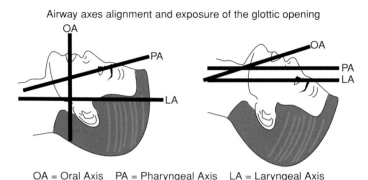

OA = Oral Axis   PA = Pharyngeal Axis   LA = Laryngeal Axis

FIGURE 67.1. Airway Axes Alignment.

the angle of the mandible to push the mandible forward (this technique may be uncomfortable for the conscious patient and may stimulate the patient with altered mental status). Given the design of the temporomandibular joint, this forward pushing of the jaw will also cause the mouth to open slightly *(Fig. 67.1)*.

Assisting the patient with ventilation via bag–valve–mask (BVM) requires careful training and may be a source of airway concerns. The opening pressure of the lower esophageal sphincter is about 20 mm Hg of positive airway pressure, and BVM ventilation pressures often exceed this level, causing patients to experience gastric insufflation. This increases the risk of aspiration, particularly during sedation-assisted or rapid sequence intubation. Once caused, gastric distension may be difficult to manage, often requiring a naso- or orogastric tube to relieve the pressure in the stomach. These tubes may induce gagging or vomiting or cause some degree of temporal or physical interference with the airway management process, and thus it is best to avoid causing gastric distension through proper mask management techniques.

Barring the presence of mid-face or basilar skull trauma, nasopharyngeal trumpets are useful in assisting ventilation and allowing more gentle ventilation.

Providers often feel that attaining a "definitive" airway will be the safest option for their patients, theoretically mitigating the risk of complications. One often hears a medic wanting to "secure" the airway or an emergency physician wanting to gain "airway control". All techniques of advanced airway management require superior training as well as constant vigilance and reassessment once applied.

Endotracheal intubation is fraught with perils, including esophageal intubation, tube displacement, tube obstruction, induction of vomiting due to stimulation of the hypopharynx, aspiration, damage to the hypopharynx or airway, patient self-extubation, and the ET tube becoming a route for over-ventilation.

Care must be taken to not over-ventilate the patient. It has been shown that even highly trained providers may substantially over-ventilate patients, which can diminish venous return and worsen shock in the setting of the hypotensive or cardiac arrest patient.

Failure to adequately manage an airway may lead to disastrous consequences. Inadequate ventilation may lead to hypoxia and hypercarbia, metabolic acidosis, aspiration, or other sequelae. The paramedic is and must be an expert in airway management, which only comes with education, clinical practice, constant vigilance, and continuous quality improvement.

SELECTED READINGS

Braude D. *Rapid Sequence Intubation and Rapid Sequence Airway.* 2nd ed. Albuquerque, NM: Dept of Emergency Medicine, University of New Mexico; 2009.

Lecky F, Bryden D, Little R, et al. Emergency intubation for acutely ill and injured patients. *Cochrane Database Syst Rev.* 2008;16(2):CD001429.

68

THE BLEEDING PATIENT: TRY TO CONTROL HEMORRHAGE IF POSSIBLE!

A.J. KIRK

EMS providers must respect the truly emergent nature of exsanguination and make all attempts to control it. There is no current technology that has been proven to replace lost blood volume better than hospital-based blood bank transfusion and preferably fresh whole blood, as recent military experience has shown. While there have been many attempts at replacing blood volume with products available during prehospital transport, there is no substitute for blood replacement in victims of massive hemorrhage.

Controlling hemorrhage where possible is critically important. Loss of intravascular blood volume—regardless if to the environment or to an internal compartment—is equally deleterious. Internal hemorrhage may or may not be slowed by intra-compartmental pressures, depending on the type of compartment and whether the source of the bleeding is arterial or venous. However, some patients may suffer from types of exsanguination for which there is no prehospital intervention available to stop the bleeding, such as in a medical patient with lower gastrointestinal hemorrhage.

Where possible, however, medics must act to slow the bleeding. Different sites of hemorrhage may be controlled in various ways. A useful way to think about approaching the management of potential sites of hemorrhage is by separating potential causes into external limb hemorrhage, internal limb hemorrhage, external thorax hemorrhage from penetrating trauma, external abdominal hemorrhage from penetrating trauma, and internal thoracoabdominal hemorrhage from any cause.

The first and primary method for controlling external hemorrhage of a limb is direct pressure at the site of hemorrhage. If the hemorrhage is arterial, pressure on a proximal portion of the artery may be effective. This is most easily accomplished at a site where the artery runs just adjacent to a bone, allowing for compression of the artery against a firm structure. Remember that blocking arterial blood flow by any means will also decrease tissue perfusion to all areas supplied by the artery. This potential anoxic insult to the extremity, however, is weighed against the risk of death from hemorrhagic shock. The old adage 'life over limb' is true, and it is with this consideration that use of tourniquets has returned to the forefront in the setting of the management of otherwise uncontrollable, severe hemorrhage from an extremity.

Tourniquets may decrease mortality from bleeding of an extremity without a significantly increased risk in the loss of the affected limb. However, patients with tourniquets placed for hemorrhage control must be transported promptly to appropriate hospitals for emergent evaluation where physicians may intervene to directly control the hemorrhage while allowing for limb reperfusion.

Internal hemorrhage in an extremity is commonly associated with a long bone fracture. Only long bone fractures are typically associated with hemodynamically significant volumes of bleeding into an extremity. Other causes of internal limb bleeding are largely located in areas where bleeding into interstitial planes is limited by the small volumes in these planes, and the surrounding interstitial pressure slows the bleeding. As this pressure approximates that of the bleeding vessel, bleeding usually stops without intervention. Bleeding from a long bone fracture, however—especially from a femur fracture—can be substantial. Long bone fractures should, at the very least, be splinted both to prevent further tissue damage as well as to minimize further pain from movement. Practitioners who reduce fractures should be well trained and familiar with the anatomy of the bony skeleton as well as the nerve locations, muscle, and vascular structures. Placing the fracture into normal anatomic position and then splinting may decrease hemorrhage. Complications of this movement into position include damage to or entrapment of nerves, tendons, arteries, and veins by the fracture fragments. Neurovascular status distal to the fracture must be assessed prior to and after reduction to ensure that no complication of the movement and splinting has occurred. Periodic rechecking of the neurovascular status of the extremity is essential.

Penetrating thorax trauma resulting in external hemorrhage generally can be divided into sucking wounds (open pneumothorax) and non-sucking wounds. Sucking wounds should be treated with a sealed wound dressing, and medics should be prepared for 'burping' of the wound periodically or placing a needle thoracostomy for decompression, should evidence of a tension pneumothorax develop. If hemorrhage exists from this wound, the removal of a corner of the dressing to 'burp' the wound and decrease intrathoracic pressure may result in a lack of adequate sealing of the dressing permitting external hemorrhage. Non-sucking chest wounds with external hemorrhage should be treated with direct pressure. The provider, however, should use care to note any crepitus and, if present, be judicious with pressure so as not to force a fractured rib into internal organs or into the provider's own hand. Overly vigorous pressure on the chest wall may limit respiratory excursion and interfere with oxygenation and ventilation.

Penetrating abdominal trauma resulting in external hemorrhage may be difficult to manage. There is not currently a general consensus as to whether these wounds should be packed. Recent developments with hemostatic agents have allowed for the possibility for prehospital providers to place packing onto various bleeding areas with some efficacy in external hemorrhage control. With regard to wounds of the trunk, however, it is very important to remember that an externally applied hemostatic agent has little to no effect on internal injuries, especially those deep to the abdominal wall involving internal organs.

While practitioners must be proficient with the techniques discussed above and mindful of the surrounding structures in areas that are treated, the slowing of hemorrhage may be lifesaving. Thus, all reasonable efforts to stop bleeding that can be stopped should be employed by the EMS provider.

Replacing blood volume with the currently available therapies, namely crystalloids such as saline or lactated ringers, serves to replace circulating volume but without correcting loss of red blood cell oxygen carrying capacity, platelet mechanical clotting capacity, or clotting factor activity. Aggressive crystalloid resuscitation will only serve to continue the worsening anemia and dilute clotting factors in the blood stream. The current consensus today seems to be that aggressive fluid replacement in the patient with uncontrolled exsanguination indeed increases mortality, though this treatment area remains the subject of intense research. Evidence has shown that minimal fluid replacement in patients with uncontrolled exsanguination—while providing prompt transport to an appropriate emergency facility—appears in fact to improve patient outcome. International EMS training standards recommend in the setting of uncontrolled bleeding that providers should only give sufficient intravenous fluids to provide for the maintenance of a peripheral pulse, while avoiding normalizing the blood pressure.

A trauma team must manage internal hemorrhage in the thoraco/abdominal/pelvic compartments. Prehospital providers can, however, decrease morbidity and mortality from these injuries. This is accomplished by early recognition of injury patterns and maintaining a high index of suspicion for internal hemorrhage based upon the history, physical evaluation, and any mechanism of injury. Considerations surrounding the mechanism of injury include speed, force, and vehicle intrusion. The transport of the patient at risk of internal hemorrhage to an appropriate facility is part of the way in which medics can best provide for these patients.

Hemorrhage control must be accomplished quickly if at all possible. Indeed, in certain circumstances, providers may need to consider controlling hemorrhage first, even before airway/ventilatory assessment. This hemorrhage control should be accomplished rapidly so that other parts of the physical assessment may be addressed. Until there is a product for the use of prehospital providers that can replace blood volume and maintain oxygen carrying capacity, clotting capabilities, and circulatory volume, then hemorrhage control will be a primary goal and concern.

SELECTED READINGS

Fowler R, Pepe P, Stevens J. Shock. *International Trauma Life Support.* 7th ed. Prentice Hall Publishing; 2011.

NAEMT. *PHTLS: Prehospital Trauma Life Support.* 7th ed. Kansas City, MO: Mosby/JEMS; 2011.

Perkins TJ. Keeping it under control. Common and effective methods of hemorrhage control. *EMS Mag.* 2007;36(6):36–37.

Sambasivan CN, Schreiber MA. Emerging therapies in traumatic hemorrhage control. *Curr Opin Crit Care.* 2009;15(6):560–568.

69

Pain hurts! Don't forget to treat it!

A.J. Kirk

Pain is a very real manifestation of tissue damage and must be treated to maintain both patient comfort as well as a normal physiologic state for the patient. The perception of pain while in a normal physiologic state is a helpful sensation and alerts the patient to an ongoing harmful and injurious condition. The central nervous system's perception of pain, however, causes a sympathetic discharge which may alter hemodynamics and vital signs. Pain also has a significant effect on both the patient's quality of life and perception of your care.

The basic tenets of medicine are to alleviate suffering and to 'do no harm'. Prehospital personnel receive training in advanced techniques such as airway management, treatment of shock, and emergency pharmacology. There are now several widely available narcotic analgesics which are highly effective in decreasing the patient's perception of pain. Medics must be familiar with each drug in their armamentarium, maintaining the skills to assess for and manage any adverse reactions from medications that they may administer. The combination of readily available pharmacological agents for treating pain—and the ability to manage side effects—means that providers should be treating their patient's pain. Providers have both the tools to supply analgesia while making it safe for the patient. Indeed, a duty exists to decrease or eliminate the patient's pain if possible.

As the philosophy of EMS medicine continues to evolve, it is accepted practice that emergency personnel have a relationship with and a duty to the citizens in their respective communities. This duty requires that standards of care must be met. Failure to provide analgesia for a patient who is in distress due to pain—as detected, for example, through a mechanism of injury or from a medical history—could be considered incomplete care of the patient, if medications are available and contraindications to medication administration do not exist. Providers must use their training and communication skills to assess the patient, determine if the patient is in pain, assess for contraindications to analgesia, and provide appropriate analgesia if allowed. Providers certainly must be allowed a significant degree of discretion as regards narcotic administration to try to determine the most appropriate medication, route of administration, and dosing of the medication. Consultation with online medical control, where available, may assist in the decision to provide more or less analgesic intervention for a given patient.

Analgesics must be administered carefully and judiciously. The experienced provider may administer them with confidence through appropriate training and experience, but all providers—from medic to physician—must be vigilant when dealing with the patient in extremis. It is important to continually reevaluate patients after medications are administered, and narcotic analgesia is no exception. For example, the perception of severe pain such as from blunt trauma to the chest and abdomen may be stimulating a patient who is in hemorrhagic shock to remain conscious. The pain indeed may be stimulating the sympathetic nervous system in a substantial manner, perhaps to some degree helping to maintain perfusion. While analgesia is not absolutely contraindicated in these patients, it is important to provide pain control while maintaining careful patient monitoring and being ready to intervene should the patient manifest signs of a worsening condition such as progressive hypotension.

The patient who appears to have pain out of proportion to what is revealed by the history and physical examination presents a dilemma for the prehospital provider. While malingering is always a possibility, that assessment should be a "diagnosis of exclusion." Pain out of proportion to clinical findings may be a sign of real and potentially devastating pathology, such as ischemic or infarcted bowel (mesenteric ischemia) or spinal cord injury. Examples of pain out of proportion to examination in the pediatric population include testicular torsion or hair tourniquet on a digit or on the penis. The vigilant EMS provider must attempt to locate these physical findings.

Many different modalities for administration of analgesia exist and should be in the medic's armamentarium. Intravenous injections are generally the most effective commonly used technique for the treatment of severe pain. Intramuscular injections and intranasal mucosal administration of analgesics are also excellent options. Care should be taken to avoid injury and exposure to providers through the use of needles. Needlestick injuries and the hazards that they present to providers give emphasis on the advantages presented by intranasal delivery of medications. Administration of medications via rectal administration is difficult in the prehospital environment and, while a historic practice, should likely be avoided in most circumstances given the considerations of access, time, patient preference, and potential exposure to body fluids that this technique presents. Administration of medications intranasally, intravenously, or via the intraosseous route in the pediatric population has essentially replaced the rectal administration route.

Medics must be masters of their pharmacologic armamentarium. They must treat the causes of pain in their patients both with direct injury management (such as splinting) and with consideration for appropriate analgesic administration. Prehospital providers, acting in the patient's best interests, and in consideration of their training, the mechanism or injury, and the physiology presented by the patient, should determine the appropriate analgesic where indicated.

SELECTED READINGS

McManus JG Jr, Sallee DR Jr. Pain management in the prehospital environment. *Emerg Med Clin North Am.* 2005;23(2):415–431.

Park CL, Roberts DE, Aldington DJ, et al. Prehospital analgesia: Systematic review of evidence. *J R Army Med Corps.* 2010;156(4) (suppl 1):295–300.

70

Examine the patient: find that penetrating trauma!

A.J. Kirk

Penetrating missile or blade trauma usually has very significant consequences and must be both recognized and assessed. These injuries are commonly missed in the patient who is found down or otherwise cannot give a history, as well as in the patient with a distracting injury. Also, prehospital assessment of the patient is often difficult compared to assessment in the emergency department.

The first steps in evaluating a patient in distress are found in the primary survey. After assessment of ventilatory, circulatory, and neurologic status, the patient should, if possible, be "exposed" to assess the entire body. It may be difficult, depending on the physical location where the assessment takes place, the environmental conditions, the safety of the scene, the number of available providers, and the patient's condition. The patient in extremis may require continuous management of the initial primary survey and never reach the exposure stage. As statistically more penetrating trauma occurs during the evening and early morning hours, injuries may be more difficult to visualize due to darkness. Efforts to achieve exposure should be made but must also be evaluated in the context of the surrounding events.

The most common locations for missed injury are axillary, perianal/perineal, and in skin folds of obese patients. Head injuries traversing the scalp and hair may be difficult to visualize, often recognized only due to the severity of the injury and its sequelae, such as a "transcranial" wound. Profuse bleeding is commonly associated with injuries to the scalp due to the great vascularity of the scalp and often the tension in the occipitofrontalis complex, which may separate the wound and increase bleeding.

Thus, it is essential when dealing with missile or blade wounds to carefully examine the axillae, skin folds, and perineal regions for injury. It is relatively common for patients running from gunfire to be shot in the buttocks or perianal region. Often untrained gunmen do not compensate for altered trajectories at close range, and patients are often running at full pace with hips fully flexing and extending while running. These positions increase the likelihood that a missile might strike the perianal regions and possibly not leave a readily visible wound or significant external hemorrhage when the patient is placed in supine position on a cot or trauma bed. The arms are similarly either outstretched during running or placed in a position of protection over the face, exposing the axillae during these events. Many patients have thick axillary hair which must be carefully but efficiently parted to examine for occult injury. Providers must be systematic and thorough while conducting their primary and secondary assessments of their patient.

Distracting injuries may be profound and visually striking. Care must be taken to conduct a uniform examination process with each patient. Most patients who sustain penetrating trauma do so under circumstances which are perilous and may be emotionally or mentally taxing to both the patient and the providers. Such stress may distract the provider and allow injury that would not have otherwise been missed to escape detection. A systematic approach will aid in decreasing human error and identifying pathology.

Penetrating trauma disrupts tissues and may lead to a host of adverse conditions. While penetrating trauma often causes readily visible sequelae—from fractures and swelling to hemorrhage or respiratory distress—penetrating trauma of the abdomen or pelvis may injure organs which are not innervated with pain fibers and thus may not directly cause pain. Penetrating perianal missile trauma will, for example, likely injure the colon and/or pelvic and abdominal vasculature. While these patients may have some component of abdominal pain, they will likely have delayed presentation of critical symptoms until they develop hemorrhage—which may be delayed in presentation—or later from peritonitis due to leaking colon contents into the abdominal cavity. Unfortunately by the time this is recognized, these patients may have developed a potentially deadly infection, suffering a substantially increased rate of mortality compared to patients who have early surgical intervention.

Tension pneumothorax is another life-threatening complication which may occur from unrecognized trauma to the chest, with delayed intervention resulting from a low index of suspicion due to lack of identification of injury. When a medic notes penetrating trauma to the axilla, for example, very close continuous assessment of the patient's ventilatory status and hemodynamics must be undertaken, and a needle decompression thoracostomy should be considered for the decompensating patient. Failure to recognize this injury may lead to a rapid decline in patient ventilation, perfusion, and mental status, and death may result if a tension pneumothorax is not treated.

Providers must recognize penetrating trauma during their primary survey as part of their initial examination and exposure of the patient. While there are variations on what is appropriate for each patient with respect to both the environment as well as the capabilities of the responding EMS agency, it is important to have a firm understanding of the primary and secondary assessment, the limitations and extent of what has and has not been evaluated, and what occult injuries may be lurking and remain to be discovered.

SELECTED READINGS

Mabry R, McManus JG. Prehospital advances in the management of severe penetrating trauma. *Crit Care Med.* 2008;36(7 Suppl):S258–S266.
NAEMT. *PHTLS: Prehospital Trauma Life Support.* 7th ed. Kansas City, MO: Mosby/JEMS; 2011.

PEDIATRIC EMERGENCIES

71

Don't wait for hypotension to diagnose shock

Brian S. Bassham, MD

A common mistake is the failure to recognize shock in the pediatric patient. Though most would agree that the tachycardic, hypotensive trauma patient is easy to recognize, those same people might fail to recognize it in the tachycardic child with poor capillary refill. As in adults, there are three main categories of shock: hypovolemic, distributive, and cardiogenic. Unlike adult patients, however, pediatric patients compensate really well until the very end, as blood pressure is the last thing to fall.

An easy mistake to make is to forget that the first sign of shock in the pediatric patient will likely be tachycardia. A child's circulation is much more dependent on heart rate than that of an adult and is therefore the primary compensatory mechanism for maintaining perfusion to vital organs. In adults, shock becomes obvious when the patient begins to become hypotensive. However, children will tolerate much higher ranges of heart rate for a much longer period of time than adults without dropping their blood pressure. If a child becomes hypotensive, they have already been in shock for some time and will be much more difficult to resuscitate.

In the pediatric population, determining "sick" from "not sick" can be difficult even for the experienced provider. A common mistake is not obtaining an adequate history, which can be very helpful in determining the severity of the illness. Most ill children will be irritable and tired, but the child who is truly difficult to arouse is a big red flag. You can learn a lot about the child's hydration status by asking about the patient's oral intake and any large volume losses from vomiting or diarrhea. Infants are often difficult to assess but you can ask the parents how many wet diapers they have had during their illness compared to their usual amount. A significant decrease in urine output is a concerning risk factor for shock so EMS providers should never forget to ask about a child's intake and output.

When examining the patient, note the presence and strength of the distal pulses. Measure capillary refill over a bony prominence such as the palm of the hand or heel of the foot and hold for 5 seconds. Diminished or absent distal pulses and capillary refill ≥4 seconds are strong indicators of shock.

As in every patient, it is imperative to continuously evaluate the ABCs. Place the patient on oxygen and provide further respiratory support as necessary. Pediatric Advanced Life Support (PALS) now teaches that as soon as shock is recognized, IV access should be obtained and fluid resuscitation begun. At least two sites of vascular access should be obtained with the largest gauge allowable. If an IV cannot be placed after three attempts or 90 seconds, place an intraosseous line.

A common mistake in both the prehospital and hospital setting is the unwillingness to want to treat shock aggressively. A goal of three 20 cc/kg normal saline boluses should be completed within the first 15 minutes of the resuscitation. This is best accomplished through either a pressure bag or through hand–pushed syringes. After each bolus, a reassessment should be done to look for improvements in the heart rate, blood pressure, and capillary refill. Monitoring for signs of fluid overload such as liver distention, a new heart murmur, or crackles in the lungs is also important.

For patients unresponsive to fluids or who are not stabilized after receiving 60 cc/kg, consideration should be given to starting a vasopressor. Most EMS units will only have epinephrine available and this can be started at a rate of 0.05 to 1 µg/kg/minute. For the rare case of cardiogenic shock in the pediatric patient, the patient will most likely not respond to rapid fluid delivery and will worsen. This occurs because of the heart's inability to pump effectively and it now being overloaded with fluid. If this occurs, discussion with medical control about the immediate initiation of vasopressors should occur.

In summary, early recognition of pediatric patients in shock is the key to the most effective management. Continuous reassessment will help the provider best anticipate the needs of the patient. Prompt and aggressive initiation of IV fluid boluses can help avoid the very late finding of hypotension.

Selected Readings

Fleisher GR, Ludwig S. *Textbook of Pediatric Emergency Medicine.* Philadelphia, PA: Lippincott Williams & Wilkins; 2010.

Han YY, Carcillo JA, Dragotta MA, et al. Early reversal of pediatric-neonatal septic shock by community physicians is associated with improved outcome. *Pediatrics.* 2003;112(4): 793–799.

Kissoon N, Orr RA, Carcillo JA. Updated American College of Critical Care Medicine—pediatric advanced life support guidelines for management of pediatric and neonatal septic shock. *Pediatr Emerg Care.* 2010;26(11):867–869.

Stoner MJ, Goodman DG, Cohen DM, et al. Rapid fluid resuscitation in pediatrics: testing the American College of Critical Care Medicine guideline. *Ann Emerg Med.* 2007;50(5): 601–607.

72

Kids with altered mental status need a glucose check

Timothy E. Brenkert, MD

The differential diagnosis of altered mental status (AMS) in infants and children is extensive and ranges from ingestion to infection. While only a few causes of AMS in children are quickly reversible, it is important to remember that some are! Thus, there is the potential for great improvement in an infant or child's clinical status by the time EMS providers arrive at the hospital with the patient.

A common mistake in both the prehospital and hospital setting is not checking the glucose on every patient with AMS. This is, however, an easily remedied problem that requires the EMS provider to always consider hypoglycemia as the potential origin of any patient's mental status changes.

Although the exact definition of hypoglycemia in pediatrics is debated, a frequently referenced figure is a plasma glucose level ≤50 mg/dL. Maintenance of sufficient levels of glucose is required for continued cellular energy production in almost all human tissue, especially in the muscle, the heart, and the brain. Hypoglycemia may result in clinical findings such as palpitations, anxiety, tremulousness, irritability, fatigue, confusion, seizures, or unconsciousness. Recognition of these clinical signs may be difficult in infants and young children; however, hypoglycemia must always be considered, detected, and corrected quickly as prolonged periods of inadequate glucose levels can result in permanent neurologic sequelae including brain damage.

EMS providers can never forget that a key to help diagnose hypoglycemia as the cause of a child's AMS is being sure to obtain a thorough history from the family. Hypoglycemia may occur in the presence of sepsis, secondary to gastroenteritis and poor oral intake, or as the result of a multitude of ingestions. Keep in mind that while adults may be able to maintain normoglycemia following days of fasting, the high metabolism of infants and young children make them potentially susceptible to hypoglycemia after as little as 24 to 36 hours of decreased intake. In addition, consideration should be given to the ingestion of common household medications such as insulin, hypoglycemics, beta-blockers, and alcohols as each can cause hypoglycemia in children. Although there is potential for any number of different ingestions, it is very important to remember to always check finger-stick glucose on children suspected to have accidentally or intentionally ingested medications or household items.

The management of hypoglycemia in pediatric patients is administration of a sugar-containing substance in some form. If the child is awake, and aspiration is not a concern, supplementation with oral glucose is sufficient. However, if any degree of AMS is present, including seizure activity or a postictal state, then proceed with dextrose-containing fluids. The concentration and dose of such fluids are dependent upon the age of the child. Never try to have a child with AMS attempt oral intake in order to avoid aspiration.

Regardless of the age of the patient, hypoglycemic children with depressed mentation should rapidly receive approximately 0.5 to 1 g/kg of dextrose intravenously or via intraosseous access. In newborns this is achieved by giving 5 cc/kg of D10W. In children over a year of age, D25 is used and given at a dose of 2 cc/kg. In adolescents (>12 years old) 1 cc/kg is given of D50. To avoid mistakes, an easy way to remember these values is to recognize that the product of the dose per kilogram and the dextrose percentage is 50 in each case (e.g., 1 cc/kg × 50% dextrose or 5 cc/kg × 10% dextrose). In each case above, the dose provided represents how to provide 0.5 g/kg. Please remember that this dose may need to be repeated as some children may require up to 1 g/kg of parenteral dextrose.

A common mistake that providers encounter is improperly making the concentration of dextrose that is needed from D50W, which is often all that is carried in the prehospital setting. To obtain D10, simply dilute 10 cc of D50 in 40 cc of normal saline. Dilution of D50 by half, in other words 25 cc of D50 and 25 cc of NS, creates a solution of 25% dextrose. These equations allow any percentage of dextrose to be delivered to the patient if ampules of D50 are the only dextrose-containing fluids available. As an example, a 4-year-old, 20 kg patient needs dextrose. Since D25 is needed, one can take an ampule of D50 and withdraw 25 cc into a 50 cc syringe. One can then withdraw 25 cc of normal saline and agitate it. The concentration is now D25 and one can administer 2 cc/kg. Having a chart written out on how to properly make each concentration should be a priority for every transporting agency.

Should intravenous access be difficult to obtain, intramuscular administration of glucagon is an option in the hypoglycemic patient. While glucagon is primarily indicated in the treatment of those patients with hypoglycemia secondary to hyperinsulinism, it may be used in the prehospital setting when the etiology of the patient's low blood sugar is still undetermined. The dosing is weight based with children <20 kg receiving 0.5 mg intramuscularly and the maximum dose of 1 mg being reserved for those patients >20 kg. Be aware that this may take up to 30 minutes to take effect.

Once the patient's hypoglycemia is corrected, continued monitoring of the patient's blood glucose at regular intervals is required as many oral hypoglycemic agents have prolonged half-lives. Dextrose-containing fluids, preferably D10, should be continued throughout the remainder of transport in an effort to maintain euglycemia.

SELECTED READINGS

Agus MSD. Endocrine emergencies. In: Fleischer GR, Ludwig S, Henretig FM, eds. *Textbook of Pediatric Emergency Medicine.* 5th ed. Philadelphia, PA: Lippincott Williams & Wilkins; 2006:1173–1175.

Glaser N, Enns GM. Hypoglycemia. In: Baren JM, Rothrock SG, Brennan J, eds. *Pediatric Emergency Medicine.* Philadelphia, PA: Saunders Elsevier; 2008:768–769.

Kleinman ME, Chameides L, Schexnayder SM, et al. Part 14: Pediatric advanced life support: 2010 American Heart Association guidelines for cardiopulmonary resuscitation and emergency cardiovascular care. *Circulation.* 2010;122(suppl 3):S882.

73

REFUSING PEDIATRIC REFUSALS: BENEATH THE SURFACE OF THE ICEBERG

ERIC CLAUSS, RN, EMT-P

LEE BLAIR, RN, EMT-P

One of the biggest and most risky mistakes an EMS provider can do is sign a refusal on a pediatric trauma patient. Spending a short amount of time on scene and not fully assessing the patient is filled with risk. Most critical care providers have some discomfort when caring for the sick and injured child because they have limited experience. These transports are best described as high risk and low frequency. Pediatric patients who are victims of trauma can have multiple injuries that can be easily missed on first glance, or after a brief assessment. Overlooking serious injuries is often due to the innate ability of pediatric patients to compensate for acute blood loss and also due to EMS providers not appreciating the etiology of a child's abnormal vital signs. For instance, how many times have you reasoned that the cause of a child's tachycardia is because they are crying? And how many times have you reasoned that the only reason they are crying is because there are strangers around, or they are in an excited environment? The only definitive way to know that the tachycardia is not due to compensated shock is by an emergency department evaluation that may include an ultrasound or CT scan.

Another mistake that can easily occur at a chaotic trauma scene is that the patient is not fully undressed and examined. If you don't see the seat belt marks across the chest and abdomen, it is hard to know that you should be concerned for intra-thoracic or intra-abdominal injuries. When a patient is brought in as a trauma to the hospital, the patient is undressed from head to toe. Every bone is palpated and moved to assess for injury. Why should it be any different on the scene if a refusal is going to be signed?

Another easy mistake to make is failing to obtain a full set of vital signs on the patient for which the parent wants to sign a refusal. Again, if you don't have all of the information on your patient, how can you decide if it is appropriate for a refusal to be signed? No EMS provider should allow a patient with tachycardia or tachypnea to have a refusal signed. There is a reason why they are called vital signs and it is because they are vital in guiding us toward the right decisions.

When the situation arises that a parent wants to sign a refusal, the medic on scene has to put all of the available information together. This includes the mechanism of the injury and if it was a motor vehicle collision, was there significant damage or was the car seat damaged? Installing and using child safety seats may appear to be easy but the National Highway Traffic Safety Administration has estimated that close to 3 out of 4 parents do not properly use child restraints. If your patient were not properly restrained, would it change your mind about signing the refusal? Last but not the least, you must take the physical examination and vital signs into account to decide if it is appropriate to have the parent sign a refusal.

A major issue prehospital care providers face is how to proceed when the parent wants to sign a refusal but the medic on scene doesn't believe that it is appropriate. First and foremost, spend time with the patient and the family to help them understand what the risks are. Most parents are reasonable when it comes to their children's health. If they are being unreasonable, ensure to the best of your ability that the parent is not under the influence of drugs or alcohol and has the capacity to make the proper decision. Always utilize medical control in difficult situations and have the parent speak with a medical control physician. Often times, a parent may not respond well to the provider on scene but will be more cooperative with the physician. These calls should be recorded so that all involved are properly medico legally covered.

The final area of potential error concerns proper and complete documentation. If you have spent considerable time on scene trying to get the patient to a hospital, clearly document your efforts and time spent. If a complaint is lodged over "your refusal to transport" or the case results in a lawsuit, proper and complete documentation will likely be the key to a successful defense. Documenting a complete set of vital signs and a full physical examination are extremely important if the patient decompensates after EMS has a signed refusal and has left the scene. Remember to document anything that the parent says in quotes when appropriate.

In conclusion, signing a refusal on a pediatric patient, especially a pediatric trauma patient, is a high-risk situation in EMS. One might even liken it to the fact that every time you get a signature of a parent signing a refusal, they are signing the document to take your license too. Be careful and document more, not less, whenever a potential transport of a pediatric patient is declined.

SELECTED READINGS

Aehlert B. *Mosby's Comprehensive Pediatric Emergency Care: Trauma and Burns.* St. Louis, MO: Elsevier; 2007.

American College of Emergency Physicians Pediatric emergencies. In: Pollak A, ed. *Critical Care Transport.* Sudbury, MA: Jones and Bartlett Publishers; 2011.

American College of Surgeons. Extremes of ages. In: *Advanced Trauma Life Support Program for Doctors.* 7th ed. Chicago, IL: Author; 2004.

Davies KL. Buckled-up children: understanding the mechanism, injuries, management, and prevention of seat belt related injuries. *J Trauma Nurs.* 2004;11(1):16–24.

National Highway Traffic Safety Administration. *Child Car Seat Inspection Station Locator.* Available at: http://www.nhtsa.gov/cps/cpsfitting/index.cfm

74

DON'T INTUBATE THAT CHILD!

PATRICK DRAYNA, MD

RULE 1: PEDIATRIC AIRWAYS ARE NOT JUST SMALL ADULT AIRWAYS

Respiratory arrest is the leading cause of cardiac arrest in children, and over half of the deaths in children less than 1 year of age are associated with respiratory failure. In order to manage a pediatric airway, it is important to know how it is different from an adult airway. A common mistake in positioning a child is failing to put a roll under the shoulders of an infant or toddler. Using one often helps better align the airway and prevent obstruction, which often occurs because of the child's large occiput and passive neck flexion. Pediatric supraglottic airways are smaller, with a relatively larger tongue and more submandibular tissue; thus a chin-lift maneuver can be extremely helpful when bag mask ventilating. Pediatric laryngeal position is always more anterior than those of adults and the epiglottis is large, floppy, and relatively large. Compared to adults, children have decreased airway reserve, are more prone to respiratory muscle fatigue and airway collapse, and have increased basal metabolic needs and thus oxygen demands. Knowing these differences and the importance of ensuring adequate oxygenation and ventilation for a child will help you manage your next pediatric airway more effectively.

RULE 2: DON'T INTUBATE IF YOU CAN MANAGE BY BAG-MASK VENTILATION

A common prehospital misperception over the years is that EMS should never bring in a patient to the ER who needs to be intubated because the intubation should have already been done in the prehospital setting. Pediatric endotracheal intubation (ETI) is a high-risk procedure that is not done frequently enough in the prehospital setting for any provider to feel completely comfortable. Major complications of ETI are common and well described in the pediatric prehospital literature such as esophageal intubation, unrecognized and recognized dislodgement of the endotracheal tube en route to the ED, right main stem intubation, multiple and failed intubation attempts, and intubation with an incorrectly sized tube. A 2001 study of a large urban EMS system found that each ALS provider only attempted a pediatric intubation once every 3 years. EMS providers should remember that current evidence is lacking to support prehospital ETI for pediatric patients. ETI gave no added benefit to bag mask ventilation (BMV) in survival or favorable neurologic outcome when studied in a randomized, prospective manner in a pediatric prehospital short-transit urban setting. When studied in a rural setting, airway complications and multiple ETI attempts were associated with transport delay, lower GCS, longer hospital stay, and lower discharge GCS. As advocates for our patients, we must remember the first rule: *Do no harm.*

In most situations (especially with short transit times), if you can manage the pediatric airway with BMV that gives good chest rise and pulse oximetry, then ETI and the risks that go along with it are not necessary.

RULE 3: DIFFICULT AIRWAYS: PROCEED WITH CAUTION!

As mentioned above, ETI may or may not be the best management option for your pediatric patient, but definitely proceed with caution with children who appear to have croup, a congenital syndrome, a suspected foreign body ingestion, a history of being intubated, or who have face and/or neck burns or trauma.

RULE 4: IF YOU NEED TO PERFORM BMV, DECOMPRESS THE STOMACH

Placing a nasogastric (NG) or orogastric (OG) tube evacuates the stomach therefore decreasing the aspiration risk and can allow for better chest expansion. If the patient does need a definitive airway to be placed at the destination facility, you will have provided an important landmark as well. Just remember, patients with facial trauma should not receive NG tubes as unintended nasocranial tubes have unfortunately been documented.

RULE 5: DON'T OVERVENTILATE

Remember to bag at an appropriate rate. Recommended rates for rescue breathing in infants and children are 20 to 24 (every 3 seconds), and 12 to 20 (every 4 seconds) for an older child. Victims of cardiac arrest are frequently overventilated during resuscitation and this can lead to reduced cardiac output.

RULE 6: USE YOUR AIRWAY ADJUNCTS—THEY ARE THERE FOR A REASON

If you are having difficulty with BMV, ensure that the child's airway is correctly positioned and reapply your grip on the mask. Perform a good chin lift and jaw thrust, and attempt ventilation again. If there is still difficulty in bagging the patient, place an appropriately sized oral airway and/or nasal trumpet. Moving beyond this, nonvisualized, blindly inserted supraglottic airway devices such as laryngeal mask airways (LMAs), King airways (for children >12 kg), or Combitubes (for older children >4 feet tall) can be placed easily, quickly, and safely as an alternative to ETI. If one of these devices is placed, you must monitor waveform capnography and secure the device in place for transport.

SELECTED READINGS

Babl F, Vinci R, Bauchner H, et al. Pediatric pre-hospital advanced life support in an urban setting. *Pediatr Emerg Care.* 2001;17(1):5–9.

DeBoer S, Seaver M, McNeil M, et al. Prehospital airway management: it's time to reconsider how we maintain pediatric airways. *EMS Mag.* 2009;38(1):42–44, 46, 48 passim.

Ehrlich PF, Seidman PS, Atallah O, et al. Endotracheal intubations in rural pediatric trauma patients. *J Pediatr Surg.* 2004;39(9):1376–1380.

Gausche M, Lewis RJ, Stratton SJ, et al. Effect of out-of-hospital pediatric endotracheal intubation on survival and neurological outcome: a controlled clinical trial. *JAMA.* 2000; 283(6):783–790.

Stockinger ZT, McSwain NE Jr. Prehospital endotracheal intubation for trauma does not improve survival over bag-valve-mask ventilation. *J Trauma.* 2005;56(3):531–536.

75

WEIGHT-BASED CARE IS ESSENTIAL IN THE CARE OF CHILDREN

CRISTINA ESTRADA, MD

Adults are often given a standard dose of medication; unfortunately, the administration of medications to a pediatric patient involves many factors. Calculating weight-based drug doses for pediatric patients is difficult and fraught with potential errors. Correctly choosing the right dose requires knowledge of the drug dose in milligrams, estimating the patient's weight, calculation of the dose per kilogram patient weight, conversion of the dose in milligrams to a volume in milliliters, and error free administration. This process is especially complicated in the out-of-hospital setting because this is a highly stressful, time-limited, and resource-limited environment. Even worse, calculating drug doses on pediatric patients is something that is rarely done by the average paramedic. A common mistake among providers caring for children is not using a weight-based system to calculate drug doses.

Medication dosages typically are based upon the child's weight in kilograms. To provide the proper dosage of a medication to the child, the practitioner must know the child's weight, the dose per kilogram, and the available concentrations of the specific drug. Pediatric resuscitation drugs are not used often enough to recall the correct dosage, and valuable time is taken to look up the correct dosage by weight. Furthermore, the dose of some medications varies with age.

Tapes with precalculated doses printed at various patient lengths are proven to work and are more accurate than age-based or observer (parent or provider) estimate–based methods in the prediction of body weight. The use of precalculated tapes makes individual adjustments in doses according to age irrelevant, thus saving the EMS provider time and not requiring any extra decision making during the evaluation and treatment process. This system of pediatric emergency treatment utilizing color-coded pathways designed to increase efficiency while reducing medical errors is the Broselow–Luten tape©.

By using a color-coded system tool, prehospital providers are able to concentrate on more important factors of care during the emergency, such as securing the airway, maintaining circulation, making a diagnosis, and rapid transport. A common mistake in using this system is not properly measuring the child. The child's length should be from the top of the head to the heels of the feet, with the child lying flat. Given lengths correspond to a weight and to color zones that provide information on appropriate drug doses, sizes of commonly used equipment, and IV fluid volumes. Therefore, each color zone can provide a guideline for treatment until the patient can be weighed. Furthermore, the practitioner does not need to rely on memory or calculations to select the appropriate size equipment or drug dosage. The color code–based system allows medical personnel to determine the weight of a child nearly instantaneously and in turn give them the proper amount of medication as soon as possible. Equipment and even medications can be organized and stored by color to permit easier access in an emergency.

Body habitus may also be an important consideration. It is unclear if an adjustment in the calculation of resuscitation medications is needed in obese children. Do not use the actual body weight of the obese child in drug dosage calculations because it may result in potentially toxic doses. Length-based tapes estimate the 50th percentile weight for length (i.e., ideal body weight), which may, theoretically, result in inadequate doses of some medications in obese patients. Despite these theoretical considerations, there is no data regarding the safety or efficacy of adjusting the doses of resuscitation medications in obese patients. Therefore, regardless of the patient's habitus, use the actual body weight for calculating initial resuscitation drug doses or use a body length tape with precalculated doses. Furthermore, the dose administered to a child should not exceed the standard dose recommended for adult patients.

In summary, medication errors in the prehospital setting can occur because of an incorrect patient weight, an incorrect drug dose calculation, or an incorrect volume for administration. Use of a system utilizing color-coded pathways can save time and reduce medical errors.

SELECTED READINGS

Deboer S, Seaver M, Broselow J. Color coding to reduce errors. *Am J Nurs.* 2005;105(8):68–71.
Deboer S, Seaver M, Broselow J. Do you know your ABCs? *Australas Emerg Nurs J.* 2005; 8:35–41.
Lubitz DS, Seidel JS, Chameides L, et al. A rapid method for estimating weight and resuscitation drug dosages from length in the pediatric age group. *Ann Emerg Med.* 1988;17(6):576–581.

76

THINK INTRAOSSEOUS NOT INTRAVENOUS

LAURIE MACPHERSON LAWRENCE, MD

A common EMS provider mistake in the critically ill or injured child is wasting time trying to get an IV. When a child needs life-saving medications or fluids quickly, an intraosseous (IO) line can be established quickly and reliably. Any drug or fluid given IV can safely be given through an IO line, including continuous infusions of epinephrine, dopamine, and other pressors. As a general rule remember that vascular access is more rapidly obtained with an IO versus the IV route, especially in the prehospital setting.

Fluids and medications given through an IO needle enter the circulation as quickly as those given IV. The inside of the long bones have a marrow cavity containing a rich blood supply that feeds into the central circulation of the body. An advantage of using the marrow cavity to access the circulatory system is that it does not collapse when the patient is suffering from shock, dehydration, or cardiopulmonary arrest.

Learning to successfully place an IO needle requires less training and experience than placing an IV catheter. One of the common mistakes with placing an IO is not identifying the proper landmarks. Many different sites can be utilized when placing an IO in children such as the distal tibia, proximal tibia, and distal femur. IO infusions can be used for all ages, including newborns. Both manual and electric devices can be utilized, though in the patient who is less than 5 kg, a manual IO may be more reliable due to the porous nature of the bone.

Do not forget that there are contraindications to placing an IO. These include infection at the site, burn at the site, inability to locate the landmarks, prior attempts at the same site, and diseases of the bone such as osteogenesis imperfecta. A common mistake is the placement of an IO in an extremity that either has a fracture or is distal to a fracture. For example, an IO should not be placed in the tibia when there is a fracture in the femur because there is a chance for extravasation of fluid at the fracture site.

After an IO is inserted, the needle should stand upright in the bone, except in young infants whose soft bones offer less support to the IO needle. Proper placement and patency of the IO should be evaluated by aspirating blood or bone marrow, followed by flushing with 10 cc of normal saline while assessing for signs of infiltration. The inability to aspirate blood or bone marrow is common and simply requires EMS providers to confirm proper placement by observing for blanching, swelling or temperature change (cold) behind the insertion site while flushing the device with normal saline.

When fluids are going to be infused through an IO, they should either be pushed or be placed on a pressure bag. Any medication that is infused should be followed by a flush. A common mistake after an IO is placed is that the site is not inspected frequently for infiltration. IO needles can become displaced during transport and while moving between stretchers. To prevent dislodgement, secure the needle in such a manner that the infusion site can be monitored for infiltration.

Complications can occur with IO infusions. The complication rate for IO infusions is estimated at 0.6%, which is much less than that seen with peripheral IVs. Infections can occur, so remember to clean the skin with chlorhexidine, betadine, or an alcohol-based solution before insertion. Hematomas or infiltration of fluid into the soft tissues can also occur. Aiming away from the knee or ankle allows one to avoid hitting the growth plates, which are located near the end of the bones.

Lidocaine 1% can be infiltrated into the skin and subcutaneous tissue prior to IO insertion to help avoid pain in children who are awake and alert. Pain can also occur during infusion of fluids through the IO. If pain occurs during infusion, administer 1% or 2% lidocaine through the IO line. A dose of 0.5 mg/kg in children weighing between 3 and 39 kg, and 20 to 40 mg for patients over 39 kg should abate any pain.

In summary, IOs should be placed first for any child in extremis or in arrest. They are a reliable way to administer fluids and medications. Special care should be taken to monitor for infiltration and dislodgement of the needle.

SELECTED READINGS

Blumberg SM, Gorn M, Crain EF. Intraosseous infusion: a review of methods and novel devices. *Pediatr Emerg Care.* 2008;24:50–56.
Deitch K. Intraosseous infusion. In: Roberts JR, Hedges JR, eds. *Clinical Procedures in Emergency Medicine.* 5th ed. Philadelphia, PA: WB Saunders; 2009:431–442.
Nagler J, Krauss B. Intraosseous catheter placement in children. *N Engl J Med.* 2011;364:e14.

77

PAIN MANAGEMENT IS NOT JUST FOR ADULTS

MATTHEW R. LOCKLAIR, MD

Providing appropriate analgesia in the emergency setting has been a hot topic during the past decade. In 2001, Congress stated, "This is the decade of pain control and research." In that same year, 2001 JCAHO set forth standards for pain management. Despite these efforts, pain control in emergency departments is still lacking, especially in children. This same lack of constant attention to pain control often applies to the prehospital setting.

There have been numerous recent studies looking at the use of analgesia for painful conditions in pediatric patients. An all-too-common mistake in both the prehospital and hospital environment is that children are far less likely to receive analgesia when compared to adults, and children less than 2 years of age are the most likely to be undertreated. There are a number of reasons why infants and younger children are less likely to have their pain controlled. Infants are expected to cry, even if not in pain, and therefore this response to pain is ignored. The fact that young children cannot verbalize the location, nature, and existence of their pain also lends to the underutilization of pain medications. Adults with a painful condition who request pain-relieving medications are rarely refused treatment; infants and young children cannot make these requests. Fear of potential side effects including hypotension and respiratory depression may also be used as reasons to avoid administering pain relief. EMS providers must remember that although it is important to consider the side effects of any intervention, the true incidence of complications from pain-relieving medications with proper dosing and administration is very small.

Pain assessment in pediatric patients with trauma or other painful conditions can be very challenging. There are several "pain scales" used in the hospital setting. Visual analog scales, number scales, and other methods of self-reporting are found to be the most effective in adolescents and adults. Unfortunately, younger children and infants cannot understand the instructions required to rate pain on these scales though the FACES pain scale and the Oucher scale have shown promise in children age 3 years and up. With all children, but especially in younger children, it is important for EMS providers to pay attention to facial expression, vocalizations, and movements. Also, the provider must be focused on physiologic markers for pain such as heart rate, respiratory rate, blood pressure, and diaphoresis. It is up to each individual agency to decide what scales work best in their setting. The key point is recognizing the very important need for assessment of pain in pediatrics.

Opiates are the mainstay of treatment for moderate to severe pain. However, a common mistake is not administering the correct dose of the opiate based on the weight of the patient. To avoid making any dosing errors in children, always use a weight-based tape to guide dosage such as the Broselow–Luten tape[©]. Although the intravenous (IV) route is the most common way to routinely administer pain medications, difficulty gaining access and the associated pain from trying to start the IV have been cited as reasons children are sometimes not treated in the prehospital setting. Intramuscular (IM) injections are not routinely used because IM medications are painful to give, doses cannot be titrated, and absorption is not uniform. Morphine 0.1 mg IV is well tolerated and offers equal to sometimes more efficacious pain control when compared to meperidine, which has many side effects such as seizures with no added benefits. Morphine when given IV has almost immediate effect and has a peak effect usually occurring within 20 minutes. Side effects can include respiratory depression and hypotension. Incremental doses ranging from 0.1 to 0.2 mg/kg with a maximum of 10 mg per dose for opioid naive patients is usually well tolerated and can be repeated q2–4h safely.

As previously mentioned, gaining IV access or giving IM injections may be painful and difficult. EMS providers should be aware that some intranasal opiate medications have been widely studied in the recent literature and have been found to be equally effective when compared to the IV route. Fentanyl, a synthetic opioid, can be given IV or by the intranasal (IN) route and has been widely studied. IV fentanyl doses range from 1 to 3 µg/kg with maximum doses of 50 to 100 µg with a rapid onset of action and shorter duration than morphine (usually 30 to 60 minutes). To avoid complications, EMS providers should remember that when giving fentanyl IV that it must be given slowly, usually over 3 to 5 minutes, to avoid respiratory depression and the development of neuromuscular blockade resulting in severe thoracic and abdominal muscle rigidity (wooden chest syndrome). IN fentanyl has been the focus of many recent studies and has been shown to be equally as efficacious as morphine in both the hospital and the prehospital setting. Doses range from 1 to 2 µg/kg with a maximum of 100 µg per dose. Onset of action is almost as rapid as the intravenous route. Many agencies have found that use of IN fentanyl allows them to control the patient's pain and avoid a difficult IV insertion in the back of a moving ambulance. Morphine and fentanyl are by no means the only choices for prehospital pain control, but have been widely studied with well-known side effect profiles and have been used frequently in patients as young as 1 year of age and some use it in infants as young as 3 months old.

One should always remember that pain control is essential in both adults and children. Many of our youngest patients cannot directly ask for their pain to be controlled. It is important for each agency to establish protocols for assessing and treating pain in pediatric patients.

SELECTED READINGS

Bendall JC, Simpson PM, Middleton PM. Effectiveness of prehospital morphine, fentanyl, and methoxyflurane in pediatric patients. *Prehosp Emerg Care.* 2011;15(2):158–165.

Borland M, Jacobs I, King B, et al. A randomized controlled trial comparing intranasal fentanyl to intravenous morphine for managing acute pain in children in the emergency department. *Ann Emerg Med.* 2007;49(3):335–340.

Fein JA, Selbst SM. Chapter 4: Sedation and analgesia. In: Fleisher GR, Ludwig S, eds. *Textbook of Pediatric Emergency Medicine.* 6th ed. Philadelphia, PA: Lippincott Williams & Wilkins; 2010:63–80.

Jennings PA, Cameron P, Bernard S. Measuring acute pain in the prehospital setting. *Emerg Med J.* 2009;26(8):552–555.

MacLean S, Obispo J, Young KD. The gap between pediatric emergency department procedural pain management treatments available and actual practice. *Pediatr Emerg Care.* 2007;23(2):87–93.

78

IF YOU ARE MISSING THE VITAL SIGNS, YOU ARE MISSING THE POINT!

JULIE PHILLIPS, MD

A common mistake is thinking that if a child is crying, they don't need to have their vital signs measured. Every child deserves to have a complete set of vital signs measured to include BP, pulse, respiratory rate, oxygen saturation and temperature. Normal vital signs are variable by age. In general, younger children have lower blood pressures but also have higher baseline heart rates and respiratory rates. Temperature and oxygen saturation norms are the same in both children and adults. It is essential that EMS providers feel a child's skin in order to better diagnose the presence of fever or hypothermia if the EMS agency does not utilize thermometers. Both extremes in temperature may be seen in sick children and may require emergency treatment.

Normal respiratory rates are inversely related to age. Infants have variations in respirations; therefore, a proper assessment of the rate should occur over 30 to 60 seconds. Respiratory rate will increase with activity and decrease with sleep. Any child breathing more than 60 breaths/min should be considered abnormal. Spontaneous ventilation should have easy inspiration, passive expiration, and be quiet. Normal respiratory rates for different age groups appear below *(Table 78.1)*.

There is a wide range of normal heart rates in children. Heart rates in children are also inversely proportional to age. Infants can have wide fluctuations i n heart rate over short periods of time. Athletic adolescents, like adults, may have low resting heart rates (as low as 40 beats/min). Common variables that affect heart rate include pain, temperature, hydration status, and activity level *(Table 78.2)*.

In children, blood pressure norms are dependent on age, height, and sex. Like heart rate, activity (crying, coughing, exercise, moving) can

TABLE 78.1 NORMAL RESPIRATORY RATE BY AGE	
AGE	RESPIRATORY RATE (BREATHS/MIN)
<1 yr	30–60
1–3 yrs	24–40
4–5 yrs	22–34
6–12 yrs	18–30
13–18 yrs	12–16

TABLE 78.2	NORMAL PULSE RATE BY AGE	
AGE	AWAKE HEART RATE (BEATS/MIN)	SLEEPING HEART RATE (BEATS/MIN)
0–3 mo	85–205	80–160
3 mos–2 yrs	100–190	75–160
2–10 yrs	60–140	60–90
>10 yrs	60–100	50–90

increase blood pressure. To accurately assess blood pressure, the proper cuff size is required. A blood pressure cuff that is too small will overestimate the blood pressure. The bladder cuff should cover approximately 40% of the mid-upper arm circumference. The cuff should cover 50% to 75% of the length of the upper arm.

A common mistake in pediatric patients is not recognizing that a fall in blood pressure is a late sign of shock; therefore, it is important to be able to recognize abnormal signs, like increased heart rate or delayed capillary refill, which may be early warning signs of shock. In children, the lowest acceptable systolic blood pressure can be estimated with the formula $2 \times$ (age in years) + 70. The diastolic pressure can usually be estimated at 2/3 of the systolic pressure *(Table 78.3)*.

In conclusion, every infant and child should have their vital signs measured. Knowing age related normals will help the provider better understand and treat all patients, especially those with abnormal vital signs. Since it may be difficult to remember normal vital signs for each age group, EMS providers should always have some way of quickly determining them such as a reference card, readily available chart, or electronic aid.

TABLE 78.3	NORMAL BLOOD PRESSURE BY AGE	
AGE	SYSTOLIC BP (MM HG)	DIASTOLIC BP (MM HG)
0–3 mos	65–85	35–45
3–6 mos	70–90	50–65
6–12 mos	80–100	55–65
1–3 yrs	80–105	55–70
3–6 yrs	85–110	50–75
6–12 yrs	95–120	55–75
>12 yrs	100–130	65–85

SELECTED READINGS

Bernstein D. Evaluation of the cardiovascular system. In: *Nelson Textbook of Pediatrics.* 18th ed. Philadelphia, PA: Saunders; 2007.

Pickering TG. Principles and techniques of blood pressure measurement. *Cardiol Clin.* 2002; 20(2):207–223.

Ralston M, Gonzales L, Fuchs S, et al. *Pediatric Advanced Life Support.* Dallas, TX: American Heart Association; 2006.

Susil G, Walker A. Emergency management. In: *The Harriet Lane Handbook.* 18th ed. St Louis, MO: Mosby; 2009:3–17.

79

NOT ALL PEDIATRIC SEIZURES ARE STATUS

VALERIE N. WHATLEY, MD

Seizures in children are common and represent one of the top three complaints that EMS responds to in infants and children. Most pediatric seizure victims will no longer be seizing by the time EMS arrives. If the patient is awake and alert, they will simply require supportive care en route to the local hospital. Expert prehospital care is required for those who are still convulsing upon EMS arrival.

As with any patient, regardless of the chief complaint, first ensure that airway, breathing, and circulation (ABC) are intact. A chin lift or jaw thrust may be required to open the airway in patients who are still having a seizure or who are postictal. A common mistake is not recognizing that many children have poor respiratory effort both during and after a seizure. They may not initially drop their oxygen saturation even though they are not taking adequate breaths. All seizing and postictal patients should be placed on a pulse oximeter and receive high flow oxygen. Bag-mask ventilation (BMV) may be required for overt hypoventilation and hypoxia. Suction should always be readily available in case of emesis. Be careful to also ensure that your patient's circulation is adequate by checking pulses and perfusion.

The prehospital focus for a convulsing patient is terminating continued seizure activity, preventing recurrence of a seizure, identifying treatable causes of seizures, and finally preventing further injury. Most seizures in pediatric patients last <5 minutes and require no intervention. When called to assess a pediatric patient who may have had a seizure, the important thing to determine is: "Is this patient still convulsing?" Remember that pediatric patients can still be convulsing without you seeing overt generalized tonic–clonic activity. Look for subtle signs such as eye deviation, nystagmus, extremity stiffening, or continued unresponsiveness. Always listen to the parents, especially in patients with a history of a seizure disorder. Parents usually know better than anyone if their child is still convulsing.

As with all aspects of medicine, first do no harm. If the infant or child is no longer convulsing and the ABCs are intact, merely transport the patient. Having intravenous (IV) access is valuable in the convulsing or postictal patient if easily obtainable. This is especially true in the patient with a history of seizures as there is a higher likelihood that the patient may re-seize.

Hypoglycemia is a common and reversible cause of seizures in all age groups, especially in the young. It is imperative to remember that hypoglycemia is the one thing that should never be missed in any patient with seizures or altered mental status. Both of these patient types must always have their glucose level evaluated in the prehospital setting.

The standard definition for status epilepticus (SE) is a single seizure lasting >30 minutes, or two or more seizures with no recovery to normal mental status in between seizures. For EMS, a simpler approach should be used. SE should be considered in any patient who continues to seize from the time of initiation of EMS to arrival on scene or any postictal patient who has another seizure while with EMS. Timely and appropriate treatment of infants and children with SE significantly reduces their morbidity and mortality.

For the patient who is continuing to convulse, treat per your service's protocol. Multiple studies have compared different medications and different routes of medication. Diazepam has always been the gold standard and can be given IV or rectally (PR). Do not mistakenly give diazepam via the IM route as it has very erratic and unreliable absorption. More recent studies have compared diazepam with midazolam and found midazolam to be equally if not more effective. Midazolam has the added advantage of being able to be given via many different routes. EMS providers may choose between IV, intramuscular (IM), PR, buccal, or intranasal (IN) midazolam administration. The IM, buccal, or IN routes of delivery are usually easier in a convulsing patient. IN midazolam is given via a Mucosal Atomization Device (MAD©) at 0.2 mg/kg (maximum 10 mg, 5 mg/nare) (see *Table 79.1*).

Finally, after necessary emergent interventions have been done, obtain important information from the family. Pertinent history can be vital in allowing the inhospital medical personnel to treat the patient optimally. Knowing what medications the patient takes and their compliance with the medications will help guide therapy at the receiving facility. A description of the event, can be very helpful to receiving medical personnel. Try to obtain information from bystanders such as length of seizure activity,

TABLE 79.1	**BENZODIAZEPINE DOSAGE BY ROUTE**		
MEDICATION	**ROUTE**	**DOSE (MG/KG)**	**MAXIMUM**
Diazepam	IV	0.1–0.3	10 mg
	Rectal	0.5	20 mg
Lorazepam	IV	0.05–0.1	4 mg
Midazolam	IV	0.05–0.15	5 mg
	IM	0.1–0.2	10 mg
	Buccal	0.2	10 mg
	Intranasal	0.2	10 mg (5 mg/nare)

whether it was generalized or focal, the presence of fever, whether there was trauma, and potential ingestion of medications or toxins.

In summary, never miss hypoglycemia as the cause of a patient's seizure. Always place the patient on a pulse oximeter and high-flow oxygen. And finally, recognize that seizures can be subtle and don't always present with generalized tonic–clonic activity.

SELECTED READINGS

Clawson J. Chapter 17: Emergency medical dispatch. In: National Association of EMS Physicians, ed. *Prehospital Systems and Medical Oversight.* 3rd ed. Dubuque, IA: Kendall Hunt Publishing; 2002.

Holsti M. Still BL, Firth DS, et al. Prehospital intranasal midazolam for the treatment of pediatric seizures. *Pediatr Emerg Care.* 2007;23(3):148–153.

Martin-Gill C, Hostler D, Callaway CW, et al. Management of prehospital seizure patients by paramedics. *Prehosp Emerg Care.* 2009;13(2):179–184.

Michael GE, O'Connor RE. The diagnosis and management of seizures and status epilepticus in the prehospital setting. *Emerg Med Clin N Am.* 2011;29:29–39.

80

ALL THAT WHEEZES IS NOT ASTHMA

ABBY M. WILLIAMS, MD

Wheezing is one of the most common pediatric complaints and reasons for EMS transport. The prehospital provider should be an expert in recognizing and treating wheezing pediatric patients and prompt treatment should be initiated in the field. It is well known that asthma is a common reason for a child to wheeze; however, it is a common mistake to think that all that wheezes is asthma *(Table 80.1)*. The age of the child, past medical history and events leading up to the respiratory complaint can provide clues as to the etiology of the wheeze *(Table 80.2)*.

Asthma is an inflammatory process that leads to repeated episodes of cough and wheezing. It is important to be aggressive in the field when treating an asthma exacerbation. Two frequent mistakes are delaying delivery of nebulized bronchodilators and neglecting to place an IV in children with severe asthma. Early treatment with albuterol (preferably with ipratropium) can help prevent hospitalization and lessen the severity of the exacerbation. For the patient in severe distress, early use of intramuscular (IM) epinephrine and intravenous (IV) magnesium sulfate has been shown to work quickly and help prevent the patient from proceeding to intubation. Don't forget that each of these medications has added benefits to inhaled bronchodilator therapy and that using IM epinephrine does not require an IV be started.

For the infant who presents with wheezing between the months of October and April, a common cause of wheezing is bronchiolitis. Bronchiolitis is a viral process that causes rhinorrhea, coughing, wheezing, and respiratory distress. A common mistake that is made is that the provider forgets to suction the nares and oropharynx to clear the secretions. As infants are mainly nose breathers, clearing the mucus from the nares will often help relieve their respiratory distress and allow for more effective delivery of oxygen. For the patient in distress, a trial of nebulized albuterol or epinephrine is worth administering; however, many patients will not respond to this. When possible, IV access should be obtained in infants in severe distress or those with observed apnea. Intubation of an apneic infant may be warranted for transport depending on the proximity of the closest hospital.

Foreign body aspiration typically presents as a sudden onset of a coughing spell followed by difficulty breathing and wheezing. The wheezing is frequently auscultated only on the side of the foreign body. A common mistake

TABLE 80.1   DIAGNOSTIC CLUES AND TRANSPORT RECOMMENDATIONS FOR WHEEZING

	DIAGNOSTIC CLUES	TRANSPORT RECOMMENDATIONS[a]
Asthma	History of cough and wheeze? Known trigger? Eczema or allergies? Family history of asthma?	Inhaled aerosols Steroids (intravenous, oral, intramuscular) Intramuscular epinephrine Intravenous magnesium sulfate
Bronchiolitis	Infant or toddler? Upper respiratory symptoms? Fever? Progressively worsening?	Suctioning with nasal saline Oxygen Inhaled aerosols (often not useful) Observe for apnea
Pneumonia	Productive cough? Dyspnea? Fever? Focal wheezing? Progressively worsening?	Inhaled aerosols Oxygen Antibiotics
Foreign body aspiration	Sudden onset? Choking episode? Unilateral wheeze?	Minimize airway manipulation Allow to sit in a position of comfort Intubation for apnea or airway occlusion Transfer to nearest hospital
Allergic reaction/ anaphylaxis	Sudden onset? Known exposure? Angioedema? Stridor? Urticaria? Hypotension? GI complaints?	Intramuscular epinephrine Inhaled aerosols Steroids Histamine blockers Fluids

[a]For all wheezing complaints, airway, breathing, and circulation (ABC) should be secured. Good airway management including placement of a nasal or oral airway may be indicated. Endotracheal intubation should be avoided when possible and reserved only for the most severe cases where signs and symptoms suggest impending respiratory failure. Intravenous access may be useful to give medications for patients with severe respiratory distress.

TABLE 80.2   DIFFERENTIAL DIAGNOSIS OF PEDIATRIC WHEEZING

Asthma
Bronchiolitis
Foreign body aspiration
Pneumonia
Allergic reaction/anaphylaxis
Anatomical malformation
Chemical/aspiration pneumonitis
Chronic lung disease
Pulmonary edema
Psychogenic

of the healthcare provider is not having a proper respect for a patient with a choking spell as they can often decompensate quickly. Another common error is the provider performing a blind finger sweep to retrieve a foreign body. If the child is able to manage his or her own airway, transporting on oxygen without airway manipulation is indicated and with the child in a position of comfort is key. However, if the child develops apnea or severe respiratory distress, emergent intubation may be warranted, depending on the proximity to the closest hospital. In cases where the foreign body cannot be removed, it may be pushed deep into the right mainstem bronchus in order to pass the endotracheal tube and properly ventilate the patient.

Allergic reactions and anaphylaxis often present with wheezing. Other signs and symptoms include urticaria, angioedema, hypotension, vomiting, and diarrhea. Common causes of anaphylaxis are stings and drug or food allergies; however, a source may be difficult to find. A common mistake that is made in treating these patients is that IM epinephrine should be administered early in patients who have two or more organ systems involved such as wheezing and hypotension or wheezing and urticaria. Epinephrine is life saving in patients with anaphylaxis. Steroids, histamine blockers, and inhaled beta agonists should also be given when indicated, but they supplement and never replace the epinephrine. Remember that some patients with anaphylaxis can present with hypotension and should be treated aggressively with IV fluid boluses and epinephrine.

In conclusion, there is a very broad differential diagnosis leading to many treatment avenues in wheezing patients. It is important for transport personnel to recognize the different etiologies of childhood wheezing and be aggressive in the treatment of any child with severe respiratory distress.

SELECTED READINGS

Baker MD, Ruddy RM. Pulmonary emergencies. In: Fleisher GR, Ludwig S, Henretig FM, eds. *Textbook of Pediatric Emergency Medicine*. 5th ed. Philadelphia, PA: Lippincott Williams & Wilkins; 2006:1141–1145.

Gadomski AM, Brower M. Bronchodilators for bronchiolitis. *Cochrane Rev.* 2010;12: CD001266.

Guill MF. Asthma update: clinical aspects and management. *Pediatr Rev.* 2004;25:335–344.

Passali D, Lauriello M, Bellussi L, et al. Foreign body inhalation in children: an update. *Acta Otorhinolaryngol Ital.* 2010;30:27–32.

Wagner T. Bronchiolitis. *Pediatr Rev.* 2009;30:386–395.

81

TRAUMA TRANSPORT: DON'T FORGET
YOU CAN DRIVE

CHRISTOPHER TOUZEAU, MS, RN, NREMT-P
BEN KAUFMAN, BS, RN, NREMT-P

BACKGROUND

The use of helicopters as air ambulances began during World War II on an extremely limited basis. Helicopters gained popularity during the Vietnam War as a method of rapidly evacuating injured soldiers. The helicopters were staffed with medical personnel so that vigorous resuscitation of the wounded could be started on the battlefield and continued during evacuation. Rapid evacuation and prompt, aggressive resuscitation proved to significantly decrease morbidity and mortality. But does this significance carry over to the civilian world in the US? Has the use of helicopters been shown to reduce mortality?

EVIDENCE

The literature suggests that delaying the transport of *some* critically injured patients is detrimental. Let's face it—helicopter evacuation is cool. It's exciting to brag about "flying one out." Aeromedical evacuation implies that the wreck was *really* bad and the patient was at death's door. The problem is that very few patients benefit from the use of helicopters, yet first-responders continue to call for aviation to evacuate patients with various degrees of injury. It is the duty of the prehospital provider to quickly and objectively evaluate whether or not use of a helicopter will decrease transport time and improve the patient's outcome.

R Adams Cowley introduced the concept of the Golden Hour in the late 1970s. He noticed a decrease in mortality in patients who reached the operating room nearest the time of injury. The concept of the Golden Hour seems logical; however, data does not support the theory for all patients. Data does show that rapid transport and helicopter evacuation actually only benefits a very small number of patients.

It is important to clearly identify the trauma patient for whom rapid transport is critical. It turns out that this patient is somewhere in the middle of the spectrum of injury severity. If injuries are minor, transport time can be delayed without life-threatening consequences. On the other hand, injuries may be so severe that even surgical intervention would be futile. For the group in the middle, helicopter emergency medical services (HEMS) can actually make a difference. But this difference does not come from sitting on the scene to immobilize the patient or place an intravenous catheter; we intervene solely by shortening the interval between injury and the operating room. When EMS activates and waits on the scene for a helicopter, the patient is in a holding pattern.

There is often no true timesaving when utilizing helicopters. Moreover, in cases where helicopter evacuation does reduce overall transport time, there is no appreciable change in patient outcome. Data suggests that helicopters are an efficient means of transport if the distance from the scene to the operating room exceeds 60 miles. Otherwise, the clear choice is ground transportation. Another study suggests that HEMS should be considered when the scene is more than 45 miles from the receiving hospital.

EMS has a tendency to significantly over-triage trauma patients and inappropriately utilizes HEMS. A significant percentage of patients transported by helicopter have only minor injuries, and many are not even admitted to the hospital. In an urban area with a sophisticated prehospital system, researchers found no survival advantage for patients transported by helicopter. Although it is accepted practice to over-triage trauma patients, providers often overlook the dangers and costs associated with helicopter evacuation.

There are countless stories of well-intentioned field providers utilizing a helicopter to evacuate a critically injured trauma patient, only to have that patient arrive at the hospital by air AFTER a less injured patient arrived by ground.

Best Practice/Considerations

There is a small group of patients who may benefit from the use of HEMS. Will your patient benefit from the skills of the helicopter crew or the service of the helicopter?

Helicopters are expensive and risky; EMS crews rarely consider this, but the risk to benefit ratio should in fact be in the forefront of our minds when deciding upon aeromedical evacuation.

HEMS is virtually never appropriate for use in an urban or suburban setting when the receiving hospital is in close proximity to the incident. HEMS may serve a role in the rural setting, but more data is required to inform this decision.

Short on-scene times (OST) are important for critically ill patients. The use of a helicopter increases OST by approximately 30%. Remember that the next time you are faced with a decision about HEMS, ground transportation may be the best option.

Selected Readings

Bledsoe BE, Wesley AK, Eckstein M, et al. Helicopter scene transport of trauma patients with nonlife-threatening injuries: A meta-analysis. *J Trauma.* 2006;60(6):1257–1265.

Cunningham P, Rutledge R, Baker CC, et al. A comparison of the association of helicopter and ground ambulance transport with the outcome of injury in trauma patients transported from the scene. *J Trauma.* 1997;43(6):940–946.

Diaz M, Hendey G, Bivins H. When is the helicopter faster? A comparison of helicopter and ground ambulance transport times. *J Trauma.* 2005;58(1):145–153.

Schiller WR, Knox R, Zinnecker H, et al. Effect of helicopter transport of trauma victims on survival in an urban trauma center. *J Trauma.* 1988;28(8):1127–1134.

Shepherd MV, Trethewy CE, Kennedy J, et al. Helicopter use in rural trauma. *Emerg Med Australas.* 2008;20(6):494–499.

82

DON'T BE AFRAID TO USE EXISTING CENTRAL VENOUS CATHETERS!

CHRISTOPHER TOUZEAU, MS, RN, NREMT-P
BEN KAUFMAN, RN, BS, NREMT-P

INTRODUCTION

Patients are frequently discharged from the hospital with indwelling vascular access devices. These devices enable patients to lead normal lives while receiving treatment as an outpatient or while at home or work. EMS providers must be familiar with different vascular access devices so that they can safely access and utilize them when needed. Central venous catheters (CVCs) are typically inserted into a large vein such as the internal jugular, subclavian, or superior vena cava.

TYPES OF PORTS/INDICATIONS

CVCs can be used for a variety of reasons. They ensure intravenous access, eliminate repeated needle sticks, and provide rapid access to the central circulation. These catheters can be used to administer chemotherapy and other medications, to provide parenteral nutrition, and to perform hemodialysis.

Central venous access devices come in a variety of shapes and sizes. The table below summarizes the type of devices, common names for each, method of access, and special considerations *(Table 82.1)*.

INDICATIONS FOR ACCESS IN THE PREHOSPITAL SETTING

Prehospital providers can access CVCs to administer medications and fluid for resuscitation. Access should be reserved for the critically ill and injured and considered only after exhausting procedures more frequently used and familiar to EMS such as peripheral intravenous or intraosseous access.

SPECIAL PRECAUTIONS

Access of CVCs increases the risk of local and systemic infection. Devices that are implanted under the skin minimize this risk by reducing the portal of entry to the diameter of the access needle. Although sterile technique is the preferred method of accessing CVC, it is impractical in the prehospital setting. Providers must use aseptic technique when accessing these devices to minimize the risk of infection. Although povidone-iodine can be used to scrub the port(s) or access site, the preferred cleaning agent is chlorhexidine. If using isopropyl alcohol, be sure to follow institutional guidelines and policies with respect to aseptic techniques. Chlorhexidine containing

TABLE 82.1	**DIFFERENT TYPES OF CVCS**	
IMPLANTED PORTS	**DESCRIPTION**	**SPECIAL CONSIDERATIONS**
Port-a-Cath, Mediport	Surgically placed under subcutaneous tissue. Catheter tunneled from port to central vein.	Must use non–coring needle. Check for blood return prior to use. Flush before and after use.
TUNNELED CATHETERS		
Hickman, Groshong, Broviac, Cook	Catheter which is tunneled under subcutaneous tissue into a central vein.	Flush before and after use.
PERCUTANEOUS CATHETERS		
Single, multiple lumen catheter	Catheter which is inserted percutaneously into the subclavian, internal jugular, or femoral vein.	Flush before and after use. All lumens can be used.
Peripherally inserted central catheter	Catheter which is inserted percutaneously into the basilic or cephalic vein in the antecubital space.	Use low pressure syringes (>10 cc). Do not use vacuum blood collection devices.
TEMPORARY DIALYSIS CATHETER		
Ash, Quinton	Catheter which is tunneled under subcutaneous tissue into a central vein.	Check for blood return before use. Flush before and after use.

solutions have been proven more effective in decreasing the incidence of catheter-associated infections.

Another risk associated with CVCs is air embolism. Providers can reduce the risk of embolism by ensuring a closed system and clamping off lines when not in use.

Totally implantable venous access devices (TIVADs) are a type of CVC with brand names such as Port-a-Cath and Mediport. These devices require the use of a special non–coring needle to prevent damage. Non-coring needles, such as the Huber needle, are designed to "push" the rubber or silicon component aside to prevent damaging the device. While some patients may have non-coring needles to access their own ports, it is recommended that prehospital providers authorized to access TIVADs stock the non-coring needles.

Some CVCs require the use of heparin to prevent clot formation inside the catheter. Heparin is incompatible with many drugs and must be removed before injecting medications. When aspirating CVCs, a 10 cc syringe (or larger) must be used to aspirate the line. Smaller syringes create larger pressures on the catheter and should be avoided. Lines should be flushed with normal saline or Ringer's Lactate before and after drug administration. Once flushed, fluid must be administered continuously to ensure catheter patency and prevent clot formation. Dialysis catheters are typically "locked" with a heparin solution. Always aspirate at least 10 cc of fluid prior to medication administration.

Percutaneous catheters and PICC lines can easily become displaced if improperly secured or accidentally pulled. It is critical for providers to properly secure IV tubing or other access devices to prevent accidental dislodgement of the catheter.

Bariatric surgery patients may also have a medical port implanted. These ports enable the surgeon to control tension on the gastric band placed during surgery. Providers must ensure that the port they are considering is a vascular access port and not being used for another purpose. If the patient or family is unable to provide information about the port, the provider should aspirate blood to ensure venous placement.

Summary

Providers must consider the indications for CVC access and the risks associated with access, including infection, air embolism, catheter collapse, and displacement. The primary risk is infection, so aseptic technique must be practiced. Chlorhexidine is the preferred cleaning agent.

In the absence of peripheral IV or IO access, EMS can safely use the CVC to resuscitate the critically ill or injured. It is paramount that providers become familiar with the various types of devices and the special equipment which may be required to obtain access. This familiarity will promote comfort and safety during future encounters with central venous access devices.

Selected Readings

Mimoz O, Villeminey S, Ragot S, et al. Chlorhexidine-based antiseptic solution vs alcohol-based povidone-iodine for central venous catheter care. *Arch Intern Med*. 2007; 167(19):2066–2072.

2010 Maryland State Medical Protocols. Maryland Institute for Emergency Medical Services Systems Website. Available at: http://www.miemss.org/home/emsproviders/emsproviderprotocols/tabid/106/default.aspx. 165–8 Accessed March 28, 2011.

83

THE DYNAMIC ENVIRONMENT OF
A HELICOPTER LANDING ZONE:
ALWAYS REMAIN AWARE!

MATT MESSINGER, RN, EMT-P, FF

Aeromedical evacuations frequently take place during dynamic and often chaotic scene environments. As an emergency medical services provider, you are simultaneously charged with managing patient care and making critical decisions. Designating a landing zone and interfacing with helicopter crews add yet another element of complexity to an already challenging scenario. This chapter emphasizes important aspects of landing zone safety and will help you to avoid distraction.

Once you have determined that aeromedical evaluation is required, you will now need to decide where the aircraft should land. One of the big errors that occur takes place while setting up, marking, and securing the landing zone. In general, a square area that measures 100 ft × 100 ft satisfies minimum requirements for the landing zone. Landing zone dimensions may vary according to aircraft size. Local air medical providers can give you detailed instructions about specific landing zone measurements and requirements. When deciding where to land the aircraft, there are several things to consider: Close proximity to the incident, the direction of travel of the responding units, and of course wires, trees, and overhead obstructions. Once you have selected an area, be sure to keep a second landing zone in mind, in case the pilot doesn't like your first choice. If no other areas suffice to land the aircraft safely, a rendezvous at an existing landing zone represents an excellent backup plan.

Large open areas, like fields, parking lots, or roadways, are all potentially good landing zones. If you are landing the aircraft in the roadway, that designated road must be shut down until the aircraft leaves. So, be sure that no other emergency responders are coming from that direction or that no one needs to depart in that direction. If you're planning to land the aircraft in a field, make sure it is firm, flat, has low cut grass, and less than a 10% grade. If time permits, someone should walk along the LZ to make sure that there are no unforeseen obstacles or debris. A dusty field or parking lot can be sprayed down with water to decrease the amount of dust created by the rotor wash. Rotor wash or, wind that is pulled through the main rotor system, can create winds up to 70 to 100 miles/hour. Keep spectators back at least 200 ft, emergency vehicles 100 ft back, and have fire equipment at the ready. To avoid loose objects being blown around in the LZ, ground personnel should wear eye protection, remove baseball caps, and securely fasten helmet chin straps during landing and takeoff operations.

After designating a suitable LZ, you must mark the area so that the flight crew can see it. During the day, the landing zone can be marked using weighted cones which are very visible from the air. At night it is important that you mark each corner with a light. Commercial produces such as strobes or LED flashers are available. Alternatively, you can utilize a hand-held light to mark the landing zone border. White lights may interfere with the optimum function of night vision goggles. Do not station personnel on the corners of the landing zone. This can be very dangerous, and if there is debris in the area, they may be hit from the rotor wash. Avoid the use of flares or scene tape. Flares can ignite fires, and scene tape could break free and be pulled into the rotor system. Use a fifth cone of light on the windward side to mark the direction of wind. When relaying information about the LZ to the flight crew, it is important to use compass direction and not

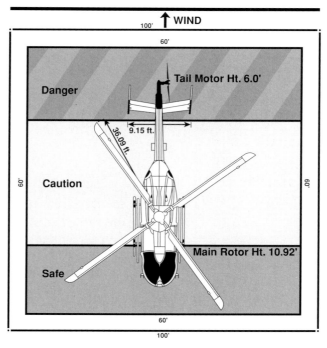

FIGURE 83.1. Diagram of a suitable landing zone.

"left" or "right." Describe the LZ's relationship to the accident scene, its surface, how it's marked, and detail any obstructions.

Once the aircraft has landed, do not under any circumstances approach the aircraft without direction from the flight crew, especially if the rotors are still turning. Never approach the aircraft from the rear. The rear tail rotor is hard to see while it's moving, and it may be at head level. It is very important that one of your emergency personnel is 30 ft behind the aircraft keeping people back and not allowing any vehicles to drive through the landing zone. This person should have radio communication with the landing zone commander and the pilot. If you are asked to help the flight crew with patient loading and transport, follow the flight crew's direction and avoid touching the aircraft. There are numerous antennas and sensitive equipment on the aircraft that can easily break off, grounding the aircraft.

As an emergency service provider you understand that your job can be extremely dangerous. Most emergency scenes are dynamic and demand close attention to detail. Working around an aircraft and establishing a landing zone involves its own set of unique hazards. Following these tips will help ensure the safety of patients and personnel alike.

SELECTED READINGS

Fromm RE, Varon J. Air medical transport. *J Fam Pract.* 1993;36(3):313–316.
Helicopter Operations, 10–2-3. Landing Zone, Special Operations. http://www.faa.gov/air_traffic/publications/ATpubs/AIM/Chap10/aim1002.html. Updated 2010. Accessed March 10, 2011.

84

Know your HEMS providers: they're not all alike!

Kevin High, RN, MPH, EMT

Helicopter emergency medical services (HEMS) in the United States have grown exponentially since 2000 with the number of medical helicopters doubling to more than 800. With this growth, there have been an increasing amount of patients being transported by air; some of these patient transports have been called into question due to the issue of medical appropriateness. To address this it is incumbent on the EMS provider not only to choose the most appropriate mode of transport but to choose the most appropriate HEMS provider to do so. This chapter will review the various types of HEMS providers and discuss general differences in education and training.

The HEMS industry as a whole is lacking in standardization and consistency. HEMS services nationwide and even on some local levels are not equivalent in capabilities. One entity offers voluntary accreditation for the air medical industry. Commission on Accreditation of Medical Transport Systems (CAMTS) is a private sector organization that offers accreditation to HEMS programs on a voluntary basis. CAMTS recognizes services that demonstrate compliance with patient safety and quality standards.

The lay public and, to some degree, EMS providers assume that all HEMS are the same; but they are not. HEMS agencies are regulated by the Federal Aviation Administration via part 135 regulations. Mere compliance with part 135 does not guarantee that each helicopter has the same level of performance or aviation safety technology. The following sections highlight factors that distinguish one provider from another.

STAFFING

Staffing patterns and personnel differ from service to service. Some may only utilize one provider while others utilize a two–person crew. Other services incorporate a two–provider, advanced life support model such as a nurse/paramedic team or more rarely a nurse/physician team. While research indicates that crew composition has little to no significant impact on patient outcomes, CAMTS requires a minimum of two providers for a program to advertise itself as providing an advanced level of care; typically this is a registered nurse/paramedic crew configuration. EMS providers should be aware of respective provider staffing of the HEMS being utilized and choose accordingly. For example, a septic patient who requires infusions of vasopressor agents may benefit from a staffing model that incorporates critical care nurses. Multisystem trauma patients may be well served by a nurse/paramedic crew configuration.

OPERATIONAL CAPABILITIES

The type of aircraft utilized by an air medical service can directly impact the service's ability to care for the patient. Some aircraft have height/weight limits and some offer very limited access to the patient (i.e., only the upper torso, head/neck, and arms are accessible in flight). Some aircraft lack the ability to maintain any type of climate control of the interior; specifically they lack air conditioning; this too can impact patient condition. Again, the lack of standards allows for wide variability between air medical services. If time permits, it is wise to select an air medical provider that is best suited to the mission's needs. For example, some helicopters are not designed to transport more than one patient at a time. Patients with multiple and complex orthopedic injuries may require transport in a helicopter with a larger patient compartment. Balloon pump, neonatal isolettes, and other specialized equipment necessitate an appropriately equipped, credentialed, and capable aeromedical provider.

MEDICAL/CLINICAL TRAINING

There is often an assumption that any HEMS crew has the capability to provide critical care interventions; this may or may not be correct. The designation of "critical care transport team" is somewhat subjective; some regulatory bodies have a standard in place such as mandatory equipment, training, and staffing patterns while others do not. Some services are able to label themselves as providers of critical care due in the absence of minimum standards. This further drives the perception that all HEMS are the same. Services capable of sophisticated critical care transport typically perform many of the following procedures.

- Intra-aortic balloon pump operation
- Extracorporeal membrane oxygenation (ECMO) transport
- Advanced invasive procedures and monitoring
- Blood product initiation, point of care laboratory studies
- High-risk obstetric transport
- Vasopressor infusion/titration

Ideally, an HEMS will furnish EMS providers with this information in order that they have the best available information when it is time to make the decision on who to call. It is imperative that regional EMS providers educate themselves with respect to the capabilities of the available HEMS and choose accordingly.

DESTINATION HOSPITAL

Air medical services should transport the patient to the closest/most appropriate facility; this may or may not happen. Hospital destination criteria vary depending on the jurisdiction. Services may have an incentive to transport to one facility over another regardless of what is most appropriate for the patient. The desire of the patient and requesting EMS agency should be communicated to the air medical service. Ultimately, the destination should be dictated by patient condition and receiving hospital capabilities.

Having an accurate working knowledge of the air medical service(s) within an EMS provider's response area is a core requisite to ensure delivery of appropriate care and transport for the critically ill and injured.

SELECTED READINGS

Atlas and Database of Air Medical Services. http://www.adamsairmed.org/

Burney RE, Passini L, Hubert D, et al. Comparison of aeromedical crew performance by patient severity and outcome. *Ann Emerg Med.* 1992;21:375–378.

Commission on Accreditation of Medical Transport Systems. *Accreditation Standards*, 8th ed. www.camts.org

The Government Accountability Office. *Potential Strategies to Address Air Ambulance Safety Concerns*, April 2009. http://www.gao.gov/new.items/d09627t.pdf

The Patient First Air Ambulance Alliance. *Position Paper—Pay for Performance: Core Measures/Never Events*, June 2009. www.acctforpatients.org

85

REQUESTING A HELICOPTER IS A MEDICAL DECISION: CHOOSE THE RIGHT PATIENT FOR AVIATION UTILIZATION

ROGER M. STONE, MD, MS, FAAEM, FACEP

INTRODUCTION

Part of the founding of EMS systems within the United States was based on scientific study pointing out the nature of a neglected epidemic in modern society caused by accidental death and disability from trauma, or the so-called "EMS white paper." This launched us in the trajectory toward formal emergency medicine and trauma systems through regionalization of resources and other specialty centers to serve as definitive care partners in the new prehospital EMS paradigm.

The shift in emphasis toward bypassing local emergency departments (EDs) in favor of direct referrals to life-saving centers was coupled to evidence that preventable morbidity and death would be mitigated by a patient's arrival to specialized, definitive care within a window of time. Specifically, "the golden hour" was established as a benchmark for trauma, and more recently a 3-hour window for stroke and 90 minutes for percutaneous coronary intervention (PCI). Specialty centers are not uniformly distributed across the country. For patients situated in remote or rural locations, these centers may not be accessible by ground ambulance. The creation and proliferation of aeromedical services has been associated with the need for the rapid transportation of critical patients to receiving facilities across large distances.

Nationwide lectures, discussions, articles, and debates have occurred over the last two decades about the benefits, limitations, and risks to patients and rescuers in the air medical industry. These have taken place against a backdrop of rapid proliferation of aeromedical services, many for profit. In addition, there is much concern over an increasing rate of aeromedical accidents. According to data from the National Transportation and Safety Board, 85 medical helicopter crashes resulted in 77 fatalities from 2003 to 2008. It stands to reason that the appropriate choice of a mode of transport must be well thought out after the triage decision that assigns specialty care.

Patient Selection for Air Medical Scene Evacuation of Critical Illnesses and Injuries. National literature has essentially endorsed the consideration of air medical evacuation for selected patients and situations that meet the following criteria, not limited to:

- **Time-critical emergencies** in need of specialty medical attention in a select window of time, examples include PCI for ST segment elevation myocardial infarction (STEMI), trauma critical care, or thrombolytic administration and/or neuro-intensive care for stroke;
- **Acute trauma with physiologic criteria** as indicated in local or national triage protocols, which implies higher likelihood of operative intervention, higher severity of injury, or need for trauma critical care.

Guiding Principles in Considering Patients for Air Medical Transport. Firstly, assignment to air medical evacuation is a medical decision. Generally, the assessing EMS provider should accurately convey the condition of the patient to incident command (IC) so that the medical disposition is driven by the medical personnel unless pressing operational factors predominate. Deciding upon the mode of transportation is an important, but separate and distinct, triage decision. Given that the greatest benefit is for emergencies that require critical intervention, air transport is indicated if clearly faster for delivering a life threat to definitive care than rapid evacuation by land. Aeromedical evacuation of a patient based solely upon the presence of mechanistic criteria is a decision not rooted in evidence. Provided that the patient is not exhibiting signs of decompensation, evaluation for mechanism can safely be conducted in time frames beyond the traditional golden hour. Long falls, ejection from a vehicle, motorcycle injuries, passenger compartment intrusion, speed of impact, and death of another passenger in a compartment are examples of such mechanistic criteria.

Pitfalls in Selection of Patients for Scene Evacuation by Air Medical Resources. One error to avoid is failing to appropriately triage a patient with a time-critical emergency. Assessments, although subject to time limitations, should never be suboptimal. Sometimes, failing to follow reasonable guidelines set forth nationally or locally can affect an appropriate triage decision for trauma patients. This might mean not differentiating physiologic criteria from mechanistic criteria and resultant over-triage, or conversely failing to recognize risk factors that make traumatic mechanisms more significant (elderly, warfarin, etc.), resulting in under-triage. Both under-triage and over-triage may lead to errant disposition of patients to the wrong destination and/or by the wrong means.

In conclusion, flying out a patient solely for mechanistic criteria when speed is not as critical a factor may not be clinically beneficial. Conversely, failing to fly a critical patient to an appropriate specialty center that is otherwise not accessible by land and the delays from deferral of the initial management to a local ED may threaten patients even more. The first step is good patient selection for patients likely to benefit from a ride in an air asset.

Selected Readings

Baker SP, Grabowski JG, Dodd RS, et al. EMS helicopter crashes: what influences fatal outcome? *Ann Emerg Med.* 2006;47(4):351–356.

Biewener A, Aschenbrenner U, Rammelt S, et al. Impact of helicopter transport and hospital level on mortality of polytrauma patients. *J Trauma.* 2004;56(1):94–98.

Bledsoe BE, Wesley AK, Eckstein M, et al. Helicopter scene transport of trauma patients with nonlife-threatening injuries: a meta-analysis. *J Trauma.* 2006;60(6):1257–1265.

Centers for Disease Control and Prevention. Guidelines for field triage of injured patients: recommendations of the national expert panel on field triage. *MMWR.* 2009;58(RR-1): 1–35.

Committee on Trauma and Committee on Shock, Division of Medical Sciences, National Academy of Sciences, National Research Council. *Accidental Death and Disability: The Neglected Disease of Modern Society.* Washington, D.C.: The National Academies Press; 1966.

Kerr WA, Kerns TJ, Bissell RA. Differences in mortality rates among trauma patients transported by helicopter ambulance in Maryland. *Prehosp Disaster Med.* 1999;14(3):159–164.

MacKenzie EJ, Rivara FP, Jurkovich GJ, et al. A national evaluation of the effect of trauma-center care on mortality. *N Engl J Med.* 2006;354:366–378.

Marler JR, Tilley BC, Lu M, et al. Early stroke treatment associated with better outcome: the NINDS rt-PA stroke study. *Neurology.* 2000;55:1649–1655.

National Transportation and Safety Board. Current issues with air medical transportation. Available at: http://www.ntsb.gov/doclib/speeches/sumwalt/sumwalt_050411.pdf Accessed on January 5, 2011.

"Tribute to R Adams Cowley, M.D.," University of Maryland Medical Center, R Adams Cowley Shock Trauma Center, University of Maryland Medical Center, 2007. http://www.umm.edu/shocktrauma/about_us/history.htm.

Trunkey DD. The emerging crisis in trauma care: a history and definition of the problem. *Clin Neurosurg.* 2007;54:200–205.

86

DON'T WAIT FOR THE HELICOPTER! PITFALLS IN AVIATION SELECTION

ROGER M. STONE, MD, MS, FAAEM, FACEP

INTRODUCTION

An essential skill of an EMS provider, especially at the advanced life support (ALS) level, is to recognize a critical complaint in addition to signs of a potentially unstable patient. The last chapter discussed the importance of accurate triage of the critically ill or injured to the closest "appropriate" facility, specifically the correct specialty center. In considering the utilization of scene air medical evacuation, a common problem is that while most EMS providers are able to correctly identify a sick patient quickly, calling for an air resource may not constitute the ideal mode of transportation on the basis of the logistics, location, and medical presentation. Medics may be led into a "knee jerk" reaction to seek aircraft activation for any triage decision toward specialty care. The reasons for this may be the widespread availability and/or marketing of air services, or the tradition in some EMS systems that establish the specialty centers as better accessible by air. Simply put, no equation should exist that automatically marries specialty center triage to air medical activation. If that occurs indiscriminately, patients will be "waiting" for helicopters for significant periods of time.

AIR MEDICAL PATIENT SELECTION: WHEN WAITING FOR AN AVIATION RESPONSE IS MOST BENEFICIAL

Summoning aviation assets is usually associated with a delay in response by definition, because on average services are spread out and coming from distances much greater than the local EMS agency. Therefore, careful thought should be given to weigh the benefits of waiting for an aircraft against the risks of that delay and even of flight. Reasonable criteria for summoning the aircraft might include:

- **Acute trauma with physiologic criteria or other time critical emergencies** were discussed in Chapter 85.
- **Inaccessible locations** for feasible land evacuation to a specialty center in a reasonable time frame; very large distances to cover, very remote locations, island emergencies, or poor topography might all be examples of situations where the air asset activation clinically benefits patients.
- **Entrapment** that creates the opportunity for aircraft to be immediately in place after rescue.

- **Special rescue situations** could represent very sound reasons for utilization.

Guiding Principles in Considering Activation

Recall that the assignment of aeromedical resources is a medical decision separate and distinct from the initial triage process. The mode of transportation constitutes a separate decision step after the destination is chosen. Air transport is indicated if clearly faster for delivering a life threat to definitive care than rapid evacuation by land. Aeromedical evacuation is not the most ideal choice for the transport based solely upon the presence of mechanistic criteria. Indeed, stable patients who are assigned to a trauma center due to "mechanism" alone may be candidates for ground transport. Since timely delivery to definitive care is a tenant of current trauma systems, each end user of aviation services should understand and factor in delays in helicopter activation and utilization. Examples of well-known time intervals include:

- Launch time
- In flight time (time en route)
- Ground travel to a remote landing zone
- Reassessment and packaging of patient by air medical crew

Cumulatively, these may exceed driving times. Some local studies show that 45 to 50 miles can be covered more quickly by land. Local data from this author's system show that average scene times for patients awaiting the helicopter are in the range of 35 to 39 minutes.

If helicopters are to facilitate arrival at definitive care, early activation via simultaneous dispatch may be helpful in shaving off several of the delay time intervals. Knowing the above, ground crews should not prolong scene times unnecessarily to await aviation assets. Providers should be conscious of scene time as the event progresses. Consequently, liberal cancellation of aircraft is a consideration if re-assessment yields that greater progress can be made by proceeding by land rather than waiting. Continuity of care by the first arriving crew is more ideal than a hand-off unless the turnover provides specific additional clinical benefit, as delays and medical errors are heightened by hand offs.

Conclusion: Avoiding Pitfalls in Waiting for Air Medical Resources

In conclusion, utilizing helicopters as a means of evacuation should never be a reflex reaction, but a separate calculation of benefit. Helicopter utilization may prolong on-scene times. In addition, HEMS activation carries a small but distinct risk of crashes. Providers should not fail to calculate known delays beyond only the estimated time of arrival (ETA) and not make the assumption that the ETA of the aircraft is the time it will depart the scene. If providers consider the above, they will appreciate when the aircraft does not represent an additional time savings. Getting a less critical patient by air to a center a few minutes earlier is a failure to maximize a clinical benefit. Allowing a single variable to dictate the reason for air asset use is also a potential error. Avoiding a drive due to rush hour, or the EMS system's convenience (in order to get back to service more quickly) is not necessarily of clinical benefit to patients, and in fact might deplete the air asset availability for a more appropriate patient. Finally, failure to cancel the activation upon re-assessment when benefit is less clear-cut and the asset is still en route might still waste time unnecessarily. Fire, rescue, and EMS departments "turn around" rescue squads, extra engines, and paramedics on a daily basis. The argument that providers might just as well "keep them coming because they are in the air" fails to acknowledge the complexities inherent in such a decision. Assignment to aeromedical transport, similar to any other treatment intervention, carries with it a list of associated risks and benefits.

SELECTED READINGS

Baker SP, Grabowski JG, Dodd RS, et al. EMS helicopter crashes: what influences fatal outcome? *Ann Emerg Med*. 2006;47(4):351–356.

Biewener A, Aschenbrenner U, Rammelt S, et al. Impact of helicopter transport and hospital level on mortality of polytrauma patients. *J Trauma*. 2004;56(1):94–98.

Bledsoe BE, Wesley AK, Eckstein M, et al. Helicopter scene transport of trauma patients with nonlife-threatening injuries: a meta-analysis. *J Trauma*. 2006;60(6):1257–1265.

Chapell VL, Mileski WJ, Wolf SE, et al. Impact of discontinuing a hospital-based air ambulance service on trauma patient outcomes. *J Trauma*. 2005;58(1):148–153.

Diaz MA, Hendey GW, Bivins HG. When is the helicopter faster? A comparison of helicopter and ground ambulance transport times. *Ann Emerg Med*. 2006;47(4):351–356.

Kerr WA, Kerns TJ, Bissell RA. Differences in mortality rates among trauma patients transported by helicopter ambulance in Maryland. *Prehosp Disaster Med*. 1999;14(3):159–164.

87

PEARLS AND PITFALLS OF INTERHOSPITAL TRANSPORT: IT'S ABOUT MUCH MORE THAN PAPERWORK!

ROBERT DICE, MS, RN, NREMT-P
KEVIN G. SEAMAN, MD, FACEP

In this chapter, pearls and pitfalls encountered during interhospital transfers are discussed. A prehospital provider may be called upon to conduct an interhospital transfer. He (or she) possesses knowledge about patient care and the tools to safely move a patient from one hospital to another. There are two main reasons for a patient to be sent to another medical facility:

1) A patient is in need of a specialized service not available at the sending facility (cardiac catheterization, organ transplantation).
2) A patient requires a level of care higher than the sending facility can provide (specialized critical care services, intensive burn care).

KEEP THE FOLLOWING "PEARLS" IN MIND WHEN RESPONDING TO A PATIENT TRANSFER REQUEST

- Document the patient's pre-transfer assessment. This is best done before transferring the patient onto your stretcher. After moving the patient onto your stretcher, conduct another assessment. Focus this assessment on any devices such as intravenous lines and monitoring electrodes. Reconfirm endotracheal tube placement and document accordingly prior to departure.
- Secure the transfer orders written by the transferring physician. Ensure that the reason for transfer is contained within these orders.
- Document any orders delivered through consultation with medical direction.
- Document reasoning that supports the mode of transfer (ground vs. air).
- Ensure that the transfer form, documenting the reason for the transfer is appropriately signed by the patient (or their medical decision maker) and the transferring doctor.
- In cases where an unstable patient is transferred to a specialty center, document treatment provided and the reason for transferring the patient (care not available at the sending hospital) and the benefit of specialty center referral outweighs the risk of transport.

It is often stated in training programs and legal proceedings alike, "*If it isn't written, it never happened.*" This premise supposes that if a care provider does not document their assessments, care, and procedures in the patient's medical record, the provider did not perform the care. Pay careful attention to documentation and list the reasons behind any interventions adjusted or undertaken during interfacility transport.

Traditional prehospital protocols inadequately address conditions encountered during interhospital and critical care interfacility transport. Patients have often been seen and treated by emergency physicians. Medications and devices encountered in the critical care setting may differ from those found on a traditional advanced life support (ALS) ambulance. The domain of "specialty care" encompasses treatment decisions, medications, and events that fall outside the normal scope of prehospital ALS practice. To that end, providers must ensure that they are (1) comfortable with rendering patient care and (2) capable of performing the requested interventions. The Emergency Medical Treatment and Active Labor Act (EMTALA) specifies that interfacility transfers must be conducted with appropriately trained and equipped personnel (2):

> Qualified personnel, with the appropriate medical equipment, must accompany the patient during transfer. The transferring physician, by law, has the responsibility of selecting the most appropriate means of transport to include qualified personnel and transport equipment.

Simply stated, it may not be acceptable for an ALS ambulance to transport a patient who is receiving vasoactive medications. It is the responsibility of the sending hospital to ensure that patients are safely transported. Should you, as a provider, feel uncomfortable with the management of a drug infusion or a chest tube, then you have the right to request the presence of qualified personnel such as a trained emergency department nurse. If your service is not qualified to administer blood products, then the sending hospital is obligated to send the patient with a professional capable of carrying out a transfusion. Critical care services typically have "expanded scope" protocols that address interventions falling outside of the usual prehospital scope of practice. Therefore, a qualified critical care transport ambulance may enlist the expertise of a nurse, respiratory therapist, or pediatric specialist.

Interhospital Transport Pitfalls

- Failure to document the care you provided as it relates to local protocol. Have copies of jurisdictional and interfacility transfer protocols available for reference. Refer to a written copy of the protocol followed so that important points are not missed. Remember, not documenting a procedure means it was not performed.

- Failure to document the source of the care provided. This is important when there is conflict between local protocol, interhospital transfer protocol, transferring physician order, or online medical direction order.
- Failure to document and justify the care you were not able to perform. For example, it may be appropriate to withhold a dose of morphine because of a significant drop in a patient's blood pressure.
- Failure to document the effects of your treatment. Did the pain medicine work? Did the anti-arrhythmic provide the desired effect? Always document patient reassessment.
- Failure to stabilize patients to the best of your ability prior to transportation.

Interfacility transport is an inherently risky endeavor. It may involve the movement of a critically ill patient outside of an intensive care unit. A moving ambulance or airborne helicopter is a less than ideal place for initiating life-saving interventions. Therefore, the anticipation of complications is in a patient's best interest. Securing the airway is of paramount importance prior to patient transport. In some cases, critical care crews possess expertise and skill sets that are superior to those found in a more remote hospital setting. Collaborate with the sending facility to secure threatened airways; endotracheal intubation may have a higher possibility of success when performed in an adequately illuminated and stable emergency department as opposed to the patient care compartment of a helicopter. Ensure adequate venous access prior to transfer and thoroughly review the sending facility's documentation.

In great measure, prehospital crews provide excellent care. Successful interfacility transport requires unique attention detail and an understanding of physiology and treatments that may be outside of a prehospital provider's comfort zone. It is imperative that the standard of care be maintained throughout all phases of interfacility transfer. The ambulance or aircraft and its crew should be capable of managing the interventions undertaken at the sending facility. Have a low threshold for consultation with medical control. Expanded prehospital protocols may assist critical care crews in the care of medically complex patients. Any service responsible for conveying critically ill patients from one hospital to another should have guidelines in place that address conditions that can and cannot be adequately managed by their transport crews.

Remember to document well the care you provide, your thinking behind the decisions, and the reasons why you provided the care you rendered or could not provide. Comprehensive documentation reflects the excellent prehospital standard of care and reduced medico-legal risk.

Selected Readings

Chapleau W. Could inadequate EMS documentation mean inappropriate prehospital care? Available at: http://www.emsworld.com/article/10319800/notes-on-trauma-poor-documentation-associated-with-increased-mortality. Notes on Trauma: Poor Documentation Associated with Increased Mortality

Leight MJ, Kupas DF. Interhospital transfer. In: *Emergency Medical Services: Clinical Practice and System Oversight*. Vol 2. Medical Oversight of EMS. Dubuque, IA: Kendall Hunt Professional; 2009:271–280.

National Highway Traffic Safety Administration. *Guide for Interfacility Patient Transfer* [Appendix D]. Available at: http://www.nhtsa.gov/people/injury/ems/interfacility/pages/AppD.htm

Swor RA, Storer D, Domeier RM, et al. Medical direction of interfacility patient transfers: policy resource and education paper.

88

SEDATION DURING TRANSPORT: THINK BEYOND PARALYSIS!

JILL D. SMITH, BSN, RN, CEN

CYNTHIA S. SHEN, DO, FACOEP, FACEP

You have intubated your patient, confirmed tube placement, and secured the tube by taping, tying, or using a tube holder. You may think your job is done, but that is just the beginning. Endotracheal intubation can be quite uncomfortable in a patient who is not comatose. No device will keep a tube in place if the patient is awake, alert, and agitated. Other detrimental physiologic responses to intubation include gagging, coughing, bradycardia, hypertension, increased intracranial pressure, and parasympathetically mediated bronchospasm. All of these conditions are detrimental to your patient and, if untreated, can lead to decompensation.

Sedation is crucial to the maintenance of proper tube placement and patient safety. By choosing the correct sedative based on your patient's condition and your transport needs, you can increase the chances of a better outcome for your patient and a safer transport for you.

There can be several reasons for the intubated patient to be agitated and it is essential that you determine the most likely causes in order to medicate most effectively. The first step is to thoroughly assess your patient including vital signs, all lines (including IVs and oxygen tubing), and any splints or restraints. Ask yourself these questions:

- First, "is my patient receiving enough oxygen?" Hypoxia leads to agitation.
- Secondly, "are all my IVs running and is my patient receiving the medications?" Underdosing or infiltration of an IV line may contribute to the lack of sedation.
- Lastly, "have injuries been addressed and injured limbs secured?" Untreated or undertreated pain can lead to agitation, abnormal vital signs, and decompensation.

There are a variety of medications available for sedation, each with pros and cons. The use of any one medication is based on the patients' condition and transportation needs. *Table 88.1* includes some of the most commonly used medications and highlights their advantages and disadvantages.

There is not enough evidence to recommend one medication or combination of medications for every situation. This is why a complete head-to-toe assessment of your patient is your most valuable tool for medication

TABLE 88.1 COMMONLY USED SEDATIVES

DRUG	LOADING DOSE/ ONSET TIME	INFUSION RATE	ADVANTAGES	DISADVANTAGES
Lorazepam[a] (benzodiazepine)	1–4 mg Onset 5–20 min Repeat dose every 6–8 hr	0.5–10 mg/hr	Potent sedative Anticonvulsant properties	Slow onset, risk of oversedation Must watch for IV line medicine compatibility/IV line precipitate
Midazolam (benzodiazepine)	0.02–0.08 mg/kg Onset 1–5 min Repeat dose every 30 min	2–8 mg/hr	Powerful amnesic and anxiolytic Quick onset and short duration	Longer time of sedation following prolonged administration Negative interactions with many common critical care drugs Not for hypovolemia or shock as it is known to cause hypotension
Diazepam[a] (benzodiazepine)	0.1–0.2 mg/kg Onset <1 min Follow with 0.03–0.1 mg/kg every 30 min	Not for continuous infusion	Rapid onset, potent sedative, and muscle relaxant	Negative reaction with many common critical care medications Seldom used for sedation of critically ill patient
Propofol (aklylphenol derivative)	No loading dose Onset <1 min	5–80 μg/kg/min	Potent sedative with immediate onset and short duration Good choice for patients needing frequent neuro checks or to reduce elevated intracranial pressures	Causes dose related hypotension, respiratory depression in bolus doses Avoid in patients with allergies to eggs, soy

(continued)

TABLE 88.1	COMMONLY USED SEDATIVES (CONTINUED)			
DRUG	LOADING DOSE/ ONSET TIME	INFUSION RATE	ADVANTAGES	DISADVANTAGES
Fentanyl (opioid analgesic)	50–200 µg Onset <30 sec Repeat every 30–60 min	0.7–10 µg/kg/hr	Potent analgesic–sedative, immediate onset, relative cardiovascular stability with little hypotension Is a good choice for analgesia and sedation of most critically ill patients due to cardiovascular stability	Accumulates with repeated dosing Possible chest wall rigidity with higher dosing, though a rare side effect
Hydromorphone[b] (opioid analgesic)	1–4 mg Onset 5–10 min Repeat every 4–5 hr	7–15 µg/kg/hr	Has no consistent advantage over fentanyl	Metabolites can accumulate in organ failure and prolong sedative effects
Remifentanil (opioid analgesic)	No loading dose Onset 1–3 min	0.6–15 µg/kg/hr	Ultrashort acting, does not build up in renal or hepatic insufficiency Good alternative to fentanyl for patients with multiorgan failure	Pain and discomfort with abrupt cessation

[a]Propylene glycol solvent may accumulate with high dosing and lead to metabolic acidosis and organ failure.
[b]Has limited use in critically ill patients due to pre-load reduction and myocardial depressive effects.

selection. It would be a wonderful world if all patients fit nicely into a single comprehensive algorithm for sedation. Unfortunately, this is not the case. The persistently hypotensive patient may require a fentanyl infusion supplemented with occasional doses of lorazepam. Trauma patients who are in extreme pain may require fentanyl and midazolam, which are short acting. An intubated patient with delirium tremens may benefit from a propofol drip. Do not be afraid to use medication combinations, as studies have shown that this strategy often reduces the required dose of the primary sedative. However, with combination drug therapy, always be sure to check line compatibility and drug interactions first.

Your post-intubation plan should address, and anticipate the need for, patient sedation. Adequate sedation reduces agitation, improves safety, and encourages compliance with the ventilator. Patients may tolerant or react unpredictably to one particular class of medication. Familiarize yourself with a variety of medications so that you can tailor a sedation plan to meet your patient's individual needs.

SELECTED READINGS

Jacobi J, Fraser GL, Coursin DB, et al. Clinical practice guidelines for the sustained use of sedatives and analgesics in the critically ill adult. *Crit Care Med*. 2002;30:119.

Mularski RA. Pain management in the intensive care unit. *Crit Care Clin*. 2004;20:381.

Ostermann ME, Kenan SP, Seiferling RA, et al. Sedation in the intensive care unit: a systematic review. *JAMA*. 2000;283:1451.

Richman PS, Baram D, Varela M, et al. Sedation during mechanical ventilation: a trial of benzodiazepine and opiate in combination. *Crit Care Med*. 2006;34:1395.

Wunsch H, Kahn JM, Kramer AA, et al. Use of intravenous infusion sedation among mechanically ventilated patients in the United States. *Crit Care Med*. 2009;37:3031.

89

UNDERSTAND THE SPECTRUM OF SEPSIS: HOW TO IDENTIFY, MONITOR, AND TREAT!

JILL D. SMITH, RN, BSN, CEN, MS, ATC
CYNTHIA S. SHEN, DO, FACOEP, FACEP

One of the buzz words in today's critical care medicine is "sepsis", as in "the patient is septic." It is often said with a sense of urgency. With that in mind, it is important to understand what sepsis is, why it is important, what to do about it, and most importantly what this means to you as a prehospital provider.

HOW IS SEPSIS RECOGNIZED?

Sepsis is actually a progression along a disease continuum; it exists in stages. Understanding the progression of sepsis helps guide therapy and prevents patient decompensation.

Systemic inflammatory response syndrome (SIRS) is a condition that reflects the widespread activation of inflammatory pathways. Two or more of the following criteria indicate SIRS:

- Temperature >100.9 or <96.8°F
- White blood cell count >12,000 or <4,000
- Heart rate >90
- Respiratory rate >20

Sepsis: Is SIRS criteria with a confirmed or presumed infection, hyperglycemia >120 mg/dl, or lactate level >2. For example, a tachycardic and tachypneic patient with pneumonia may actually meet sepsis criteria.

Severe sepsis: Sepsis-induced organ dysfunction or tissue hypoperfusion.

Indicators include cool vasoconstricted skin, decreased or no urine output, lactic acidosis, and altered mental status.

Septic shock: Severe sepsis plus hypotension persistent despite adequate fluid resuscitation.

HOW IS SEPSIS MANAGED?

First and foremost is the stabilization and maintenance of the airway through positioning (i.e., head tilt, jaw thrust), nasal trumpet, oral airway, or possibly intubation. Once an airway is established the patient should receive supplemental oxygen to maintain adequate oxygen saturation. If the patient is intubated, it is important to maintain adequate sedation. The sedated patient will have a decreased demand for oxygen and utilize less cellular energy reserves. Studies have shown that the earlier the resuscitation is begun, the better the outcome for the septic patient. Parameters for adequate resuscitation:

■ Central venous pressure of 8 to 12 mm Hg
■ Mean arterial pressure >65
■ Arterial oxygen sat >92%
■ Urine output ≥0.5 mL/kg/hour

Clearly, an improving mental status and normalizing vital signs also indicate a successful ongoing resuscitation.

Septic patients will often be hypotensive due to hypovolemia caused by fluid shifts (the so-called "third spacing") and fluid losses (sweating due to fever, water loss due to tachypnea). Acidosis and hypoperfusion cause blood vessels to dilate; this further decreases the circulating blood volume. Hypotension is initially addressed with aggressive, high-volume fluid boluses. It is not unusual for a septic patient to receive more than 5 L of fluids during the first 24 hours. During this initial phase of resuscitation, fluid input will be far greater than urine output.

If the patient has hypotension that is resistant to fluid resuscitation, it will be important to add a vasopressor: "Pressors" work through different channels and it is helpful to understand how each medication works.

■ Dopamine works on the heart to increase BP by increasing stroke volume and heart rate. At higher doses, dopamine causes peripheral vasoconstriction. See the chapter on "Don't Fear the Pressor!" for more detailed discussion.
■ Levophed (norepinephrine) and phenylephrine augment blood pressure through increasing peripheral vasoconstriction with little increase in heart rate.
■ Dobutamine, an inotrope, increases heart output and BP by increasing heart muscle contractility. It is not a true "pressor" in that it has no direct action on the vasculature.

Specific patient conditions inform vasopressor selection. For example, a patient with tachycardia is more likely to be treated with levophed than with dopamine. An elderly patient in cardiogenic shock may be a candidate for prehospital dopamine administration.

Another important aspect of treatment for the septic patient is the administration of antibiotics. It is likely during early stages that the patient will be treated with broad spectrum antibiotics to cover the most likely sources of infection. Antibiotics administered early in the patient's course have been shown to improve outcome.

In summary, the treatment for septic shock involves: Establishing an airway, providing adequate oxygenation, monitoring blood pressure, addressing hypotension, and treating the source of infection. Septic patients require aggressive initial and ongoing care. Be prepared for large volume fluid administration and for the administration of vasoactive agents like dopamine or levophed. Pay close attention to hemodynamic parameters and reassess them frequently.

SELECTED READINGS

Balk RA. Severe sepsis and septic shock. Definitions, epidemiology, and clinical manifestations. *Crit Care Clin.* 2000;16:179.

Dellinger RP, Carlet JM, Masur H, et al. Surviving sepsis campaign guidelines for management of severe sepsis and septic shock. *Crit Care Med.* 2004;32:858–873.

Dellinger RP, Levy MM, Carlet JM, et al. Surviving Sepsis Campaign: International guidelines for management of severe sepsis and septic shock: 2008. *Intensive Care Med.* 2008;34(1):17–60.

Hynes-Gay P, Lalla P, Leo M, et al. Understanding sepsis: From SIRS to septic shock. *Dynamics.* 2002;13(1):17–20.

90

DON'T FEAR THE PRESSOR!

SAM MATTA, RN, CEN, CCRN, NREMT-P

Vasopressors in the prehospital environment can be some of the most intimidating medications; however, they can also be some of the most useful. For example, early and aggressive initiation of vasopressor therapy can benefit septic patients who may be unresponsive to fluid boluses. It is common knowledge that a patient's blood pressure rises following vasopressor infusion. What is less clear is which vasopressors augment blood pressure most efficiently and minimize untoward side effects. This chapter furnishes the prehospital provider with an overview of some of the more commonly utilized vasoactive medications *(Table 90.1)*.

DOPAMINE

Dopamine is a widely used vasopressor both in prehospital and critical care medicine. The medication takes advantage of three distinct mechanisms of action. The drug's mechanism is directly related to the dose administered. At low doses (2 µg/kg/minute) dopamine binds to dopamine (D1 and D2) receptors and moderately increases renal blood flow. Dopamine promotes blood flow into coronary, renal, mesenteric, and cerebral vascular beds through localized vasodilatation. At intermediate doses (5 to 10 µg/kg/minute) dopamine promotes the release of norepinephrine. This results in increased cardiac contractility, chronotropy, and a hint of increased systemic vascular resistance. Finally, at higher doses, (10 to 20 µg/kg/minutes) the vasopressor properties of the medication dominate as a result of alpha-mediated vasoconstrictor effects.

NOREPINEPHRINE (LEVOPHED)

Norepinephrine is another widely used and highly selective vasoactive medication. The drug is a potent alpha agonist and has little effects on beta receptors. Norepinephrine's alpha agonism causes peripheral vasoconstriction. Though

TABLE 90.1	SELECTED VASOPRESSORS AND RECEPTORS		
	ALPHA (α)	BETA (β)	D1/D2
Dopamine (low dose)	+	+	+++
Dopamine (medium dose)	++	++	+++
Dopamine (high dose)	+++	+++	+++
Norepinephrine	++++	++	N/A
Epinephrine	++++	+++	N/A

predominantly an alpha receptor agonist, norepinephrine is a catecholamine and causes increases in heart rate and cardiac contractility. Norepinephrine may be beneficial in cases of severe septic shock or for patients with refractory hypotension. The dose range of the medication varies according to setting with the average dose being 4 to 30 μg/minute with doses as high as 100 μg/minute being required for some patients (0.01 to 3 μg/kg/minute). As with all vasoactive medications, norepinephrine should be administered through a large central vein. Invasive blood pressure monitoring is recommended for patients dependent upon vasopressors.

Epinephrine

Epinephrine is the "sledge hammer" of the vasopressor family. Where the other agents have an increased affinity for one receptor over another, epinephrine targets all receptors. Epinephrine has a strong affinity for alpha and beta receptors alike. As the infusion dose is increased, the alpha-1 (vasoconstrictor) effects of epinephrine predominate. Though related to norepinephrine, epinephrine is less alpha receptor selective. Epinephrine infusions cause increases in heart rate, contractility, and systemic vascular resistance. Indications for intravenous epinephrine infusion include refractory symptomatic bradycardia, anaphylactic shock, and septic shock unresponsive to crystalloid infusion. Epinephrine drips are started at 1 to 4 μg/minute.

Decisions, Decisions

So how do we decide which agent is right for our particular patient? In the world of critical care medicine, it is exceedingly difficult to come up with an answer that works for every patient encounter. Part of the answer to the question begins with identifying the cause resistant hypotension and shock. A patient in anaphylactic shock, for example, benefits from both bronchodilation and vasoconstriction. Epinephrine may be a wise choice given the drug's ability to act on beta-1 and beta-2 receptors. Furthermore, the drug's alpha receptor effects mitigate the widespread vasodilation that accompanies a profound allergic reaction. The first thing to remember with all vasopressor therapy is that the patient must have an adequate fluid volume status for vasopressors to be effective. In general, it is always wise to begin with filling the "tank" whenever possible. Septic patients lose significant amounts of fluid due to fever, high respiratory rate, and capillary leakage. Septic patients may require large volumes of isotonic crystalloid prior to the initiation of vasoactive agents. Patients in cardiogenic shock pose significant challenges to the selection of adequate "pressor" agents. A weakened heart is already irritable and may not respond well to agents that stimulate the sympathetic nervous system. Dopamine has the advantage of increasing inotropy and chronotropy via its effects on the beta-1 receptors.

Furthermore, its alpha agonist properties cause peripheral vasoconstriction which may be beneficial for the hypoperfused patient in cardiogenic shock. There is not one simple algorithm to assist the provider with making decisions about vasopressor administration. However, it is imperative that providers credentialed to use these agents remain familiar with their indications and mechanisms of action.

SUMMARY

In summary, there are several vasopressors available today, with the three mentioned in this chapter being among the most popular. There are only a few hard and fast rules when it comes to their use:

- Fill the tank! Septic patients may be extremely volume depleted. Their fluid deficit may be profound and vasopressors may be less effective if circulating volume is not restored.
- Understand the mechanisms! Dopamine, for example, may not produce a measurable increase in cardiac output until it is infused at doses of at least 5 to 10 µg/kg/minute. That drug, like epinephrine, acts on both beta and alpha receptors.
- Titrate adequately! Administration of vasopressors requires that the pre-hospital professional pay close attention to end-organ perfusion. Invasive blood pressure monitoring is preferred. Other markers of perfusion such as mental status and urine output are also important to track.

Finally, don't fear vasopressors, get to know them: They truly are some of the most effective medications we carry.

SELECTED READINGS

Marx JA, Hockberger RS, Wallls RM, Adams JG, Barsan WG, Biros MH, Danzel DF, Gaushe-Hill M, Ling LJ, Newton EJ, eds. *Rosen's Emergency Medicine Concepts and Clinical Practice.* 7th ed. Philadelphia, PA: Mosby Elsevier; 2010.

Overgaard CB, Dzavik V. Inotropes and vasopressors review of physiology and clinical use in cardiovascular disease [Supplemental material]. *Circulation.* 2008;118:1047–1056. Retrieved from circ.ahajournals.org/cgi/content/full/118/10/1047

Sanders MJ. *Mosby's Paramedic Textbook.* 3rd ed. St. Louis, MO: Elsevier; 2007.

91

AVOID BEING THE MODERN DAY CANARY: ENSURE SCENE SAFETY WHEN RESPONDING TO A MASS CASUALTY EVENT

FREDERICK W. SMITH, EMT-P

Years ago, before Incident Command Systems (ICS) were fully developed, many first responders followed the "Modern Day Canary" principle: Its simplicity was borrowed from the canary used by coal miners to identify dangerous levels of methane when working in the mines. If the canary died, it was assumed the mine wasn't safe. In the "Modern Day Canary" role, medical first responders gauged the safety of the disaster scene by watching the police officers who entered first. If the police officers did not become immediately ill, it was assumed safe for all EMS responders to enter. Of course, the police officers had a similar system and utilized the medical first responders as their canaries. Disaster response systems have evolved considerably beyond the use of canaries. The best emergency responders will remember the following key pearl:

- *Avoid entering a scene before responder safety has been secured and the response is coordinated. Failing to do so can jeopardize an entire response operation.*

To avoid mistaking scene safety and duplication of efforts, the capable first responder will undertake their response in coordination with the Emergency Operations Center (EOC) within the ICS. The EOC is the hub where all command and support staff assemble to coordinate the response. The EOC can be established anywhere identified by the Incident Commander to be a safe distance from the scene accounting for wind direction, elevation, and distance.

To avoid confusion at the start of an MCI, incident command structures, roles, and responsibilities are delineated for appropriate individuals to assume an active role in the response. The Incident Commander is the highest ranking official and the first person to begin filling the positions that form the command staff. Developed from "lessons learned" following the 2004 outbreak of Severe Acute Respiratory Syndrome (SARS) in Canada and the US. Gulf Coast hurricanes in 2005, pre-identifying four or even five candidates qualified to fill each command and general staff position will significantly aid your agency's ability to respond rapidly and appropriately during "off" hours or when the senior authority is unable to respond immediately. When disaster strikes, individuals chosen to fill command staff position assemble to form the "Incident Planning Team" which coordinates the Incident Commander's directives.

Members of the command staff who comprise the Planning Team are identified on an organizational chart. It is important to understand that an ICS is a management system, not an organizational chart. It is imperative that a prominently displayed organization chart be developed to limit inefficiency and duplication of efforts and resource assignment for your specific jurisdiction.

The National Incident Management System (NIMS), through "lessons learned" and best practice evidence stresses the importance of a strong ICS, and at times the need to develop a Unified Command between coordinating multi-jurisdictional agencies. EMS providers and their leaders must always remember that when planning for large scale mass casualty incidents that there will be multiple agencies responding, and each agency will have its own inherent command. Leadership from each agency must assemble to develop a Unified Command that allows different agencies to work together with one cohesive goal and purpose. This prevents or limits duplication of personnel assignments, resource allocation, media control, victim transport, and other essential elements required when dealing with any large scale incident.

The "lead" commander in a well organized Unified Command will be determined by the "type" of response incident. Unified Command should establish multiple staging areas in large scale incidents. This is a critical step in maintaining close personnel accountability as it provides areas where arriving personnel must check in with a Staging Officer. This record of staged personnel is frequently relayed to the EOC, and ensures that essential staff is available when Operations at the incident site requests additional personnel resources. Maintaining constant communication between the Labor Pool and the EOC allows Incident Command to request additional off duty resources or mutual aide before exhausting valuable essential responders. Transportation Officers maintain written records of all personnel who leave the incident and their destination (if transporting patients). This information is frequently reported to Incident Command. Personnel who "rotate out" of their initially assigned zone report to a rehabilitation area and are accounted for on their arrival. This information is frequently sent to the EOC so that no part of the organizational command and planning structure is void. When a replacement is determined for any role, the organizational chart is updated to reflect the changes. This is all part of a unified effort to maintain strict accountability of all assigned participants.

To avoid confusion it is imperative that when one is relieved from a position or assignment that the "oncoming" individual receives a face-to-face report from the "outgoing" person. Being sure that personnel formally check-in and check-out ensures that planning strategies are not compromised.

Finally, accountability of personnel is never limited to persons designated as command staff, but every EMS provider must be accountable for everything he or she does including the recording of the final destination of any victim they transport. An effective MCI planning team is one that accounts for all services, personnel, victims, equipment, and miscellaneous needs.

In closing, mass casualty events have the potential to easily become filled with confusion and disorganization. It is essential that every EMS responder regardless of agency or rank follow a formalized, pre-agreed upon, and coordinated MCI response plan.

SELECTED READING

The Federal Emergency Management Agency, www.fema.gov offers multiple free training opportunities in the National Incident Management System. Suggested courses include:

ICS-100 Introduction to Incident Command Systems
ICS-200 Basic Incident Command Systems
ICS-300 Intermediate Incident Command Systems
ICS-400 Advanced Incident Command Systems
and can be found at: FEMA Emergency Management Institute. 2011. 22 April 2011
http://www.training.fema.gov/IS/NIMS.asp

92

Prepare, prepackage, and pre-plan the disaster pack you need

Brian Froelke, MD, FACEP

A key mistake we frequently make in EMS is reflexively responding to a disaster after it strikes. In some ways, this is inevitable since we can't plan for every disaster. But there are areas we can do better. One such area is gear organization.

■ The responsible first responder will have a generic and pre-staged disaster pack with gear that is effectively used when responding to any disaster.

When preparing for a disaster there are several available lists that can help provide an outline of equipment for personal response. From wilderness medicine websites, Boy Scouts of America and the Red Cross, to Federal Emergency Management Agency (FEMA), the National Disaster Medical System (NDMS N-2060 Personal Gear for Deployments), and individual Disaster Medical Assistance Teams (DMATs), each list of recommendations has its own unique focus, and one should review several of these when preparing a disaster kit. The following are a list of experience-driven observations and recommendations.

Prepackage Equipment and Make It Easily Portable

No matter what the disaster, personal equipment should be packaged and prepared to be portable. Avoid large unwieldy bins and boxes. Use a two–bag system and be prepared to carry the equipment for long distances over unstable terrain, even if the plans are for home or office. Expect possible plane travel and adhere not only to personal physical limitations but also to Transportation Security Administration (TSA) regulations for weight and prohibited items. Plan the first bag as a carry-on bag and try to pack it with supplies that will last 24 hours. Plan the second as a checked bag. Use caution if purchasing wilderness or military surplus supplies as many contain matches, sharps, or gels that are prohibited for flight. Use lightweight and durable bags with backpack design and consider an optional roller attachment. Use plastic zip seal baggies to organize and provide some weather resistance for the contents. Two disposable plastic bottled waters will round off the list and can be emptied and refilled from tap water inside airport security to save a buck or two on essential drinkable resource. This is the most versatile all-hazards packing approach.

Prepare Basic Clothing for Three Days

Whether traveling to help in a disaster, or sheltering in place for a disaster close to home, anticipate any likely weather extremes. Dress in layers, especially two layers of socks that can wick water and reduce friction blisters. Weatherproof and comfortable boots are critical. Break them in and use them before they are needed. Do not keep them in a box on the shelf. Mechanic's gloves offer some protection while remaining nimble enough for finer activities. Choose clothing with plenty of pockets. A hat with a brim can offer some protection from the elements as can water resistant over-pants and a hooded sweatshirt.

MAKE SURE TO ALWAYS PACK A FEW CERTAIN ESSENTIALS

Pack a flashlight small enough to attach to a belt, and preferentially choose an LED battery for long battery life. Pack another flashlight headband for hands-free use. Bring a bicycle lock with cable. Find a multi-tool utility knife and remember to put it in your checked bag of supplies. A few yards of quarter-inch nylon cord and some duct tape will help with almost any makeshift project that will arise. Pack a few comfort items such as an inexpensive MP3 player or a deck of cards. Remember to bring nothing with you into a disaster that you are not willing to lose!

In conclusion, the most important pearl is simple: *The most important piece of your disaster preparedness pack is YOU. Disasters are hard on the body, so remain vigilant with a healthy lifestyle.* Avoid addictive habits, such as tobacco, for the objects of your addiction may not follow you into the disaster. Remain well hydrated and avoid over use of caffeinated products. Keep any chronic medical conditions well controlled and keep a couple of weeks' supply of essential medications. Avoid the prepackaged salty/sugary foods that can wreak havoc on conditions such as hypertension and diabetes. Instead, select energy bars and other simple pocketable foods. Try them out before having to depend on them, and rotate them through your daily lunches to keep them from getting stale. Due to the limited resources, the changing environment, and the surge of patient needs, prepare for difficult medical decisions, and the lack of routine. If you plan on using your professional expertise in disasters, be prepared to make some errors due to sleep deprivation and the long hours of strenuous work. Use a team approach and a preset system of response for professional disaster assistance, both for the mental health and for the logistical support, as well as the security that such a group can offer.

In summary, failure to pre-plan for a disaster can be disastrous, both for you and for those you are trying to assist. By following the advice provided above you have a much higher likelihood of providing expert and much-needed assistance to disaster victims.

SELECTED READINGS

The Federal Emergency Management Agency. www.fema.gov
Jaslow D. Operations and Logistics. In: Ciottone et al., eds. *Disaster Medicine*. Philadelphia: Mosby Elsevier; 2006:203–206.

93

DON'T FORGET THE SPECIAL POPULATIONS THAT REQUIRE SPECIAL RESPONSE

BRIAN FROELKE, MD, FACEP
HAWNWAN PHILIP MOY, MD

Pairing appropriate resources with the right patients and anticipating medical needs and staffing requirements are essential for running any medical system. One can group certain populations into a "special needs" category referring to patients such as pediatric or geriatric patients and those with psychiatric disease. These specific groups are anticipated to require greater resources to provide the standard level care.

■ In a disaster setting, these special populations will require special response capabilities that must be planned for in advance.

In disasters and mass casualty events, resources are limited. By planning for "special needs" patient preparedness around an all-hazards and resource availability model, one can obtain a more accurate and robust plan than preparing solely for more common patient categories. Some areas may also have facilities that deal with a significant number of patients with certain disabilities such as neuromuscular diseases or developmental abnormalities. Each of these relatedly unique populations will have very specific needs that are beyond the scope of this chapter. There are, however, several common potential events or disasters for which it's possible to preplan in order to assist the largest groups of "special needs" patients. EMS providers and services should always plan around likely resource gaps such as power loss, communication deficits, social support network collapse, and environmental hazards.

■ Once likely gaps are identified, create a list of patients who will have increased problems due to these gaps and you have successfully identified both your "special needs" and likely surge categories.

PLAN FOR THE LOSS OF ELECTRICAL POWER

Power loss will especially affect patients with susceptibility to environmental extremes such as the very young and very old. Children are more vulnerable in that they may deteriorate more quickly, may have fewer defenses against temperature variability (i.e., newborns), and may have different clinical presentations and treatment options than their adult counterparts. The elderly have even less physiologic reserve to tolerate any disturbance from their equilibrium as well as chronic diseases that require supportive care. If significant numbers of elderly are affected, this will likely create surges of patients who are dependent on oxygen, dialysis, and home ventilators. Hearing and visual impairment, while a hallmark of the aging process, can also stem from excessive noise and confusion from disasters or tympanic membrane damage from explosives. Brightly colored signs, LARGE BLOCK PRINT, and roped off areas can help both at-risk patients and unfamiliar staff navigate the complicated triage system.

DISRUPTION OF NORMAL ROUTINES AND CIRCADIAN RHYTHMS WILL FURTHER STRESS SURGE CAPABILITIES FOR PEDIATRIC, ELDERLY, AND PSYCHIATRIC POPULATIONS

The loss of routine and social support networks will likely affect children who may be without parents to pick them up. As a result, the pediatric population will require close psychiatric and parental counseling to aid in the understanding of events. Psychiatric patients may also have difficulty with the loss of routine. It is of paramount importance that this latter population receives early psychiatric support to prevent a mental breakdown that may cause harm to both the patient as well as others. The loss of routine and familiar surroundings may also exacerbate dementia or cause delirium in the elderly. Thus with all three of these special needs populations, close attention needs to be paid to their psychological status.

THE SPREAD OF INFECTIOUS DISEASE IS LIKELY TO COMPLICATE SHELTER AND MASS GATHERING CARE

As shelters are opened, those patients with infectious wounds or diarrheal diseases that are normally self-confined to their homes may be a risk for rapid disease spread. This is especially true in close quarter environments and may force providers to deal with end-of-life care in the elderly who may rapidly develop overwhelming infections. The uncertainty of each patient's wishes and the lack of family to provide a power of attorney can further complicate this issue. A familiarity of the state's protocol for which the decision should fall to should be reviewed before such issues were to arise. On-site family assistance and child care become essential not only for displaced victims but also for the families of the staff who may be working longer and unscheduled hours during an event.

LISTEN TO YOUR INTERNAL STOPLIGHT

From a system and resource utilization perspective, a "stoplight approach" can be used to build a robust personal and agency-wide situational awareness. Green designates "business as usual," yellow indicates a surge or particularly trying day, while red indicates an overwhelming or failing situation.

Know whether your personal level is green, yellow, or red. Be aware of your fellow colleagues' levels, and maintain a situational awareness by keeping apprised of one level in front and one level downstream from your place in the triage chain. No one should be operating in the red when someone else, or some other care area, is in the green.

In conclusion, when disasters occur, it is easy to get distracted by the emotional assault of disaster and tragedy. Subsequent organization using an all-hazards approach can aid in further organization and add a more robust plan than preparing solely for common "special needs patient" categories. In addition, foresight from a system and resource perspective may prevent one link in the triage chain from working in the red while others work in the green. Even though each disaster has its unique set of challenges, using these protocols can help initiate the most important aspect of dealing with disasters, preparation.

Selected Readings

Becker B. Children and disaster. In: Ciottone et al., eds. *Disaster Medicine*. Philadelphia: Mosby Elsevier; 2006:51–58.

Federal Emergency Management Agency. www.fema.gov

Halpern P, Larken G. Ethical issues in the provision of emergency medical care in multiple casualty incidents and disasters. In: Ciottone et al., eds. *Disaster Medicine*. Philadelphia: Mosby Elsevier; 2006:63–70.

Wimbush T, Courban C. Psychological impacts of disaster. In: Ciottone et al., eds. *Disaster Medicine*. Philadelphia: Mosby Elsevier; 2006:59–63.

94

FROM THE HOT ZONE TO HOSPITALS: TRANSPORT YOUR PATIENTS SAFELY AND EFFICIENTLY

FREDERICK W. SMITH, EMT-P

According to Murphy's Law, "If anything can go wrong, it will." It has even been said, "if you perceive that there are four possible ways in which something can go wrong, and circumvent these, then a fifth way, unprepared for, will promptly develop." When your disaster hits, Murphy's Law will be in full effect: There will be no warning, no perfect weather, no midday sun to illuminate the destruction. Regardless of the climate, personal schedules, or time of day, all disaster responses begin at incident onset and continue until all accounted victims have been transported from the scene. *Your job, as a first responder, is to help make order out of the chaos.*

It is important for responders arriving on the scene of an unknown incident to pay particular attention to their surroundings for any clues that might help identify the cause of the incident. EMS administrators should develop First Responder Arrival checklists to assist in identifying scene dangers, causes, and ongoing threats to other responders. These guides also help remind first responders that other agencies may need to respond (fire, law enforcement, mutual aid, etc.). Their assistance may be needed to maintain order, secure evidence, and assist in victim care and movement.

First responders entering a hot zone should have hazardous material training and wear appropriate personal protective equipment.

- Victims of chemical, biological, radiological incident who are brought to the appropriate victim staging area must already have been decontaminated. Carelessly allowing a contaminated victim to be placed into a transport vehicle jeopardizes the medical transport crew, contaminates the first receivers, and takes a much-needed response vehicle out of service until it can be thoroughly decontaminated.

Alternate transportation modes must be considered early in any event. The geographical location of the incident will determine the transportation assets immediately available. When developing response plans, consider your city's transportation infrastructure including air, sea, and rail. Other potential sources of transport include air ambulances, city buses, private ambulance services, and mutual aid medical services from surrounding counties.

First responders tasked with triage of victims must work rapidly, tagging and moving victims to staging areas for transport. Appropriately prioritizing victims from immediate, delayed, minor, and expectant/dead and placing them in the correct staging area will greatly facilitate victim transport from the scene to the most appropriate treatment facility. *Remember the golden hour begins when the injury occurred, not when you arrive on the scene.*

With any mass casualty incident, Incident Command may initiate a Medical Branch. A Medical Branch structure is designed to provide the Incident Commander with a basic, expandable system to manage a large number of patients during an incident. Under the guidance of the Medical Group Supervisor are the triage units, treatment units, patient transport units, and Ambulance Coordinators. These teams work independently yet report all actions to the Medical Group Supervisor. This Supervisor reports to the Medical Branch Director who in turn reports to the Operations Chief. The Operations Chief speaks directly to the Incident Commander. This structure allows for a manageable distribution of authority.

Within the Medical Branch, supervisors, leaders, and managers will assess victim injuries, coordinate transportation resource needs, and identify ambulance staging areas, helicopter landing zones, and even the alternative transport methods noted above (rail, sea, etc.). As victims begin arriving at appropriate staging areas, the Victim Transportation Unit leader working with the Ambulance Coordinator should begin requesting transportation resources.

At the onset of the incident's first operational period resources are likely to be minimal.

■ It is important to "size up" the incident and request additional resources early.

The Medical Branch Director must communicate these needs up the command chain to the Incident Commander as soon as possible. By staging transportation resources, the Transportation Leader and Medical Branch Director are able to maintain resource availability and a regularly updated needs list that allows for efficient patient transport. The Victim Transportation Unit Leader is responsible for the maintenance of records related to victim identification, condition, and transport destination. This information is frequently reported to the Medical Branch Director who reports it to the Incident Commander.

It is crucial that the medical branch director, operations chief, and liaison officer work together to ensure that receiving hospitals are capable of receiving and treating the victims. This will change often as hospital resources are rapidly utilized. You can expect that level 1 hospitals will become rapidly overwhelmed with victim surge; therefore, there should be thoughtful consideration to initially transporting noncritical victims to level 2 and level 3 medical facilities. Hospitals will communicate their availability to receive victims on the basis of their available beds, available surgeons, and resources.

If your city or county has an established committee of first receiver and first responder members, it is of tremendous benefit to your service to become an actively involved member. Pre-event communication and information sharing cannot be overstressed in importance. In developing your response plans consider the number of different emergency medical resources immediately available to you.

- It is important to remember that medically based 911 demands will continue to occur separately from the incident.

If your city has 50% to 60% of its 911 ambulances busy as a norm, then you must consider that at best you will only have 40% to 50% of your city medical response and transport resources immediately available. Having preplanned agreements and arrangements with private ambulance services and mutual aid agreements with surrounding counties are imperative to your success.

In closing, it is essential that every community and every EMS have a pre-established disaster response. Once victims have been triaged, a well thought out and executed transportation plan must be known to all EMS providers and area hospitals.

SELECTED READINGS

Emergency Management Institute Web site. http://www.training.fema.gov/IS/NIMS.asp. Accessed April 22, 2011.

Kellams CL. Homeland Security Field Guide: A Pocket Reference for WMD & Terrorism Response [book review]. *J Homel Secur Emerg Manag.* 2005;2(4):1–2.

Murphy's Laws site. http://www.murphys-laws.com/. Accessed April 26, 2011.

95

UNDERSTAND HOW YOUR PPE WORKS BEFORE THE BIG DAY

MICHAEL T. LOHMEIER, MD, EMT-T

Personal protective equipment (PPE) is a nebulous term that refers to all of the specialized equipment designed to protect the wearer from a wide variety of injuries. It generally involves specialized helmets, goggles, respiratory barriers, protective clothing, and footwear that can protect against blunt injury, electrical shock, splashes, airborne dangers, and infectious exposures. These pieces of equipment help shield the wearer from the hazards in an environment that are known or expected to be encountered. In the prehospital setting, the most common PPE encountered is the turnout clothing or, "bunker gear" used during firefighting activities and the specialized suits used in hazardous materials incidents. All EMS providers must also remember that PPE also includes the facemasks and nitrile gloves used during patient assessment.

- One of the most common mistakes we can make includes possessing large amounts of gear without a complete understanding of what the different levels of protection entail or how to don and doff PPE quickly and efficiently.

Turnout clothing generally consists of a helmet, jacket, trousers, and boots and is standardized by the National Fire Protection Association (NFPA). NFPA 1975 requires that the garments worn during firefighting activities be able to withstand temperatures of 500°F for 5 minutes without igniting, melting, or separating. NFPA 1971 requires that all turnout clothing consist of an outer shell, a thermal barrier, and a moisture barrier, which serve to protect the wearer from heat and steam injury as well as exposure to contaminated water. The addition of a self-contained breathing apparatus (SCBA) with positive pressure ventilation allows firefighters to enter structure fires that are likely to contain hazardous byproducts of combustion in order to complete their missions.

Hazardous materials gear is designed to protect the wearer from hazardous chemicals, biological agents, or radioactive materials. They serve as barriers against liquids, splashes, and gases and are classified into Levels A, B, C, or D based upon their degree of protection.

Level A suits are the highest level of protection and guard against liquids, vapors, airborne particulates, and gases. They consist of a fully encapsulated chemical entry suit with puncture resistant boots and chemical resistant gloves worn outside of the suit. A full-face piece SCBA worn inside the suit provides full respiratory protection.

Level B suits guard against liquids and splashes from a hazardous material. They consist of either a one- or two-piece hooded suit with puncture resistant boots and chemical resistant gloves worn outside of the suit. Respiratory protection is through a SCBA that may be worn outside of the suit and is therefore not protective against vapors or gases.

Level C suits provide the same splash and liquid protection as Level B but have a lower level of respiratory protection than the SCBA.

Level D protection includes clothing and footwear that guard against injury but do not protect against chemical or liquid exposure. Most of the "bunker gear" worn during firefighting activities is Level D. In addition, all of the body substance isolation protection worn on routine EMS calls is, in fact, a level of hazardous materials protection. Latex gloves, face shields, and masks all serve to protect the wearer from intentional or accidental exposure to potentially dangerous body substances.

- It is essential that every person on the team not only knows what is included for each level of protection but also knows how to properly don, use, and doff the equipment quickly and efficiently. Waiting for disaster to strike to practice with your gear puts you and your teammates at risk.

All of the levels of protection listed above are considerably heavier and more cumbersome than standard work clothes. Because of the limited air supply when using a SCBA, the awkward nature of the protective equipment, and the increased physical exertion, active time working an incident is generally limited to 15 to 20 minutes. Regular training exercises using the actual equipment that may be used during a "real-world" event will help familiarize personnel with the common problems that are encountered with its use and prevent confusion or potential injury during an actual incident.

The most important thing to consider when selecting the type of PPE for a scene is the highest-level hazards that are known or expected to be encountered so that the most appropriate level of PPE may be selected in advance. The first personnel responding to a scene should report all aspects they encounter, including placards on vehicles, scents noted, and wind direction. Situational awareness is key for an effective, appropriate response to any EMS scene. No provider should enter a hazardous environment alone, and everyone should always be diligently monitoring for unexpected or hidden dangers. *Before all else, personal and team safety should be every responder's primary concern.*

SELECTED READINGS

National Fire Protection Association Codes and Standards. http://www.nfpa.org/aboutthe-codes/list_of_codes_and_standards.asp. Accessed April 26, 2011.

U.S. Department of Labor, Occupational Safety and Health Administration. *Personal Protective Equipment.* http://www.osha.gov/SLTC/personalprotectiveequipment/. Accessed April 26, 2011.

U.S. Department of Transportation. *Emergency Response Guidebook: A Guidebook for First Responders During the Initial Phase of a Dangerous Goods/Hazardous Materials Transportation Incident.* Baton Rouge, LA: Claitor's Law Books and Publishing Division; 2008.

96

KNOW THE VALUE OF STAKEHOLDER COMMUNICATIONS

MARK D. LEVINE, MD
JACOB B. KEEPERMAN, MD

Previous chapters have noted the importance of pre-event communication among first response and public safety personnel. Beyond these communities, however, are the important stakeholders who are putting on the event. The importance of including these stakeholders in all aspects of planning cannot be understated. It is of vital importance to understand who these stakeholders are and what each of them would consider a successful event. The reasons for this can be summed up in a single pearl:

- Effective mass gathering security and medical response have to be integrated into the background of an event so as not to be intrusive and overbearing on the larger events of the day.

It is important to remember that although public safety is our primary interest, it is not the primary interest of the event sponsors. Our challenge in EMS is to effectively support a large event that allows the stakeholders to carry out their goals. The main sponsor of the event is usually the primary stakeholder. They will measure event success in various forms including the production of a high-quality event, monetary success, a happy public, a return invitation for the event, and/or positive media coverage. Thus, it is essential that EMS representatives be involved early and throughout the planning process. Competent committee members and open minds are also very important for a successful outcome.

The value of undertaking detailed study of similarly sized prior events cannot be overstated. Although it is impossible to forecast the future, the study of prior events may clue the team into issues that occurred in the past and possible suggestions for change. In addition, minor aspects should not be overlooked. Is the weather service involved for outdoor events? Who is going to collect garbage on site and how often? Are there special needs from a utilities standpoint (electrical outlets, extension cords, generators)? A collection of data from prior events will also help with the planning aspect of attendance records, injury patterns, and what specialized services might be needed. From an EMS standpoint, remember that staging is a very important consideration. The most important issues to be sure to address are: where and how are crews going to be staged; is a single first aid station adequate, or are multiple "first aid" stations required; will mobile EMS responders be involved; where will the ingress and egress for ambulances be located in both regular transport and mass casualty incidents (MCI) situations; and will all of the supplies be easily available?

Communications are vital in any EMS activity and are of paramount importance whenever supporting a mass gathering. Decisions must be carefully made concerning where the command posts are going to be located and how they will communicate with each other. Radios must all be on shared frequencies, and if cell phones are going to be used, everyone needs to have the available numbers. The lead stakeholder should have someone available to be the liaison between fire, police, EMS, and city planners. If they do not, your job as a first responder is to offer them that suggestion. Before any meetings it is essential to know if there are any issues that have to be kept confidential or only discussed with the senior leaders of the agencies involved. From a public safety standpoint, separate communication channels may have to be in place to not interfere with the daily running of the locale.

The media is an important aspect of communication, as that is their primary role within society. The media can be used for sending out important information to the community in the event of unforeseen issues or hazards. Social media is a growing method of online communication and may also be used within the confines of planning groups for discussion and immediate group-wise notifications.

The important stakeholders should also have a command and communication structure within the top echelon. Everyone should know their responsibilities and limitations in this command structure. If there is an unsafe situation, the incident commander may need to overrule the corporate stakeholder if public safety is involved. This decision must be discussed and agreed upon before an actual event occurs.

Finally, redundancy needs to be built into planning with special concern given to the potential for breakdown in communications. Situations that must be addressed include response to problems with the internet or a breakdown in radio communications. EMS providers and leaders must have a plan to deal with cell phone failure should a cell tower stop working or there is a reception problem. How the necessary parties discuss and solve issues must also have a backup plan.

These issues are all important to discuss with the primary stakeholders. These should be discussed during planning meetings prior to the events. Timetables should be laid out, important members of the community should be invited, and their input should be taken seriously. A tabletop exercise should be put together and, if possible, should be observed by a neutral outsider. Conflicts should be resolved early and consensus should be reached if not actual decisions. Easy-to-read information should be handed out early leaving plenty of time for correction. A worst-case play-by-play manual may be put together and should be in every command area. Phone numbers, and other contact information, should be given out and tested beforehand, so all necessary parties will know who to contact and what chain of command they should follow.

In summary, it is vital that information be shared in a transparent manner as possible with the end goal being a successful event for all parties, with the least amount of inconvenience, damages, injuries occurring, allowing everyone to enjoy the planned event.

SELECTED READINGS

Ennis-Holcome, K. Disaster communications. In: Ciottone et al., eds. *Disaster Medicine*. Philadelphia: Mosby Elsevier; 2006:229–230.

The Federal Emergency Management Agency. www.fema.gov

Noltkamper D. Media relations. In: Ciottone et al., eds. *Disaster Medicine*. Philadelphia: Mosby Elsevier; 2006:232–237.

97

KNOW THE PRINCIPLES OF DISASTER MANAGEMENT BEFORE AN EVENT OCCURS

MARIO LUIS RAMIREZ, MD, MPP*

One of the biggest mistakes we can make in prehospital medicine is being unfamiliar with the principles of disaster management before an event occurs. A key strategic mistake made all too often is failing to preplan and just waiting for a disaster to strike. The job of the first responder and paramedic is to be one of the very first safety officials on scene. By understanding the role of the medic in the incident management and command systems, the ability to provide high quality life saving care for injured victims can be improved dramatically.

Planning for incident management has come a long way since officials first began developing a systematic approach in the 1970s. Currently, the Federal Emergency Management Agency (FEMA) is responsible for developing and updating the guidelines known as the National Incident Management System (NIMS). By using the term "system" to describe NIMS, FEMA has attempted to create a scheme that meets two goals: Flexibility and standardization. Essentially, the concept is that NIMS is an "approach" to incident management, rather than a set of actual instructions that are automatically applied to every disaster no matter how large or small. This approach uses a set of guidelines and creates roles through a construct named the Incident Command System (ICS) to manage disasters. Once the ICS is instituted, a specific set of predefined job assignments and titles is used to manage the response.

To avoid making many of the common mistakes during a disaster, the most important points for the medic to be aware of are the following:

- When an event occurs that overwhelms an agency's response capabilities, the medic should expect that the ICS will be utilized and will guide the response.
- Since all agencies will be using the NIMS and ICS approach, different organizations should now be able to integrate their responses using the same terms and definitions.

One error to avoid is not being familiar with the chain of command in the ICS structure. "Incident Command" is the overall incident coordinator.

---

*The following statements represent the views of the author and not necessarily the view of the Department of Defense or its respective components.

It may be a single person or a group of representatives working under the title "Unified Command." This Commander has the responsibility for preparing the action plan to respond to the incident. Under this Command position, there are also four functional areas: Operations, planning, logistics, and finance/administration. The Incident Commander may also choose to establish additional command staff as they see fit. Within each functional area are separate functions known as Emergency Support Functions (ESFs):

- Transportation
- Communications
- Public works and engineering
- Firefighting
- Emergency management
- Mass care, housing, and human services
- Public health and medical services
- Urban search and rescue
- Oil and hazard materials response
- Agriculture and natural resources
- Energy
- Public safety and security
- Longer community recover and mitigation
- External communications

It is important to understand that regardless the size of the incident, when the ICS/NIMS construct is being used, the response is being coordinated across these areas. If the incident is small scale, one or two persons may be able to assume multiple responsibilities and direct the entire incident. But, if the incident is of larger scale, there may be only one person in charge or each functional area which creates a large command hierarchy.

In your jurisdiction, there should be continuing, ongoing preplanning about creating the ICS if it becomes necessary. If you are unfamiliar with these plans, a responsible medic should contact their supervisors to understand how the system will work in your community. There may be community specific provisions about where EMS control will be in the incident command hierarchy, and by understanding the provisions before an event strikes, the medic will be able to understand their chain of command structure during the response. Failing to do so, however, can lead to role confusion and poor communication that has been shown to inhibit response capabilities and could lead to poor patient outcomes.

Paramedics and first responders have some of the most difficult jobs in a disaster: They must provide quality care and comfort in austere conditions. By understanding the ICS and NIMS constructs above, and undertaking some pre-event planning and study of their community's response plans, the medic can achieve these goals with greater success.

SELECTED READINGS

FEMA Emergency Management Institute. 2011. 6 March 2011 http://www.training.fema. gov/IS/.

FEMA National Preparedness Directorate. 2011. 6 March 2011 http://www.training.fema. gov/.

NIMS Resource Center. 2011. 6 March 2011 http://www.fema.gov/emergency/nims/index. shtm.

98

KNOW HOW TO INTERACT WITH THE MEDIA

GREGG TAGGARD, EMT-PARAMEDIC

Large-scale panic and confusion among the public often follow large-scale disasters. The flow of reliable information following a mass casualty incident is of utmost importance in mitigating this problem.

- *The release of accurate information after a disaster, delivered in a timely manner from a reliable source, is paramount in ensuring successful response and recovery efforts.*

This is the role of a Public Information Officer (PIO). Most, if not all, public safety or response agencies have a designated PIO. If your agency does not have a dedicated PIO, or they are unavailable, the duties of the PIO are usually assumed by the Incident Commander or Deputy Commander.

The PIO is defined as "a member of the Command Staff responsible for interfacing with the public and media or with other agencies with incident-related information requirements" according to the Incident Command System (ICS). The PIO reports directly to the Incident Commander in the ICS chain of command. If multiple agencies are involved in the incident response recovery and each is represented by a PIO, it may become necessary to appoint a lead PIO.

"But where do these public information officers get their training?" The National Information Officers Association (NIOA) conducts an annual conference hosting both basic and advanced PIO courses. The Federal Emergency Management Agency (FEMA) has several online courses as well. Training may also be conducted by in-house personnel (a dedicated news/public affairs department) and/or in conjunction with local media. The latter is usually the most effective tool of all as it typically combines lecture with practical exercises (taped video/audio interviews followed by feedback from faculty and peers).

- *It is important to realize that if you do not hold the PIO position, your job is to refer the media and others to the designated PIO. Doing so is vital to maintaining a unified and coherent message for the public.*

Once on site the PIO begins to develop the information needed for the initial press release. Before building a release, the PIO needs to determine from the Incident Commander if there are any limits on what information can be shared with the public. Once the limits, if any, have been established the PIO then starts gathering some initial information. This should include:

Incident type, area affected, responding agencies, and status of the response efforts. Remember, all information gathered must be first verified, and then approved by the Incident Commander prior to release.

There are several ways that information can be released. Traditionally, information is released through media sources including radio, television, and newsprint. A PIO will usually have pre-established contacts and methods of submitting the information to the media. Alternative sources for release can include social media (Facebook, Twitter, blogs, etc.), text messages, or even a dedicated website (usually only established for events requiring long-term response and recovery efforts). Information can also be released using the Emergency Action System (EAS, formerly known as the Emergency Broadcast System [EBS]) and amateur radio operators using Amateur Radio Emergency Service (ARES). Once the information has been shared with the media, the PIO will then monitor the release to ensure both accuracy and timely delivery.

Often times, the media will request direct access to the incident site and/or personnel for interviews. Approval for this access must come from the Incident Commander through the PIO.

■ *Again, it should be stressed that if you are approached by a member of the media or any individual not part of the response effort, always refer them to your* **PIO** *or Incident Commander if they are asking questions about you, your work, or the incident in general.*

Following a disaster, the Incident Commander or PIO may ask you to give an interview. Don't be afraid to participate. One of the greatest tools in ensuring the transparency and understanding of the response/recovery effort is through interviews with the responders. Should you accept the request, your PIO will brief you before the interview begins on what information may or may not be shared during the interview. The PIO will also be present to monitor the interview and help you with any questions you may not have been prepared for.

The keys to a successful interview include these things:

1) Be sympathetic—having a friendly and understanding responder instills public confidence.
2) Avoid technical jargon—plain language works best.
3) Don't guess or fake an answer—if you don't know, tell them you'll find the answer and respond to the question later.
4) Keep your answers short and simple (great for "sound bites").

On occasion, a media team may also become embedded with you as part of the interview process. Again, your PIO or Incident Commander will brief you ahead of time before this occurs. Any photography or videography obtained during this time will be reviewed and approved prior to use by the media team.

In summary, it is important to remember that the media plays a key part in any unfolding disaster. Do not make the mistake of providing off the cuff responses, and be sure to refer them to the PIO for official statements. If you are asked to address the media, do so honestly and sincerely with fewer words rather than more. If asked a question for which you cannot adequately answer, let the questioner know that you do not yet have that information.

SELECTED READINGS

Amateur Radio Emergency Services 26 April 2011 http://www.ares.org/.

FEMA Public Information website. 26 April 2011 http://www.fema.gov/emergency/nims/PublicInformation.shtm.

The Federal Emergency Management Agency, www.fema.gov offers multiple free training opportunities in the National Incident Management System. Suggested courses include:
G-290: Basic Public Information Officers course
E-388: Advanced Public Information Officer
IS-702: National Incident Management Systems, Public Information Systems
and can be found at: FEMA Emergency Management Institute. 2011. 22 April 2011 http://www.training.fema.gov/IS/NIMS.asp.

National Information Officer Association 26 April 2011 http://www.nioa.org/site/.

99

Ensure optimal communication between all parties

Jacob B. Keeperman

When planning for the medical aspects of a mass gathering event, communication between all those involved is not only essential, but also a frequently neglected aspect of good pre-event planning. The key pearls are simple:

- *Effective communication must occur between all stakeholders far in advance of the event.*
- *Effective communication must include ensuring that a cohesive and resilient contingency strategy has been developed.*

There are some key lessons that should guide mass gathering event planning. *Pre-event information collection needs to start with establishing some basic data about the event.*

This includes the type of event (i.e., rock concert, sporting event, symphony, presidential visit, papal visit, marathon, etc.), the venue for the event (stadium, school, motor speedway, street, etc.), the expected crowd size for the event (thousands to hundreds of thousands), the expected demographics of the crowd (young and healthy people who may use too much alcohol/illicit, highly educated young adults, special needs spectators or event participants, children, elderly, etc.), and anticipated weather (cold/ice/snow, hot/humid, etc.). Once these variables are known, organizers can start to make predictions about the potential medical needs and develop plans for the provision of medical care. The medical care provided at mass gathering events requires coordination amongst several entities, from those within the event and those external to the event.

Information sharing is essential to ensure that all entities are operating in concert with one another as opposed to working against one another.

Event management must be kept informed of all medically related planning, and they must also provide access to all information potentially needed by those providing the medical care. It is the medical team's responsibility to get buy-in from the event leadership (including sponsors, organizers, management, etc.), and this can be facilitated by providing regular updates and offering a free flow of information.

It is imperative that a pre-event jurisdiction agreement is in place before the event occurs.

Local EMS agencies must be informed of the event medical plans and included in the planning for which patients will be treated by the internal medical teams and which will require assistance from external EMS. A frequent mistake is failing to establish pre-event agreements that outline where different EMS agency's jurisdictions begin and end. At many events the internal medical teams are responsible for anything on the immediate venue grounds (stadium, concert hall, etc.), but local EMS is responsible for all areas outside of the event structure (parking lots, surrounding streets, etc.). Failing to plan for such contingencies is frequently a weakness in mass gathering medical response and can put providers in very difficult situations.

The public safety answering point (PSAP), better known as 911, should also be informed of the medical plans for all events. With the proliferation of cellular telephones, PSAPs are often notified by people dialing 911 about potential emergencies inside of event venues. The PSAPs must have a way to notify the event communications/command team so that internal medical teams can respond to emergencies. Similarly, the event medical staff must have a way to let the PSAP know when to dispatch outside resources.

Area hospitals and emergency departments should be included in the event planning, and should be kept informed of the medical protocols for patients coming from the event.

Open communication about which patients will be transported to hospitals needs to be established prior to the event. Event organizers must have pre-identified which facility should receive certain patient populations (i.e., trauma, pediatric, burn, STEMI, OB). Public health agencies may also need to be included in event planning including plans for surveillance of potential public health emergencies such as food-borne sickness. The local emergency management agency must be included in planning for the event and comprehensive plans should be made for potential mass casualty incidents (MCIs). This may include involving local Disaster Medical Assistance Teams (DMAT) and others involved in providing MCI care.

Those involved with security at the event have to be intimately involved in the planning of medical services.

Medical personnel require access to all areas of the venue in which they are required to provide medical care. Credentials must clearly delineate each individual's role, but also ensure them access to all areas. The security staff will also serve as the eyes and ears of the medical staff and are often the ones who notify the medical team of potential emergency situations.

In conclusion, event communication is a complicated task with multiple aspects that can be easily overlooked. Remember to give it thoughtful consideration and constantly revisit your communication plan to minimize the potential for any errors.

SELECTED READINGS

Ennis-Holcome K. Disaster communications. In: Ciottone et al., eds. *Disaster Medicine*. Philadelphia: Mosby Elsevier; 2006:229–230.

The Federal Emergency Management Agency. www.fema.gov

Noltkamper D. Media relations. In: Ciottone et al., eds. *Disaster Medicine*. Philadelphia: Mosby Elsevier; 2006:232–237.

100

USE AN APPROPRIATE TRIAGE SYSTEM TO GUIDE DECISION MAKING IN THE MASS CASUALTY SETTING

MICHAEL T. LOHMEIER, MD, EMT-T

When most people think of a mass casualty incident (MCI), they think of hundreds or thousands of people who have been critically or fatally injured at once. This is however not the case at all.

■ *Any situation where emergency medical resources are overwhelmed by the number, or severity, of injuries is termed a "mass casualty incident."*

A MCI may occur whenever there is a shortage of available responding personnel or when there is a lack of essential equipment; regardless, the common thread is that resources are overwhelmed. In these situations, it is essential that responding medical personnel do their best to triage, or sort, the casualties so as to offer the greatest amount of assistance to the largest number of victims possible.

As difficult as it may be, triage does not afford the time to stop and provide prolonged interventions for each individual person.

■ *The purpose of triage is to rapidly assess the patient's condition, determine the urgency of the patient's injuries, and to assign a treatment priority.*

If there are more victims than there are rescuers, all victims must be triaged before the person or team performing the initial assessments may begin providing prolonged care for any patient.

The most widely used system of sorting in the United States is the Simple Triage and Rapid Treatment (START) system, which divides patients into four categories based on the severity of their injuries. This system is preferred not only for its simplicity, but also for the fact that the cards need not necessarily be present on the scene to begin triage. This system quickly assesses the breathing, circulation, and level of consciousness for victims on scene, and then assigns them to one of the four color-coded groups based on severity; green, yellow, red, or black. Here is a brief review:

First and most importantly, call for additional resources. If you are first on scene, you must ensure that additional support is on the way. Next, call out to the victims present and begin issuing color-coded tags. Those with minor wounds who are able to follow commands and self-extricate to a treatment area are given a green tag, and are the second-lowest treatment priority. When many sick and injured await you, do not make the mistake of spending time doing any additional examination of patients who can walk and do not appear to have obvious serious injuries, Red tag victims are those with treatable but life-threatening injuries such as: Uncontrolled bleeding, airway or breathing problems, altered mental status, and shock or severe burns. Yellow tag victims are those with serious but not life-threatening injuries, such as burns without airway involvement, and major bone or multiple joint injuries. Black tag victims are those who are dead or non-salvageable due to the extent of their injuries or anticipated need for extensive rescuer involvement. Examples of these victims are those with exposed brain matter, victims in cardiac arrest for more than 20 minutes (except hypothermia or cold water drowning), and victims who have been decapitated or incinerated.

While moving through the scene and identifying patients, individuals may perform several basic maneuvers during their assessment to assist with severity assignment. For each patient encountered, follow these simple steps in evaluation:

1) Check the airway. If the airway is not open, perform a simple jaw thrust to open it. If the victim begins to breathe on their own, move on to the next step in evaluation.

2) Check the victim's level of responsiveness. If they are unresponsive, check for breathing and a pulse. If they have neither, they receive a black tag and you should not provide any further care for this patient. Move on to the next victim.

3) Check the victim for a pulse. If they have a pulse, quickly assess for large or exsanguinating bleeding. If there is a large amount of bleeding present, apply a pressure dressing and move on to the next patient.

Finally, scene size up and responder safety should be carefully monitored by all rescuers involved. If the scene has the potential to become dangerous, patients should be moved to a safe location regardless of their injuries.

Depending on the size and complexity of the incident, consideration should also be given to establishing a temporary treatment facility as well as an on-site morgue for victims pending transport to definitive locations. Interim treatment facilities are generally chosen based on their size and capacity to safely house large numbers of people. In general, pre-existing buildings such as gymnasiums and recreation centers are preferable because they usually have electricity, running water, and provide a safe and secure shelter. These locations may also allow for temporizing treatments to be initiated until patients can be transported safely to a hospital, or even for definitive care and discharge from the scene.

In summary, triage requires EMS providers to rapidly move from patient to patient without providing definitive care to each. When triaging, EMS providers must avoid the impulse to "just get to work saving lives." If you do not take time to call for help and then begin rapid assessment of all patients, more, not less will suffer or die.

Selected Readings

American College of Surgeons. *Resources for the Optimal Care of the Injured Patient: 2006.* Chicago, IL: American College of Surgeons; 2006.

Burstein JL, Hogan D. *Disaster Medicine.* Philadelphia, PA: Wolters Kluwer Health/Lippincott Williams & Wilkins; 2007.

Centers for Disease Control and Prevention. Guidelines for Field Triage of Injured Patients: Recommendations of the National Expert Panel of Field Triage. April 26, 2011. http://www.cdc.gov/mmwr/preview/mmwrhtml/rr5801a1.htm.

The JumpSTART Pediatric MCI Triage Tool. April 26, 2011. http://jumpstarttriage.com/.

START Triage. April 26, 2011. http://www.start-triage.com/.

CUSTOMER SERVICE/MEDICOLEGAL

101

NEVER FORGET: EMS IS MOSTLY ABOUT GREAT CUSTOMER SERVICE!

KEVIN G. SEAMAN, MD, FACEP

Think back to when you decided to go into EMS. Were you motivated by the possibility of being able to help others? A large number of EMS providers, as well as medical directors, attribute their decision to select health care to the value of wanting to help others. EMS providers do a tremendous job, at times under the most difficult circumstances. What experience in EMS teaches is that the opportunities to truly save a life are few and far between. And in the larger group of patients, in whom saving their life is not in the cards, there are a number of challenges.

As providers, we all have one or more specific complaints that "push our buttons"—the alcoholic, the frequent flier, the chronic pain patient are some examples. Perhaps a number of years have intervened and the enthusiasm born of the desire to help others may have waned. In times like this a renewed focus on customer service can help the majority of your patients and provide a renewed sense of job satisfaction. Let's focus on an old medical saying; starting here can provide a good perspective as well as a dose of humility.

Medical maxim—10% of patients get better because of what you do, 10% get worse no matter what you do and 80% get better on their own.

Interpreting this saying closely matches the EMS patient care experience—it's rare to save a life. On the other hand, some patients get worse no matter what you do. The important lesson is that most patients get better on their own, not because of the medical (or prehospital) care provided. Two important points: First, be humble because our efforts don't save lives very frequently and, more importantly, for the 80% that get better on their own, it's how you treat them that they will remember. Patients and their families may never have met you before and their interaction with you typically lasts less than 30 minutes; their perception of the care is formed far more from the empathy and personal care we provide than from the actual medical treatment. So, to get rave reviews from patients and their families act as a patient advocate. This powerful technique can be applied to all patients, comforting them and making their family confident that you are caring competently for their loved one.

Five tips to attain great customer service and avoid complaints

Always Advocate for the Patient

Following first patient contact, what is your approach? Is the patient always the top priority? Though we try our best to avoid it, we sometimes place greater importance on ourselves than our patient. Instead, ask yourself: Have I considered the "worst case" cause of these symptoms, worked it up properly and recommended transport and ED evaluation? Inadequate assessment and treatment, delay in patient transport, and provider initiated refusal to transport patients are commonly associated with EMS-related litigation.

Practice the Golden Rule

Treat patients as you want to be treated, or as you'd want your family to be treated. As health care workers, everything we do is under constant scrutiny. Everyone is listening to what we say and how we say it and watching our every move. In a sense, our behavior is "on stage" for all to see. Our patients are often under tremendous stress, may be in pain, or sleep deprived, causing them to react inappropriately. We must be keenly aware of the patient's needs and modify our own actions to put them at ease and de-escalate the situation. When faced with a difficult patient encounter, ask yourself this: "If this were my family member, how would I want them to be treated?" Remember to consider the family's needs as well as the patient's. If at the end of the call the family and patient feel as if they were treated with kindness and respect, you will be golden!

Be a Role Model for Your Peers

Individual actions impact all of those around us. Actions speak louder than words! Think about who's watching and emulating your every move. Would your actions pass the front-page-of-the-newspaper test? Take this one step further and try to model caring, patient-centered behavior for your co-workers, especially students.

Avoid Provider Initiated Patient Refusals

Patient refusals constitute one of the highest risk complaints in prehospital care. We are far better off transporting the patient than leaving them on the scene. In some cases, the patient persists in refusing transport. In these cases, there is plenty of risk to go around. Be generous and share it! First involve the family in the discussion. Advocate for treatment and transport and ask a family member (whose opinion the patient seems to trust) to do the same. If this doesn't work, consider a consult with the base station physician. This allows a summary of the important facts of the refusal and the second opinion provided by the consult physician can, at times, influence the patient to accept transport. By doing all of these steps, and documenting them accurately, you will have done the best you could. In every refusal-related encounter, be sure your documentation accurately and completely reflects the circumstances on-scene.

SEAMLESSLY TRANSITION FROM DOING EVERYTHING FOR THE CARDIAC ARREST VICTIM TO CONSOLING THE FAMILY WHEN CARE IS FUTILE

Calling 911 elicits our response much like hitting a patellar tendon produces a predictable knee reflex. As EMS providers, we are well practiced at maximal resuscitation in cardiac arrest. In addition, we also recognize when the patient has not responded to our maximal efforts. We have had less (if any) training in counseling the family when a loved one dies. If the patient does not respond to adequate BLS and ALS resuscitation efforts, our attention should turn to the survivors. EMS educators and Medical Directors need to develop more training for prehospital providers on how to provide support to families in circumstances where they have lost a loved one.

SELECTED READINGS

Jazwiec, Liz. *Eat That Cookie.* Gulf Breeze, FL; Fire Starter Publishing, 2009.

Morgan DL, Wainscott MP, Knowles HC. Emergency Medical Services Liability in the United States: 1987 to 1992. *Prehosp Disaster Med* 1994;9(4):214–220.

102

Don't forget to keep an open mind with each new call

Roger M. Stone, MD, MS

Although generally very skilled, EMS providers both develop skills and use experience that enhances their future performance. That very same practice experience can be a double-edged sword. How many times has the station discussion involved speaking of the "BS" calls they run daily? Depending on multiple factors, human and otherwise, a given provider may be lulled into a false sense of security or complacency about the encounter in real time or in advance. This is the classic potential customer relations mishap caused by letting one's guard down.

Patient Populations at Risk of a Vigilance Lapse

Classic areas of potential conflict occur in similar patient populations that may often fool the emergency physician and the emergency medical technician alike:

- **Inebriates:** The consumption of alcohol not only hampers the judgment of patients with respect of refusing care, but is fraught with occult (hidden) pathology or diagnoses. In addition, these patients often have very concerned—but under-resourced—family members who maximize efforts to advocate for their loved one before a 911 call represents a crisis they cannot handle. On EMS arrival, the last frustration expected by family is one coming from their dealings with the crew.
- **Inmates:** This population represents a heterogeneous group of patients that are tempting for some to dismiss, both for skepticism associated with criminal culture and perhaps our own personal biases. Inmates however also have tricky occult conditions, and even do not divulge traumatic mechanisms, leaving them with similar medical needs as any other sick patient. Avoidance of bias is difficult, and it is imperative for providers to conduct a thorough patient history and examination.
- **Psychiatric** patients may have by definition a condition challenging their interaction with the environment around them; that fact makes differentiating between functional and organic illness very difficult to impossible in a single EMS encounter. Moreover, advocates for mental health are frequently present as the internal customers for allied health care providers. Consider the observations of mental health professionals

(social workers, case workers, caretakers) throughout the processes of patient assessment, treatment, and transport.

■ **Frequent flyers:** Patients who rely on EMS more than average, many not close to being amongst the true 911 system abusers, will often have multiple episodes yearly of a non–life-threatening condition; the possibility of an exacerbation of truly critical illness still exists. It is usually more effective to deal with the challenging issues of system misuse when not actively engaged in incident response. Discussing these patients with a departmental quality assurance or community outreach officer helps reduce distraction and ensures adequate follow up of concerns.

CUSTOMER RELATIONS PRINCIPLES: AVOID THE PITFALLS OF A CLOSED MIND

Firstly, failure to keep a general open mind with each new call is the set-up for occasional but recurrent customer relations disasters. All events have a risk of their own. Specifically, the common sub-theme is judging the validity of a new call based upon previous EMS utilization, when in fact the "not so frequent flyer" may still be sick. Next, failing to mitigate judgmental tones in the presence of family or advocates jeopardizes subsequent trust and encourages confrontation. In fact, EMS crews should look to all persons as resources for extenuating history and coax the patient to cooperate and submit to care. Enlisting patient family members as allies helps alleviate tensions during a difficult patient encounter.

In a related twist on a theme, allowing less relevant issues to play a role in the medical assessment, such as lamenting the time of a call, pre-judging a neighborhood, or even getting caught up in a patient's sub-optimal personality serves as a "trap" for well-intentioned providers. Deploying a "distraction filter" is a way to ensure that the focus of any response remains on the delivery of excellent, high-quality patient care.

Underestimating the severity of a complaint by or about an inebriate or chalking any mental status change as being due to drinking, as well as dismissing the incarcerated patient or arrestee because of any of the above lapses have similar risks as Russian roulette applied to EMS. The resultant bullet in the chamber equates to a complaint against providers. Chalking up all symptoms of a mental patient to a psychiatric process, cutting corners in the physical assessment of a psychiatric patient, or dismissal of symptoms given by advocates is frustrating at best, or offensive at worst. Keep in mind the sensitivity associated with mental illness: It becomes painful or infuriating for patients when somatic complaints are automatically brushed off as being "all in your head." The medic who is sucked into this stereotype should be warned that the failure is not only a customer service failure, but might represent a huge medical error. The opposite strategy, one of additional empathy and insight, is the guiding principle for the short time EMS has to be engaged with patients.

Clearly, the reality of our every day practice in EMS mirrors that of the emergency physician and nurse. It is well known in the risk management and error literature that the types of patients or situations addressed in this chapter pose a huge challenge to our vigilance and need for rapid assessments and decisions. The avoidance of problems is predicated upon maintaining excellent communication skills and exercising sound clinical judgment. The pitfalls of succumbing to a weakened sense of readiness are self-evident, and part of the solution starts with an open mind on every call.

Selected Readings

Bigham BL, Buick JE, Brooks SC, et al. Patient safety in emergency medical services: A systematic review of the literature. *Prehosp Emerg Care.* 2012;16(1):20–35.
Colwell CB, Pons PT, Pi R. Complaints against an EMS system. *J Emerg Med.* 2003;25(4): 403–408.
Doering GT. Customer care. Patient satisfaction in the prehospital setting. *Emerg Med Serv.* 1998;27(9):71–74.
Ludwig G. Up at night? An EMS manager's concerns, from safety to politics. *JEMS.* 2011; 36(8):24.
Persee DE, Jarvis JL, Corpening J, et al. Customer satisfaction in a large urban fire department emergency medical services system. *Acad Emerg Med.* 2004;11(1):106–110.

103

DON'T FAIL TO MANAGE THE DIFFICULT, BUT STILL MANAGEABLE CONSUMER

ROGER M. STONE, MD, MS

Earlier in the section and elsewhere in this text, we spoke of the concept of patients and their advocates utilizing our services as customers. Using the analogy of any organization providing services or selling goods, there are always those more difficult to satisfy, or with lower thresholds to be critical of our efforts. By the same token, good agencies train a workforce that makes dealing with these customers a part of their skill set. Although we would all agree that extremely rude, abusive, or violent behaviors by patients towards EMS is completely intolerable and our safety is paramount, the majority of "difficult" patients are still manageable using our best human relation skills.

TYPES OF DIFFICULT CUSTOMERS

Common situations serve to exemplify difficult encounters. Accordingly, certain patients can exhibit frustrating behavior. The following scenarios may result in challenging encounters for EMS personnel:

1) Providers greeted with initial hostility from callers/patients
2) Being immediately questioned about "why it took you so long to arrive"
3) Having actions questioned or critiqued in the setting of what a previous provider did for the patient, or being berated by a layperson's expectations of what care should be given
4) The immediate or unreasonable demand to be transported to a more remote ED or facility
5) The patient calling for an ambulance with a very benign medical concern, or malingerer
6) The patient with sub-acute complaint waiting until overnight shift to call for help; this occurrence, however frustrating to EMS, might be viewed differently from a patient's perspective.
7) A patient selectively refusing parts of our proposed therapy we think are important
8) A patient posturing to refuse transportation even with a life-threatening condition
9) A patient who is a very poor historian and lives alone, with either sporadic or overbearing family support
10) An out of town advocate or family member making requests from a remote location that differ from a patient's desires or refusal of care (usually the elderly or family conflict)

Customer Relations: Common Pitfalls in Managing Difficult Patients

In the face of starting on the wrong foot with a patient, losing our cool is not a viable option in salvaging the recovery of the call. It is a relative failure to not de-escalate tensions in the early stages. Meeting belligerence with more belligerence only accomplishes the opposite; unless the degree of hostility by the customer amounts to an unmanageable or unsafe situation, it is often more constructive to meet belligerence with kindness. Another solution is letting a partner try a different approach.

If at all possible one should not fail to initially use benign apologetic skills to address circumstances beyond one's control, such as mechanical issues or traffic. Appearing to make excuses for actions or results within our control often backfires. A common distraction is letting irrelevant factors dictate our posture or demeanor with given patients. Poor attitude during a "middle of the night" call for a possibly not so serious complaint or judgmental behavior about previous EMS utilization might be at best not helpful, but at worst, prejudicial. Imagine the call from a citizen's perspective. Clearly, a tax paying, law abiding, and non–system-abusing citizen has the right to expect professional and courteous emergency care—at anytime. Frustration during early morning hours is a natural and understandable coping mechanism. However, it is best to re-redirect one's own and the patient's thoughts to the medical issue at hand.

Before failing to honor a reasonable request for an alternative destination to a closest hospital, the provider should understand the degrees to which patients frequently have reasonable rationales. These may include doctors and records of all care there, anxiety of a transfer, or complications from specialized procedure done there before. It is not worth a fight to protect an over-rigid interpretation of closest hospital.

If a conversation starts suggesting patients be transported in a private car or cab, each provider should stop to pause. Judging a social situation and declaring a disapproval that there is a car outside and it was not being used instead of the ambulance, or actually being on record as helping a patient into a car for someone else to drive to the ED is at very high risk for either medical or public relations sequelae.

Enlisting the patient's family in advocating the very best disposition for patients is often underutilized. The family's concern is actually a tool to get patients to accept services. Dismissing the input of the third party caller who knows the patient ("Dad is not acting right!") or failing to let a third party caller/family know about efforts to get the patient to submit, may not only be an opportunity lost, but may catch family off guard so that they cannot make arrangements to attend to the patient at home.

SELECTED READINGS

Bourdreax E, Mandry C, Brantley PJ. Stress, job satisfaction, coping, and psychological distress among emergency medical technicians. *Prehosp Disaster Med.* 1997;12(4):242–249.

"The Difficult Patient Lesson Plans: Lubbock EMS." Available at: http://www.lubbockems.org/CE%20Articles/The%20Difficult%20Patient%20-%202-06.pdf. Accessed on January 1, 2012.

Kusima M, Maatta T, Hakala T, et al. Customer satisfaction measurement in emergency medical services. *Acad Emerg Med.* 2003;10(7):821–815.

104

THE BUCK HAS TO STOP AT THE QUALITY ASSURANCE/LEADERSHIP OFFICES

ROGER M. STONE, MD, MS

In addition to delivering quality emergency care, public safety agencies must also establish a culture of accountability. Citizens and members of the medical community should be able to articulate concerns about their medical care. Furthermore, they have the right to expect prompt follow-up and if necessary, corrective action. The Quality Assurance (QA) Office is therefore a gateway to accountability for those who express a good faith concern about their care. In that spirit, a range of sophistication exists in processes for fielding complaints, from the line officers of a volunteer fire or rescue company, to a single employer supervisor, to a true QA Office. Whichever the process, the individuals assigned thereto each have by definition a mission in customer relations, and the need for good habits and skills in that arena.

Many challenges exist for a QA Office. The first is a universality of input: The QA staff must consider all potential callers, either internal or external customers, to include patients, families, co-workers, and even bystander witnesses. Next, accessibility should be user friendly. The QA or leadership staff must have a contact number for any complainant, and cultivate a robust method of referral by any in the chain of command to the correct person(s). Once input of concerns is made, all subsequent exchanges should be courteous and professional. Cordial communication must extend to both the public and any scrutinized EMS provider or their representatives.

Impartiality must dominate as the tone in any initial stages of inquiry. The office must be able to look into facts before drawing interim or later permanent conclusion, deferring any tone either in the complainant or target's favor.

Confidentiality must be maintained in compliance with Federal (e.g., HIPAA), State and local records and/or personnel statutes and regulations. Interviewing skills acquired in training and through experience must be sustained over phone and personal meetings to elicit facts, and explain processes to customers or EMS providers. Risk Management techniques are mandatory in all communications that balance transparency of the investigation with risk, and mitigate any mistrust and its resultant increase in scrutiny.

Finally, maintaining a minimal set of data analysis skills and a culture of improvement round out the list of challenges.

With the basic leadership skills needed, the first pitfall for any EMS system is failure to have adequate quality mechanisms in place to begin with. If a citizen has a difficult time finding out how to register an initial concern, or multiple people have to be called, then corrections should be made. Next, failing to appropriately field complaints as envisaged should be addressed. There should never be an unreasonable timeliness to call a complainant back after an initial referral. Another shortcoming might be the failure to give an explanation of the process and limitations of what can be divulged going forward (subject to due process, personnel regulations, etc.). That skill might help mitigate unreasonable expectations by an allegedly aggrieved party, and protect a targeted or accused provider. In fielding the initial call, failure to express regret that the customer felt a shortcoming in the service and all concerns are seriously investigated may be an opportunity lost for customer recovery.

Impartiality being key, appearing to take sides right away when fielding the complaint is a potentially adverse and unnecessary strategy. Neither making any critique of the provider, nor defending the provider prematurely is productive, outside of a factual misunderstanding about a universal process that can be fed back immediately to the complainant as a possible explanation (e.g., Our service does not diagnose). Doing so might give false impressions to the caller that the system is admitting fault, or conversely dismissing the complaint without caring.

Every QA system should look for improvements. Failure to utilize data to find system concerns from the complaint is another opportunity lost. Blaming only "the bad apple" rather than looking at "the tree" is failure to correct systemic causes that might prevent the next customer problem or even adverse outcome. If found by investigation, it is a failure to inadequately address the specific shortcomings of an errant provider, using remedial training for attitudinal, sensitivity, cultural, or medical breaches, or more severe action as indicated. Finally, pre-empting the other providers at risk through training is ideal.

In conclusion, failure to follow-up on initial concerns hampers customer recovery.

Omitting thanks for interest in the process and concern, or feedback of limited information allowed to be divulged unnecessarily fails to show good faith and transparency. For example, we can let customers know that a review is complete and appropriate action can include many corrective processes, even if laws prevent the discussion of individual personnel actions.

SELECTED READING

Cone DC, OConnor RE, Fowler RL. *Evaluating and Improving Quality in EMS,* 1st ed. Dubuque, IA: Kendall Hunt Publishing; 2009.

105

DON'T LEAVE HIGH RISK CHIEF COMPLAINTS ON THE SCENE

ROGER M. STONE, MD, MS

Individual cases cross the desks of the Quality Assurance Offices in EMS systems every day. Most of the time, education is the solution to avoiding the pitfall of underestimating medical problems. One essential skill of an EMS provider, especially at the ALS level, is to recognize a high risk chief complaint. While we are able to spot a sick patient from across the room, we may be victims of "tunnel vision" with respect to how a patient looks in real time, without the perspective of the natural history of a complaint. Medics may first infer, and then give a patient a sense of security based on the present. The posture of the provider can easily trickle down to the patient or a lesser trained emergency medical service professional. Risky situations include those where patients are "talked out" of going to the hospital or downgraded by ALS personnel to BLS for transport.

RECOGNIZING HIGH RISK CHIEF COMPLAINTS

Our jobs as astute medics involve much more than the correct application of protocols and performance of skills. Providers sort through complex medical decisions and cultivate a sense of hindsight and foresight on the basis of our didactic funds of knowledge. Recognition of **high risk complaints** and our limitations in detection or diagnosis are essential. These complaints are those that point to dysfunction in a major organ system or its blood/nerve supply:

- **Breathing trouble** can be progressive, or fluctuating.
- An **altered mental status** has a HUGE differential diagnosis, and represents a stress or damage to the brain or its blood supply.
- **Syncope** (transient loss of consciousness) implies an interruption of blood supply to the brain. Concerning causes for a syncopal episode include structural heart disorders, dysrhythmias, and neurologic abnormalities.
- **Chest pain** not only represents high risk if cardiac, but other causes can be fatal as well, such as pulmonary embolism and aortic dissection.
- **Focal neurological signs** (weakness on one side, spinal sensory deficit) imply either peripheral or central nervous system damage or interruption.
- **Back pain** or **abdominal pain**: Back pain can represent something as serious as a spinal epidural abscess or as common as a musculoskeletal strain. These complaints mandate careful and thorough evaluation.

- **Fever in the elderly and children.**
- **Seizure** can also reflect injury or insult to the central nervous system.

GUIDING PRINCIPLES IN RESPONDING TO COMPLAINTS

High risk chief complaints demand a cautious approach. Advising patients to seek evaluation and treatment at a healthcare facility is always consistent with sound medical advice. Dismissing the timeframe leading up to the 911 call itself, in favor of focusing only on the conditions on scene, might ruin the opportunity to appreciate the natural history of complaints. Good faith third party input into the call, such as family calling in because they are worried, or bystanders, should be taken into consideration. Providers should take a positive approach to the value of a hospital evaluation and stress the emergency department's ability to accurately rule out a life threatening diagnosis. Any activity that can be perceived as "milking" or "coaxing" a patient refusal cannot be tolerated.

COMMON PITFALLS IN MANAGEMENT OF THE HIGH RISK CHIEF COMPLAINT

Failure to encourage patients with high risk complaints to seek treatment or transport is not putting forth our best efforts. Opening the encounter with something like "Do you want to go to the hospital?" is projecting a medical decision on the layperson, as though being evaluated might be medically elective. Only casually offering to take high risk patients to an ED may falsely give patients the impression that they were screened by a medical authority and might be safe to delay or seek follow-up attention electively. Downplaying the value of an ED visit or emphasizing negative aspects of the visit such as long wait times will discourage compliance, and might even be argued as coercing an EMS refusal of care.

Failure to capture the information prior to the 911 activation as part of the history or failure to listen to information provided by family or bystanders—including callers from remote locations—may miss details that indicate high risk in the first place. Dismissal of information is frustrating to customers who wanted its consideration, but underestimating their concerns becomes infuriating when the outcomes are sub-optimal.

Once discussion of a refusal takes place, suggesting a patient proceed to a hospital by car and/or helping a patient into the car does not necessarily get the crew off the hook.

Pinning any refusal on the patient using their signature has limitations. Patients, family, and their attorneys retroactively will blame the refusal on any provider failing to (1) outline the foreseeable risks and (2) provide an informed decision.

- Doctor's office or surgery centers are not geared towards handling urgencies.
- Physicians may display a lack of respect for, or knowledge of the capabilities of, EMS.
- Staff may not show up at the bedside to greet EMS, in favor of attending other patients.
- The code status or advanced directives of patients are not well known by staff.

PITFALLS IN HEALTH CARE FACILITIES RESPONSE

Despite challenges described above, displaying poor will in a Doctor's Office, Urgent Care, or Skilled Nursing Facility is fraught with pitfalls and helps no one. Failure to practice restraint on a given call in light of previous problems with over-utilization, or starting debates with nurses and doctors about patients' dispositions or mode of transport may only distract the provider from medical vigilance and cause the dismissal of a sign or symptom. Failure to keep disagreements with medical staff away from patients or their families, or allowing attitudinal, emotional or judgmental overtones to be picked up by customers is merely an invitation for complaints, or worse yet lawsuits if there are bad outcomes. If there is a disagreement, the inappropriate documentation of irrelevant factors or implicating guilt in the medical record (engaging in "chart wars"), instead of filing a confidential quality assurance incident report is another recipe for legal peril that sucks in rather than exonerates the provider.

Whenever possible, EMS providers should view physicians or other HCF staff as allies in the delivery of emergency health care. The general tone of all encounters should start out as attentive and welcoming of input, even if the medic is the better person. Dismissing physicians' working diagnosis or failing to offer a collaborative approach with the physician, with an explanation of EMS protocol, might create rather than avert a misunderstanding, and thus undermine smooth handoffs and continuity of care.

After all the justified frustrations EMS providers may have about HCFs in certain encounters, some fail to constructively engage the quality leadership in writing at a later date when input about system issues may actually lead to quality improvement for future calls. This is ironically a pitfall after the fact, when venting those frustrations is actually appropriate.

BEST PRACTICES

Responding to HCFs is a daily routine and presents unique challenges for the EMS responder. On the one hand, many of these facilities might be expected to have better capabilities to care or provide first response for, or information about, patients they serve. On the other hand, many are less familiar with triaging patients in need of acute care, or discriminating between the types of prehospital services most appropriate to move patients given their complaint. Consummate professionals should use all medical information from facilities to their and the patients' benefit, avoid conflict about 911 utilization in real time, be poised to use physicians and nurses as allies, and address system issues later in a constructive manner.

SELECTED READINGS

Becker LJ, Yeargin K, Rea TD, et al. Resuscitation of residents with do not resuscitate orders in long-term care facilities. *Prehosp Emerg Care.* 2003;7(3):303–306.

Benkendorf R, Swor RA, Jackson R, et al. Outcomes of cardiac arrest in the nursing home: Destiny or futility? [see comment]. *Prehosp Emerg Care.* 1997;1(2):68–72.

Davis CO, Rodewald L. Use of EMS for seriously ill children in the office: A survey of primary care physicians. *Prehosp Emerg Care.* 1999;3(2):102–106.

Guardian EMS Statement of Quality Mission: http://guardian-ems.com/.

Johnson A. The customer's always right: Steps you can take to ensure customer satisfaction. http://www.jems.com/article/administration-and-leadership/customers-always-right-steps-y From Journal of EMS, March 2010.

Life Care EMS Serves Medical Facilities: http://www.lifecare-ems.com/.

Santillanes G, Gausche-Hill M, Sosa B. Preparedness of selected pediatric offices to respond to critical emergencies in children. *Pediatr Emerg Care.* 2006;22(11):694–698.

Shah MN, Fairbanks RJ, Lerner EB. Cardiac arrests in skilled nursing facilities: Continuing room for improvement? *J Am Med Dir Assoc.* 2007;8(3) (suppl 2):e27–e31.

Don't fail to consider the family

Jeff Beeson, DO, EMTP

"Medic 70, respond code 3 to 100 Main Street for a 60-year-old male in cardiac arrest." You begin to run the possible causes in your mind. Is it a coronary occlusion, is there an underlying cardiac condition, is there some reversible cause I can identify? You pull out of the station clearing traffic to the left. Main Street is just a few miles from the station. The controller advises CPR is in progress by a family member. The crew discusses the role each will provide upon arrival. What equipment are we going to take in with us? As you approach the address, the house is dark, and no excitement is visible.

You arrive on the porch and open the door. Your partner loudly announces EMS is here. You hear an excited middle-aged women yelling, "We are in here!! PLEASE HURRY!!" You walk into the room to find a middle-aged man in his recliner. His wife is attempting to perform chest compressions while he is in the chair. Your partner rudely asks why she didn't get him onto the floor. With tears in her eyes she advises she was unable to move him to the ground, "I did the best that I could, I am so sorry!" she says.

As you move him to the ground and take over CPR, your partner attaches the cardiac monitor. "Asystole," he states. You both inquire to how long he has been like this. The wife says, through tears and sobbing, "He told me he wasn't feeling good after dinner and was going to sit in his chair to watch the news." She says, "I was washing the dishes, and I heard a weird sound coming from the room. I went in and found him foaming at the mouth, and he wouldn't respond to me so I called 911." Your partner asks if the man has any advanced directives. The wife is unsure what that means. He then asks if her husband ever told her what his wishes were about life support. She replies, "He has a will, and it says that if there was no chance of him waking up, he didn't want to be on a breathing machine or have a feeding tube." She is now distraught and crying loudly as you continue compressions and resuscitation.

Your partner then says, rather sharply, "We need to call our doctor because your husband doesn't want anything done, so we need orders." You feel uncomfortable with this but your partner has been doing this longer than you, so you keep quiet. A minute later your partner returns to the room and says, "Dr. B at County Hospital gave us a termination order at 2145." The wife asks what that means, and your partner replies, "Your husband has died."

While you are picking up your equipment, the son arrives at the home and asks what is going on. Your partner advises him his father has died. The son screams at your partner, "WHY ARE YOU NOT DOING CPR ON HIM?!?!" The son hurries past you and starts chest compressions on his father. Your partner goes over and wrestles the son to the floor. You get on the radio and state, "Medic 70 needs a police officer code 3 for a family member fighting with EMS!" Police arrive and the situation escalates. You get your equipment out of the house and return to the station. This call does not sit well with you. Your partner keeps stating, "How dare that man fight with me. We should have had him arrested for interfering with a medical examiner case!"

Customer service seems to be intuitive in EMS. It is not all that difficult to treat people the way you want to be treated. But is it? We all have been part of similar cases to the one above. Statistics on survival from cardiac arrest are not great. Many groups have been studying this for years and no one magic bullet has been found. So why do we not give everyone the same chance? Why does a 60-year-old man who was witnessed by a family member, with bystander CPR in process, only get a termination order, when a 1-month-old child last seen hours ago who is cold with rigor mortis gets a full resuscitation with transport to the hospital? Who are we to remove loved ones from the room where we are attempting to resuscitate their family member? After all, they have known each other for years, and we have known them for only a few minutes.

Many studies have shown that family presence during resuscitation improves satisfaction. When family members witness a crew of individuals—working feverishly on their loved one—they often ask if efforts to resuscitate can be stopped. Many providers feel, however, that there is some liability risk if family members are present, that they may not understand what is being done, and that when or if their loved one dies, they will sue us. There is no evidence to support this, even though stories exist. It is simple: Resuscitation should be very fluid and practiced. It should look like a smooth pit stop at a NASCAR race with the handling of all four tires and a tank of gas. It should not look like a bunch of keystone cops running around the car looking for the door. The pitfall for the EMS provider here is not being practiced and prepared.

The focus should be to first ensure that a resuscitation appropriate for the clinical situation is being performed. We should then turn to the family: Bring them in the room. Explain everything that is going on, even what the monitor is showing and what that means. An experienced provider can tell if a family member is not going to maintain composure before being taken in to the resuscitation area. If the provider has any question, the family members should be asked if they would prefer someone else to go instead.

Communication is the key. From the initial 911 call to the transport, we should explain everything, and the pitfall is in not doing so. We set the tone for everything we do. Providing good customer service is the same as being a patient advocate, and the pitfall is in failing to do so. No matter what type of call you are on from the worst trauma you have seen to the sore throat, patients are persons, and we should treat them and their family with the utmost respect. Do unto others as you would have them do unto you.

Medicine is a science, but dealing with patients and their families is an art. Some artists are born with talent, but they still must practice to improve their skills. We must do the same. We must take each situation and improve upon it. We would never allow a paramedic to treat our family like the lead provider in the beginning of this chapter. We must not allow it to happen to anyone.

SELECTED READINGS

Holliday S. EMS Customer Service. In *Fire Engineering,* 2009: http://www.fireengineering.com/articles/print/volume-161/issue-10/departments/fire-service-ems/ems-customer-service.html, last accessed 12/29/11.

Kuisma M, Määttä T, Hakala T, et al. Customer satisfaction measurement in emergency medical services. *Acad Emerg Med.* 2003;10(7):812–815.

Porter W. It's about customer service. In *EMS World,* 2005: http://www.emsworld.com/article/10323479/ems-its-about-customer-service, last accessed 12/29/11.

109

DON'T POST PATIENT OR FAMILY INFO ON SOCIAL MEDIA

JEFF BEESON, DO, EMTP

Medic 12 responds to a car crash on the South Freeway. When you arrive, you find a minor crash with two victims, complaining of neck and back pain. You begin to evaluate the patients and place them in spinal precautions. The police officer comes over to inform you that this wreck is not in your service area, and you are actually in an adjacent town. As the ambulance from that town arrives on scene, you quickly recognize the paramedic. She used to work for your service, but left under not so comfortable reasons. She gets out of her ambulance and quickly starts to verbally attack you for "jumping their call." She says she used to work for your company and "knows what kind of games you play."

You and your partner apologize and give her a report on what has been done so far. You attempt to assist her and her partner in getting the patients into their ambulance but her verbal attacks continue. You have had enough. You begin to stand up for yourself and your company. You remind her of what got her fired and state your company is better off without her. All the time the patients are asking you both to stop yelling at each other.

Later in your shift as you continue to fume over this interaction, you make an online post to update your status and let everyone else know what happened. Soon after an online discussion begins with many employees, both current and previous. Then the paramedic from the other town chimes in. She is a friend of a friend who saw your post and is now letting it all out. You *BOTH* look quite like fools as it seems that almost everyone on the Internet now knows the situation. And worse: You both have your identities linked to your current employers!

The next day, on your day off, you get a call from the operations supervisor who needs you to come in. This can't be good. You run the story through your mind. You remember the company's new policy on social media, so you quickly go online and delete every post you made about the call.

The next day you go into the office and are escorted to Human Resources. You think you are cleared because there is no record of your conversation: After all, you deleted it. Then it happened. Your supervisor hands you a printed copy of the posts and asks about it. You quickly inform him you already deleted the posts and begin to deny everything. The meeting does not go well, as you can imagine.

Social media has changed the face of medicine. We now have patients posting things on the Web even as we do them, including photographs. Co-workers live their lives, and all of their movements seem to be on Facebook within moments. The pitfall for the EMS provider here is to remember that all posts to any public place could end up on the front page of the newspaper very quickly, even email! It is critical that providers understand and remember that companies today are usually staying one step ahead of their employees with strict policies regarding the utilization of social media by their staff members. The rules change and technology advances, but we are still playing catch up.

Stories abound of EMS professionals who have taken pictures or videos of victims and have posted them online. It has been reported that a photograph of an accident involving a fatality was posted online and then subsequently viewed online by one of the victim's parents. Such a posting is a violation of patient privacy and most certainly puts the provider and the employing EMS agency in great jeopardy for litigation.

EMS providers must look their best and always strictly obey company policy as well as ask themselves how they would feel if their own private information were shared in a public forum.

Who is the customer? The best definition is that it is everyone with whom we come in contact. Whether providers work for a contract company or city employees, they represent the employer to everyone. They must take pride not only in their profession but as well as with the agencies for whom they work. Customer service is treating others like you would want to be treated. It is not only the patients and their families, but also co-workers, those of other companies, and even competitors. In doing so, the EMS provider can optimize the work environment, make the practice of EMS medicine much more enjoyable, and especially avoid the risks inherent when the customer's trust is violated.

SELECTED READINGS

Berndtson K. What does your social media policy say? Posted July 31, 2010, at http://www.emsworld.com/article/10319404/what-does-your-social-media-policy-say, last accessed 12/29/11.

Lugwig G. Social media dilemmas one employee's public opinion could tarnish your agency's image. *JEMS*. 2010;35(5):26.

MedStar Internet Communications & Social Networking Policy, posted on April 11, 2010, at http://www.jems.com/article/administration-and-leadership/medstar-internet-communication, last accessed 12/29/11.

110

CONSENT AND CONFIDENTIALITY IN EMS:
MISTAKES THAT YOU SHOULDN'T MAKE

R. Jack Ayres, JD, LP
Chris Ayres, JD, NREMT
Wendy Ruggeri, MD

Most people wouldn't argue with the premise that paramedics and attorneys occupy very different professional realms. They wouldn't prefer the typical attorney to be the sole provider of emergency care to their children after a traumatic accident anymore than they would prefer the typical paramedic to represent them in a court of law. The two disciplines are not entirely without overlap, however. There are some situations in which a little bit of basic EMS-related state law goes a very long way towards keeping the field medical provider out of a heap of trouble, and the following discussion highlights some of the more common instances where field providers can get into trouble.

DNRs and the Termination of CPR

The basic rule of field resuscitation is simple: Every patient who is a candidate for CPR should be resuscitated to the best of the practitioner's ability, or until the patient is resuscitated or is pronounced dead: *Unless* there is a medical or legal reason not to do so. The legal reasons to withhold resuscitation include the presence of court orders, "living wills," and "powers of attorney." Medical reasons include conclusive evidence of death (as defined by the agency Medical Director), and valid out-of-hospital do not resuscitate orders.

Upon encountering reasons to withhold care, the provider should confirm the identity of the patient and make contact with a medical control physician where available in a region. CPR should be performed while this contact is being made. A copy of any documentation regarding patient request for withholding of care *must* be presented. The directions of the medical control physician—or EMS agency policy as authorized by the Medical Director—to terminate or continue efforts take precedence from here. It should go without saying that the need for thorough documentation in these cases is of utmost importance.

A conscious patient who has a written DNR order in hand can still choose to revoke that document at any time. If the patient is unconscious, a document may be revoked if a qualified representative with power of attorney of the patient—or a legal guardian—states the intent to revoke the DNR. It can also be revoked if the patients themselves communicated desire to revoke the order before becoming unconscious.

In the event of the revocation of a DNR order, the provider should record the time, date, and place of the revocation for relay to the medical control physician. If possible, the revoked document or device should be retained and transported with the patient.

LIMITED USE OF COURT ORDERS: FIRST TRY SPEAKING SOFTLY. IF THAT FAILS, USE THE BIG STICK

EMS has clearly proven its worth to society, but just within the generation that EMS has existed there have been many factors that have begun to strain the resources of EMS. Among these stressors are the patients that we occasionally encounter who clearly need medical assistance but refuse this treatment for a variety of reasons. Many EMS systems have sought to use court intervention—at appropriate times—to legally assist medics in the field with these types of patients who clearly need intervention.

The first most common issue that will require court intervention is one in which patient consent cannot be obtained. After attempts for express, involuntary, and implied consent, the paramedic may have been unsuccessful, but treatment is still obviously necessary. State laws can often allow for the obtaining of a court order to provide treatment to patients without their consent, but several problems may arise with this action.

Primarily, the EMS agency and/or medical control physician must have direct and immediate contact with an attorney who has *the appropriate legal and medical training to analyze the situation* and who can promptly contact a court to obtain the order. This requires both immediate access to an attorney, and also access to a judge. It is also necessary to *immediately communicate* with medical control while this court order is being obtained, as the process typically takes at least five to ten minutes. In the interim, the field providers should be instructed to stand by to provide appropriate care through implied consent principles, should a patient lose consciousness or the ability to communicate.[1]

PATIENT CONFIDENTIALITY AND EMS REPORTING REQUIREMENTS

The general premise for every EMS provider is that patient confidentiality must be strictly observed. Absent specific legal exceptions, an EMS field

---

[1]This is, obviously, subject to the provisions of medical, legal rationale that prohibits care or resuscitation.

practitioner is strictly limited to discussing a patient's medical information with someone else within the continuum of medical care or for quality assurance purposes only. Reports circulate of strict confidentiality having been ignored in a patient care scenario, a matter of increasing concern with social media outlets regularly and quickly available to EMS staff (Facebook and Twitter being examples of these outlets). A failure to have protocol in place regarding patient confidentiality has the potential to result in significant embarrassment for not only the patient, but the EMS agency as well.

All information and records obtained while providing EMS services is confidential and privileged.[2] Confidentiality is not only claimed by the patient, it should also be asserted by the physician or provider *on the patient's behalf* in any civil, criminal, or administrative proceeding.[3] Likewise, EMS providers are "covered entities" in the eyes of the Health Insurance Portability and Accountability Act (HIPAA) of 1996. HIPAA provides limited exceptions that allow for a healthcare provider to disclose a patient's confidential health information.[4] Both state and federal law generally provide severe penalties for violation of these confidentiality laws, as well as criminal penalties for any intentional violation. There are *very few* exceptions to this law.

EMS agency protocol should be very clear in its language. There should be an absolute prohibition against any EMS provider providing any pictures, posts, tweets, or any patient information on any social media site. This *includes* any identifiable patient information, documents, or case information even when patient features or names are taken out. It is imperative that there is zero tolerance within the agency for doing so.

In short, protocol should state that an EMS provider is only afforded the ability to reveal patient information to the hospital team receiving the patient during continuity of care, or upon advice of counsel and receipt of subpoena. Interdepartmental or interagency gossip and war stories are highly inappropriate and should be discouraged.

At the end of the day it would be counterproductive for the field paramedic to be constantly paranoid about the threat of litigation, as this would likely impair his or her ability to be decisive on scene, and this is often critical. It does a lot of good, however, to have at least some basic working knowledge of the relevant state statutes and keep a few of these in mind when rendering and transferring care in the field. As the old saying goes, "An ounce of prevention is better than a pound of suffering."

---

[2]Tex. Health & Safety Code § 773.091(a)
[3]*Id.* at 773.091(e)
[4]*Id.* at 160.203

Selected Readings

Ayres RJ. Legal considerations in prehospital care. *Emerg Med Clin North Am.* 1993;11(4): 853–867.

Meador SR, Slovis CM, Wrenn KD. EMS bill of rights: What every patient deserves. *JEMS.* 2003;28(3):70–75.

Shanaberger CJ. Case law involving base-station contact. *Prehosp Disaster Med.* 1995;10(2): 75–80.

Sherbino J, Keim SM, Davis DP. Clinical decision rules for termination of resuscitation in out-of-hospital cardiac arrest. *J Emerg Med.* 2010;38(1):80–86.

Weaver J, Brinsfield KH, Dalphond D. Prehospital refusal-of-transport policies: Adequate legal protection? *Prehosp Emerg Care.* 2000;4(1):53–56.

111

DON'T BE GUILTY OF SHOWING NEGLIGENCE

R. JACK AYRES, JD, LP

CHRIS AYRES, JD, NREMT

WENDY RUGGERI, MD

In this day and age of extensive litigation, one of the easiest ways for plaintiffs to win their cases (and we in EMS to lose them) is for medical responders to behave in a negligent manner. Systemically speaking, providers in EMS systems can show carelessness when it comes to accountability, and thus get in trouble that way, too. Take a few of the examples below as food for thought:

"YOU'LL BE FINE. YOU DON'T NEED TO GO TO THE HOSPITAL"

A decision to not transport a patient is the most dangerous decision an EMS provider can make, both medically for the patient, and also legally for the providers themselves. Providers should strongly consider including the medical control physician in such a decision. The vast majority of EMS lawsuits stem from a decision by a field provider not to transport a patient to the hospital. The EMS practitioner must recognize his or her limitations, technologically and experience-wise, and realize that asking for help or guidance should not be perceived as a sign of weakness, but a wise move by a medic who gets the "team" concept of an EMS agency.

One major reason that decisions are made not to transport an EMS patient is sometimes related to a practitioner's inappropriate and subjective assessment of a patient's "nonmedical features." While disturbing to consider, some EMS providers are willing to lessen their focus on some patients for various reasons such as lifestyle. Such behaviors may include the fact that the patient is homeless, a drug addict, or any number of other characteristics perhaps felt to be "unsavory" by the provider. Making treatment decisions on the basis of such impressions can cause a deadly mistake to be made, one that cannot be tolerated in EMS.

The take-away point is this. There should be but one standard for a practicing EMS provider in this country: To provide the same treatment that that provider would demand and expect of someone taking care of a family member of that provider. Anything short of that standard betrays the EMS mission.

"WHO CARES, NOBODY READS THESE REPORTS ANYWAY!"

The EMS run sheet is either the practitioner's greatest ally or worse nightmare, depending on how seriously they take its completion. Simply put, *if something isn't documented, it didn't happen.* Does this sound familiar? It should. A complete run sheet is the foundation for insuring continuity of care, and truly sets the table for all subsequent providers. This continuity of care depends on every subsequent provider's ability to rely on the accuracy of the documentation of the field crewmembers.

Electronic patient care records have been helpful in improving documentation, but can also be detrimental to record keeping. It is important that the individual medics do not become dependent on the software program and assume that the software will notify them if there is a problem with their documentation. Many programs offer such features, and it is safe to say that they are all *very* far from foolproof. Each individual practitioner must take personal responsibility for the content of their documentation and not rely on a computer program to complete all documentation steps.

Quality assurance and routine audits of EMS providers are also an important component in insuring proper documentation. If it is well known throughout the EMS agency that there are staff members assigned to review all or portions of the patient care records, then this will add to the standard of accountability that will ultimately boost both the quality of patient care and documentation.

In short, documentation gives valuable insight into a method and manner of practice by the individual in the field. If a practitioner is lazy, incomplete, and sloppy in his documentation of a patient encounter, it is very likely that he or she exhibits those same traits when actually caring for the patient.

The Drug Enforcement Administration (DEA) Is Serious about Accountability for Narcotics!

Not so long ago, a highly respected EMS Medical Director had heard great things about the use of fentanyl for pain control in the field. He established policies and procedures for all logistical aspects of the clinical use of the controlled substances within his small, rural agency, and authorized its use in his protocols. When he went back to audit his agency, he had a shocking revelation: The Paramedic Director of this agency had "diverted" (the DEA's polite term for stealing) fentanyl, ultimately taking more than 200 ampules of this schedule II drug over about a year's time. Upon discovering the "diversion" of this astounding quantity of fentanyl, the Medical Director took all appropriate action. He fully investigated the matter at the local level, satisfying himself that the paramedic appeared to have acted alone in this. He notified the state licensure board and worked to have the paramedic's license revoked. He also notified the DEA, and even outlined his plan for preventing future diversions. He truly felt he had taken all appropriate steps.

Apparently, the DEA did not share this view. The total of fines sought by the government against the Medical Director due to the paramedic's theft of medications approached three million dollars. To make matters even worse for the Medical Director, the State initiated an action to revoke his medical license. Following extensive discussion between the Medical Director, the DEA, and legal counsel, the case was resolved, though a fine was still levied.

What is clearly evident from the experience is that the DEA requires *absolute accountability* by an EMS agency that carries controlled substances authorized by the Medical Director. Records must be completed and stored by the agency consistent with the DEA requirements. Often these regulations are not fully known or understood by many Medical Directors, and it is important that the EMS agency and the Medical Director fully understand the DEA regulations regarding ordering of controlled substances, the receipt into inventory, inventory control and "distribution" of medications within an agency to vehicles, wastage, possible DEA registration of individual stations, and records maintenance. Those affected by the need for individual registrations of both emergency vehicles and central inventory systems should carefully monitor upcoming developments in the interpretation of DEA regulations.

In summary, these are not the only ways to "let things get lax" and get in trouble, but certainly a few of the easiest and most visible. EMS organizations must avoid inattention to detail, especially in the critical areas discussed above, to avoid injuring a patient and to avoid becoming a target for litigation.

SELECTED READINGS

The Drug Enforcement Administration Regulations. http://www.deadiversion.usdoj.gov/21cfr/index.html. Accessed May 29, 2012.

Texas Administrative Code Title 25, Part 1, Chapter 157, Subchapter C, Rule 157.36.

112

Don't confuse roles in the EMS

R. Jack Ayres, JD, LP
Chris Ayres, JD, NREMT
Wendy Ruggeri, MD

EMS is the perfect environment for disagreements to surface. On many emergency calls, there is plenty of stress to go around. Add to this the fact that there are a lot of "type A personalities" and differences of opinion on how to handle a certain situation, and there the perfect storm of factors is created for a good healthy debate. While some debate is good for the soul and the brain, the emergency scene is hardly the place for technical or tactical disagreements to drag on. For the patient's sake primarily—but often also for the safety of the responding crewmembers—these differences must find a workable solution, and quickly. Some of the more common turf issues begin to repeat themselves, and though the solutions are often easy to see, it may be challenging sometimes to implement them.

The Buck Stops *Here,* and not Anywhere Else!

Now that EMS is its own subspecialty of medicine, it is very important for medical directors to have appropriate policies in place to allow them the ultimate control of the agency with regard to hiring, training, supervision, and retention decisions. Remember that the "buck stops" with the Medical Director. This can be challenging when dealing with agencies that have their own hierarchy, oftentimes with the EMS personnel reporting directly up the chain to high-ranking fire department officials, for example. Sometimes these officials are EMS attuned, and sometimes they aren't.

Responsibility begins with the hiring of providers, as the Medical Director is ultimately responsible for the clinical actions of anyone who works under that Medical Director's license. EMS agencies should assure that a system is in place to evaluate the education, skills, and qualifications of the candidate *prior* to that individual being hired. Agencies should determine if provider candidates should have maintained certification by the National Registry of Emergency Medical Technicians, and, if not, do candidates need to go through the process of recertification. Also, how they are trained (not just officially certified) by the State and the cognitive and skills knowledge base of a new-hire candidate should also be given extensive consideration.

Areas of significant liability for EMS agencies are found in both inadequate field supervision of clinical care as well as in the ongoing training of employees. Liability is created by failure to adequately enforce clinical protocols and to address through ongoing training those who fail to adhere to it. Agency protocol should be in place to give the Medical Director complete control over adverse disciplinary action for clinical reasons—from verbal or written warnings or reprimands to more aggressive discipline. An additional policy consideration must be provided that any employee of the EMS agency must notify the Medical Director immediately of anything that might affect the practitioner's ability to operate under the Medical Director's license (such as complaints against them, etc.). In short, the best way to prevent an adverse patient outcome is by education, training, and supervision of all field paramedics and EMTs.

JUST EXACTLY WHO IS IN CHARGE HERE?

EMS Medical Directors and agencies must remember at all times that their medics are not independently licensed or certified to practice elsewhere without proper medical direction. Many local governments allow for mutual aid agreements to exist between jurisdictions to assist with EMS response when necessary. It becomes the agency and Medical Director's responsibility to clearly define how all agency practitioners should perform when assisting in another jurisdiction, and it is of critical importance to coordinate this matter with the agency's lead legal counsel or ultimate decision maker and have input in these agreements.

Another issue stems from how a scene should be handled when an outside physician arrives and offers to assist in patient care. The primary concern here is which physician's direction will control the scene and patient care. The first step in this process is always to identify the physician. The physician must produce identification and a current license from the State Medical Board. There have been numerous examples of individuals who impersonate physicians, so the provider should not merely accept the word of a person claiming to be a physician who offers assistance. After identifying the doctor and the patient's relationship to the physician, field practitioners should then consult their online medical control, if available, for assistance. At this point, the physician on scene and the online control physician should communicate to determine the role the on-scene physician will have with the patient's care.

Generally, another physician may assume responsibility for the patient's care and the medics should defer to his orders unless those orders conflict with their medical guidelines. Any orders given by the private physician should be documented in an acceptable manner. If the orders conflict at all with the medical guidelines of the EMS agency, then the field provider should request that the physicians communicate to determine a proper course of treatment. If that is not possible, then the private physician must be willing to accept full care and be willing to *accompany the patient to the hospital.* Otherwise, a medic should return to their established protocols. Providers should always use caution in the setting of having received medical orders from an on-scene physician that are outside of the agency medical guidelines. If there is a disagreement between the two physicians, the EMT or paramedic should follow the orders of the online medical control physician or, if this resource isn't available, then follow the EMS agency medical guidelines for care. If the intervening physician is delegated any responsibility, all orders provided by that intervening physician should be checked with their medical control physician.

Setting up the Pyramid of Responsibility

Relevant law requires that EMS practitioners must stay strictly within their scope of practice when caring for a patient. Without proper qualifications, anyone who tries to practice medicine without a medical license is subject to both civil and criminal penalties.[1] Physicians may "*delegate*" their authority to various EMS providers, and State law creates a branch of the government to monitor and to supervise licensure of all EMS practitioners.[2] It is therefore incumbent upon the provider to operate *only* in the scope of the tasks delegated to them.[3]

A common problem in many EMS organizations is actually the *way* in which the system is organized. EMS agencies should resemble a pyramid with a Medical Director at the top of the clinical aspects of the pyramid, having responsibility over all aspects of the organization relative to patient care. Below them there should be appropriate levels of supervision and support to insure that the frontline EMS providers provide adequate care. Careful attention must also be given to provide direct contact between the field practitioner and the online medical control physician where available as soon as appropriate, so as not to delay vital communications.

In any situation where there is a lot on the line and not a lot of time to weigh all the options, it helps to be decisive, and the side effect of this decisiveness is often conflict. Along the lines of "An ounce of prevention…" it is generally a wise course of action to address these turf battles early on, preferably before they materialize out in the field and on the scene of an actual emergency. This requires clear, concise, and proactive communication on these matters, but just a few conversations or training sessions will go a long way toward adequately clearing up any misunderstandings before they get out of hand and potentially jeopardize patient outcomes.

---

[1] *Id.*
[2] *Id; See* 25 Tex. Adm. Code 157.1 *et seq.*
[3] *Id.*

SELECTED READINGS

Alcorta R, Manz D. EMS scope of practice. In: *Prehospital Systems and Medical Oversight.* Vol 1. Dubuque, IA: Kendall/Hunt Publishing; 2009:321–331.

Ayres RJ. Legal considerations in prehospital care. *Emerg Med Clin North Am.* 1993;11(4): 853–867.

Margolis G, Murray J, Swankin D. Certification, licensure, and credentialing of EMS personnel. In: *Prehospital Systems and Medical Oversight.* Vol 1. Dubuque, IA: Kendall/Hunt Publishing; 2009:332–339.

113

DON'T MAKE THESE ERRORS IN MANAGING MEDICATIONS, AND KEEP THAT PATIENT AREA CLEAN!

BRAD LONDON

Many errors can be made by field providers regarding the management of medications. Providers have to be really careful with the handling and administration of medications or one or more of a number of things can happen that can be adverse to the patient.

FAILING TO PERFORM A DAILY INSPECTION OF INVENTORY

Of all errors that could be prevented, this one is at the top. It is the duty and responsibility of each individual provider to make sure that all supplies are fully stocked each and every shift/day that they work. This includes making sure that each ambulance has the proper amount of each drug, that each drug is in proper date, and that none are expired, and that each container has not been tampered with. Some drugs should be stored in certain places, and that should be taken into consideration during the inventory process. Some drugs are not supposed to be exposed to light, some are supposed to be kept in cool environments, and others are not to be shaken prior to administration. It can be difficult to comply with such considerations when it is in the middle of a hot summer afternoon after a bumpy lights and sirens response through congested traffic. During daily inventory, if the EMS provider makes sure the drugs are accounted for, stored, and secured in the right place, then this can help prevent field errors.

FAILING TO CHECK FOR PATIENT ALLERGIES

This is a simple error to fix, yet it can happen in the field at any time. The EMS provider can get rushed during the examination and treatment of a critically ill patient, and it is possible to make the mistake of administering a medication without asking patients if they are allergic to any medications. A simple question to the conscious patient could prevent this error, and avoid creating a potentially life-threatening problem. If there is an unconscious patient, then checking with a family member or bystander who might know the patient should be attempted. Also checking the patient for any type of medical ID jewelry could be beneficial. Some people carry a list of their known allergies in their wallets, and some have them printed on the back of their driver's licenses.

Along with allergies there are other medicines that might not necessarily produce an allergic reaction, but certain medicines should not be administered with other medicines already in the patient's system. One such example is asking if a patient is on sexual performance enhancement drugs prior to the administration of nitroglycerin for an acute cardiac emergency. This particular question in this clinical setting should be asked along the same lines when asking about medical allergies.

These two simple quick questions—if asked during the initial assessment of the patient—could help in the outcome of the patient. Failing to do so could have fatal effects on a patient who is already in need of medical attention.

FAILING TO KNOW SPECIFICS OF CERTAIN MEDICATIONS, INCLUDING DOSING AND ADMINISTRATION

This error is mainly due to a lack of education which could arise from two different areas: One would be the provider passing training courses and passing board examinations by either guessing or getting lucky, and the other way is by a provider not staying up-to-date on his or her continuing education courses. Whether it's computer classes, live continuing education (CE) classes, or attending classes individually, each provider should be accountable for his or her knowledge. Even though providers might be away from work for an extended period of time for some reason, they need to be responsible enough to maintain their CEs and their proper certifications. The field of medicine is ever changing, and it's a job in itself to maintain the highest level of education to which providers have committed themselves.

FAILING TO MONITOR THE STATUS OF PATIENTS AFTER MEDICATION ADMINISTRATION

Once a medicine is given, it is imperative to continue monitoring the status of the patient. Patients may react differently to many medications. Even if a medication has a standard anticipated reaction—such as improvement in wheezing in an asthmatic who receives albuterol—patients must be watched carefully to determine how they will respond to these administrations.

One example would be in the application of continuous positive airway pressure (CPAP). When using CPAP on a patient in respiratory distress, the patient is either start feeling better or will not improve, perhaps even deteriorating clinically. Thus, it is critical that a provider carefully monitor a patient when CPAP is being administered. Another example might be adenosine. Even though it has a very short half-life in the system, it could cause a person to become asystolic. Carefully observing the patient following the administration of any medication is thus extremely important.

The critical point is that patients must be watched closely after they have received any medications in the prehospital setting.

Failure to Maintain Sterility of Equipment during Drug Administration

During an emergency in the field, each provider is responsible for providing the highest level of care possible. This care includes assisting the patient all the while maintaining a high level of cleanliness in the back of the ambulance and keeping all supplies and instruments clean according to recommended handling instructions. This is a hard feat to accomplish when times are difficult during the care of a patient in the back of an ambulance, but every effort must be made to do so.

Maintaining a sterile technique includes the provider wearing gloves while performing his or her duties and using appropriate sterile precautions during procedures that call for such technique. Maintaining a clean environment means preventing cross-contamination and putting used needles in the sharps container. Sterile technique includes the cleaning of intravenous ports properly with alcohol before needles are inserted and cleaning the skin with Betadine before administering an intraosseous needle insertion. Maintaining sterile technique includes not attempting to use the same intravenous catheter more than once.

Such errors can be prevented in the prehospital area, and providers must avoid forgetting the possibility of these errors. In the middle of a crisis in the back of an ambulance while taking care of a critical patient, it is hard to maintain a sterile environment, but the goal is to do the best that one can.

If sterility is not kept, then both the patient and the provider may suffer.

Selected Readings

Lifshitz AE, Goldstein LH, Sharist M, et al. Medication prescribing errors in the prehospital setting and in the ED. *Am J Emerg Med.* 2011 July 7 [Epub ahead of print].

McManus JG, Sallee DR. Pain management in the prehospital environment. *Emerg Med Clin North Am.* 2005;23(2):415–431.

Park CL, Roberts DE, Aldington DJ, et al. Prehospital analgesia: systematic review of evidence. *J R Army Med Corps.* 2010;156(4 suppl 1):295–300.

114

KNOW THE PROS AND CONS OF CHEMICAL RESTRAINT

C. CRAWFORD MECHEM, MD, FACEP

EMS providers frequently encounter patients who are violent or agitated as a result of an underlying medical or psychiatric illness. Such behavior makes care difficult and may also lead to injury to the patient and the providers. In one review of injuries to paramedics and firefighters in a metropolitan fire department, 4% resulted from assaults, almost all of which occurred during patient care activities. Some examples of medical conditions that can lead to combative behavior include hypoxia, hypoglycemia, acute drug or alcohol intoxication, stroke, CNS infection, brain trauma, heat stroke, thyrotoxicosis, and a postictal state. Causative psychiatric conditions include, but are not limited to, schizophrenia and bipolar disorder, borderline personality disorder, and antisocial personality disorders, often in the context of medication noncompliance. If verbal attempts to de-escalate the situation are unsuccessful, it may be necessary for EMS providers to restrain the patient to ensure the safety of all involved and to facilitate the patient's care. Options include physical and chemical restraints. Physical restraints may limit range of motion but do not always control agitation. Patients who continue to struggle despite physical restraints are at risk of exacerbating underlying or precipitating medical conditions. The act of struggling against restraints may also result in metabolic acidosis, hyperkalemia, rhabdomyolysis, and sudden cardiac arrest. Chemical restraint may minimize these risks and complications.

The most frequently used pharmacologic agents for chemical restraint include benzodiazepines and neuroleptics. Commonly employed benzodiazepines are diazepam (5 to 10 mg), lorazepam (1 to 2 mg), and midazolam (1 to 5 mg). All three can be administered by the intravenous (IV), intramuscular (IM), or intraosseous (IO) route. Lorazepam and midazolam can also be administered intranasally using a mucosal atomizer device. Neuroleptic agents used in this setting include the classical antipsychotics, haloperidol (2.5 to 10 mg IM) and droperidol (5 mg IM); and the newer, atypical antipsychotics, ziprasidone (10 to 20 mg IM) and olanzapine (10 mg IM). In addition to these classes of drugs, ketamine (4 mg/kg IM or 2 mg/kg IV), a dissociative anesthetic and analgesic, may be used as a second-line agent.

While benzodiazepines, neuroleptics, and ketamine have been safely used for many years, they are not without risks. Benzodiazepines may cause respiratory depression, made worse in patients who have ingested alcohol or other sedating agents. Oversedation and hypotension may also be noted. Droperidol and haloperidol may cause acute dystonia, manifested by involuntary, painful muscles contractions. Akathisia, an unpleasant sensation of restlessness, may also result. These are effectively treated with diphenhydramine or benztropine. A more concerning adverse effect of classical antipsychotics is QT prolongation, which may result in torsades de pointes. In 2001, the Food and Drug Administration (FDA) issued a black box warning for droperidol, stating that prior to administration an ECG should be obtained to assess for underlying QT prolongation. If QT prolongation is present, droperidol should not be used. The FDA warning also recommended that patients be placed on a cardiac monitor before and for 2 to 3 hours after administration. Given the realities of the prehospital environment, compliance with this FDA warning may be extremely difficult. In 2008, the FDA also issued a warning regarding the use of haloperidol in the elderly with dementia-related psychosis, because of an association with increased mortality. Therefore, while both agents may be effective for controlling agitated patients, the EMS must assess whether their benefits outweigh potential medical and medicolegal risks.

The atypical antipsychotics, ziprasidone and olanzapine, are generally safer than the classical antipsychotics. They are also more effective as tranquilizers and less likely to cause sedation, acute dystonia, and akathisia. However, olanzapine may cause hypotension, and ziprasidone may cause mild QT prolongation.

Another potentially fatal adverse reaction to all antipsychotic agents that EMS providers should know about is the neuroleptic malignant syndrome (NMS). This is characterized by a combination of fever, altered mental status, muscle rigidity, and autonomic disturbances such as severe hypertension and tachycardia. NMS is uncommon and treatment is supportive and includes aggressive cooling measures.

Ketamine is generally safe in commonly used doses. It has a rapid onset and produces minimal respiratory or cardiovascular depression. It may cause increased secretions, transient hypertension, tachycardia, and emergence hallucinations as the patient wakes up. It may also rarely precipitate laryngospasm, which is treated with supportive measures. However, ketamine is another agent to consider for one's armamentarium.

It is not uncommon for paramedics to encounter violent or agitated patients in the field. They can be challenging to manage and often have serious underlying medical illness. It is important to gain prompt control so that these patients can be evaluated and transported without compromising patient or provider safety. This can be done with physical or chemical restraint. Agents used for chemical restraint can facilitate care but may also lead to serious, and at times fatal, complications. Regardless of which agent is used, it should be administered in accordance with established patient care protocols and service policies. Protocols should include the involvement of law enforcement officers to assist with placement of physical restraints. Once the patient's behavior is controlled, a search should be made for readily treatable precipitants, such as hypoxia or hypoglycemia. When EMS providers reach the emergency department, they should give the accepting staff a full report on the medication administered and any adverse reactions that may have developed.

SELECTED READINGS

ACEP Excited Delirium Task Force. White Paper Report on Excited Delirium Syndrome, September 10, 2009. http://ccpicd.com/Documents/Excited%20Delirium%20Task%20Force.pdf. Accessed March 25, 2011.

Brice JH, Pirrallo RG, Racht E, et al. Management of the violent patient. *Prehosp Emerg Care.* 2003;7:48–55.

Coburn VA, Mycyk MB. Physical and chemical restraints. *Emerg Med Clin North Am.* 2009; 27:655–667.

Kupas DF, Wydro GC. Patient restraint in emergency medical services systems. *Prehosp Emerg Care.* 2002;6:340–345.

Martel M, Sterzinger A, Miner J, et al. Management of acute undifferentiated agitation in the ED: a randomized double-blind trial of droperidol, ziprasidone, and midazolam. *Acad Em Med.* 2005;12:1167–1172.

Mechem CC, Dickinson ET, Shofer FS, et al. Injuries from assaults on paramedics and firefighters in an urban emergency medical services system. *Prehosp Emerg Care.* 2002;6: 396–401.

115

CONSIDER PHYSICAL RESTRAINT AS A LAST RESORT OPTION FOR THE COMBATIVE PATIENT

SABINA BRAITHWAITE, MD, MPH, NREMTP
JON E. FRIESEN, MSOD

EMS providers care for combative patients frequently. These providers must therefore be skilled at using all available methods to determine the reason for the patient's combative behavior and to manage it in a way that is as safe as possible for both the patient and the provider.

CAUSES OF COMBATIVENESS

Behavioral problems and combativeness are seen with acute and chronic organic diseases, substance abuse, and psychiatric problems. Often the definitive cause of the patient's combativeness can be difficult to determine, particularly in the field, and may be a combination of the above. The priority for EMS providers is to safely transport the patient to a site with the appropriate resources for further evaluation and treatment. To accomplish this, EMS providers should do a medical assessment, gather a history, and provide context for the treating facility on how events unfolded, and provide information from witnesses or law enforcement to aid in treatment and appropriate patient disposition.

APPROACHES TO RESTRAINT

The goal in managing the combative patient is to prevent harm to self and others, and to allow for necessary evaluation to determine the cause and facilitate management of the underlying problem. Physical restraint has been identified as a quality focus because of a pattern of deaths in such patients. There have been numerous deaths linked to the syndrome of excited delirium (addressed elsewhere in this book) in patients who were restrained during EMS transport. Because of this, a staged approach to the combative patient in any setting should begin with verbal de-escalation and similar non-contact measures. In EMS settings, it may become clear in a matter of seconds that these techniques are not viable, but they should still be considered first. Physical restraint and chemical restraint are the other options for management of the combative patient. Depending on the situation, either of these may be the next step when non-contact measures fail.

Physical Restraint

Physical restraint should be considered a high-risk intervention where skill is needed to apply the intervention safely and appropriately. The decision to use physical restraints should be carefully weighed against the risks to both the patient and the provider.

If physical restraint is needed, it should be done with an organized approach, using adequate personnel to rapidly and safely neutralize the threat. Most authors recommend at least five people for effective initial physical restraint (one for each appendage and one for the head). The patient should be searched for weapons (including needles). Each limb should be secured using soft restraints in a way that can be rapidly released by the provider should the patient deteriorate. Be certain you know the proper method of restraint application, as improper application may result in injury to both the patient and the provider. An additional soft restraint across the thighs to limit bucking may be useful. The chest or abdomen should not be restrained to avoid respiratory difficulty. Hard restraints such as leathers are not recommended, nor is hog tying (also known as hobble restraints). Ideally, the patient should be restrained on their side to minimize aspiration risk. A quiet environment with limited external stimuli is preferred (limit sirens, enabling "friends" and family). Patients should never be restrained in a prone position, nor should they ever be left unsupervised and unmonitored. Once initial restraint is accomplished, physiologic monitoring appropriate to the situation should be initiated, potentially including cardiac monitor, noninvasive blood pressure, oxygen saturation, capnometry/capnography, and glucometry. Medical management as dictated by the assessment should be provided promptly. If the patient calms down sufficiently, consideration may be given to releasing one appendage at a time.

Ideally, physical restraint should be used as a temporizing measure that allows EMS to chemically restrain the patient who continues to be severely agitated. Patients who continue to fight against physical restraints are at risk for exacerbation of underlying disease processes as well as significant metabolic acidosis.

Pearls

- Be sure you understand and know how to apply your agency's policy or medical protocol for physical and chemical restraint.
- Restrain the patient on their side whenever possible to avoid aspiration. Do not restrain a patient in the prone position.
- Thoroughly document:
  - the circumstances surrounding the encounter with the patient,
  - the reason physical restraint was required,

- what other measures were attempted and failed,
- exactly what method(s) were used to restrain the patient and for how long,
- initial and frequent reassessments of patient's physiologic and mental status.

- Maintain continuous observation of the restrained patient and a high index of suspicion for excited delirium.

Pitfalls

- Not providing adequate assessment or monitoring to discover and manage urgent medical problems.
- Taking it personally. Resist the urge to take your displeasure out on the patient, tempting as it may be.
- Lack of an adequate agency policy or medical protocol for physical and chemical restraint that is aligned with state law and in sync with local law enforcement practice.

Selected Readings

Cheney PR, Gossett L, Fullerton-Gleason L, et al. Relationship of restraint use, patient injury, and assaults on EMS personnel. *Prehosp Emerg Care.* 2006;10(2):207–212.

Coburn VA, Mycyk MB. Physical and chemical restraints. *Emerg Med Clin North Am,* 2009; 27(4):655–667.

Kupas DF, Wydro GC. NAEMSP position paper: Patient restraint in emergency medical services systems. *Prehosp Emerg Care.* 2002;6(3):340–345.

Reich J. Behavioral Emergencies. In: Krohmer J, Sahni R, Schwartz B, Wang H, eds. *Emergency Medical Services: Clinical Practice and Systems Oversight.* Vol. 1. *Clinical Aspects of Prehospital Medicine.* Dubuque, IA: Kendall Hunt; 2009:360–372.

116

DO NOT OVERDIAGNOSE ANXIETY

DAVID PERSSE, MD, FACEP

Anxiety disorders are the most common, most frequently occurring mental disorders, and patients with anxiety-related issues are frequently encountered by EMS providers. Many patients with anxiety disorders will experience physical symptoms related to their underlying anxiety. They often will seek medical attention through the emergency care system for physical symptoms, not always recognizing their anxiety is the cause of their symptoms. Conversely, emergency care providers often incorrectly assume that a person's physical symptoms are due to anxiety. It has been estimated that among emergency center patients, panic and anxiety disorders are found in 2.7%. Despite the high prevalence rates of anxiety disorders, they often are underrecognized and undertreated clinical problems. The most common anxiety disorders that were formerly classified are listed below:

- Anxiety due to a general medical condition
- Substance-induced anxiety disorder
- Generalized anxiety disorder
- Panic disorder
- Acute stress disorder
- Post-traumatic stress disorder (PTSD)
- Adjustment disorder with anxious features
- Obsessive–compulsive disorder (OCD)
- Social phobia, also referred to as social anxiety disorder

Anxiety disorders appear to be caused by an interaction of biopsychosocial factors, which interact with situations, stress, or trauma to produce clinically significant syndromes. Each patient's symptoms will depend on the specific anxiety disorder and the level of stressor. Long-term non-EMS therapy, usually consists of a combination of pharmacotherapy and/or psychotherapy. It is estimated that the risk of getting an anxiety disorder, including post-traumatic stress syndrome, is as high as 10% over a patient's lifetime.

The biggest pitfall in the care of patients is to assume that their complaint is a result of an anxiety disorder. Other organic causes of the patient's presentation must be ruled out before that determination can be made. The diagnosis of one of the anxiety disorders is complex and time consuming. Symptoms can include muscle tension, trembling, twitching, aching, soreness, cold and clammy hands, dry mouth, sweating, nausea or diarrhea, or urinary frequency. Anxiety attacks can mimic or accompany nearly every acute disorder of the heart or lungs, including heart attacks and angina (chest pain). Conversely, nearly every acute disorder of the heart or lungs, including heart attacks and angina, can induce anxiety. A complete history and physical examination along with laboratory and often times, imaging studies, as well as a detailed psychiatric interview is required to make the diagnosis. This is primarily because so many other illness and pathologic conditions can induce anxiety. Anxiety is often a natural symptom of an unrecognized underlying illness. The definitive diagnosis of anxiety is significantly beyond the ability of most emergency centers and certainly the out-of-hospital environment.

The differential diagnosis of anxiety is long and diverse. There are other psychological disorders including post-traumatic stress, OCD, major depressive disorder, schizophrenia, etc. As mentioned, many cardiac and pulmonary disorders can also present with anxiety symptoms. These include hypoxia, hypotension, hypoglycemia, myocardial infarction, pulmonary embolism, left ventricular failure, right ventricular failure, etc. In the acute, emergency setting the EMS provider must consider symptomatology of other medical disorders, which may present with anxiety as the patient's primary symptom. These will include, but not be limited to the diseases and symptoms listed in *Table 116.1*.

EMS providers should NEVER determine that a patient's acute anxious behavior is due to an anxiety disorder of any type. All other possibilities must

TABLE 116.1   **SERIOUS DISEASES PRESENTING WITH "ANXIETY"**

DISEASE	RELATED SYMPTOMS
Angina and myocardial infarction	Dyspnea, chest pain, palpitations, diaphoresis
Cardiac dysrhythmias	Palpitations, dyspnea, syncope
Mitral valve prolapse	Palpitations, chest pain
Pulmonary embolus	Dyspnea, hyperpnea, chest pain
Asthma	Dyspnea, wheezing
Hyperthyroidism	Palpitations, diaphoresis, tachycardia, heat intolerance
Hypoglycemia	Anger, confusion
Pheochromocytoma	Headache, diaphoresis, hypertension
Hypoparathyroidism	Muscle cramps, paresthesias
Transient Ischemic Attacks	Confusion, syncope, weakness
Sepsis	Hyperpnea, fever, weakness
Seizure disorders	Confusion, disorientation

be considered more likely, and the patient managed in that light. A patient, or their family member, may tell you the patient has an anxiety disorder diagnosis. In that case, the patient or perhaps their family member may even be able to tell you that the signs and symptoms the patient is exhibiting are consistent with their anxiety disorder, and that may be helpful. However, even in that setting it is still the responsibility of the EMS provider to treat the patient with a high degree of suspicion for the long and varied differential diagnoses listed above. Patients with anxiety disorders can still suffer from any of the other pathologies and as a result trigger an anxiety or panic reaction. Remember, anxiety disorders are caused by an interaction of biopsychosocial factors, which interact with situations, stress, or trauma to produce clinically significant syndromes. The hypoxia resulting from a pulmonary embolism could certainly be the trigger for anxious behavior in a patient with a previous diagnosis of anxiety disorder, just as in you!

SELECTED READINGS

Karno M, Golding JM, Sorenson SB, et al. The epidemiology of obsessive-compulsive disorder in five US communities. *Arch Gen Psychiatry.* 1988;45(12):1094–1099.

Kessler RC, McGonagle KA, Zhao S, et al. Lifetime and 12-month prevalence of DSM-III-R psychiatric disorders in the United States. Results from the National Comorbidity Survey. *Arch Gen Psychiatry.* 1994;51(1):8–19.

Klein E, Linn S, Colin V, et al. Anxiety disorders among patients in a general emergency service in Israel. *Psychiatr Serv.* 1995;46(5):488–492.

Magee WJ, Eaton WW, Wittchen HU, et al. Agoraphobia, simple phobia, and social phobia in the National Comorbidity Survey. *Arch Gen Psychiatry.* 1996;53(2):159–168.

Stein MB, Stein DJ. Social anxiety disorder. *Lancet.* 2008;371(9618):1115–1125.

Wittchen HU, Fehm L. Epidemiology, patterns of comorbidity, and associated disabilities of social phobia. *Psychiatr Clin North Am.* 2001;24(4):617–641.

Yates WR, Bernstein BE, Bessman E, et al. Anxiety disorders. Accessed at http://emedicine.medscape.com/article/286227-overview.

117

Don't assume the intoxicated patient is just drunk

Corey M. Slovis, MD

"He is just drunk" is so easy to say, but unfortunately diagnosing someone with alcohol intoxication and blaming alcohol for a patient's alterations
in mental status can be a potentially fatal error. Yes, most times, drunks
are just drunk—but this always needs to be a diagnosis of exclusion. Paramedics must be very vigilant to rule out all other obvious causes of altered
mental status (AMS) and must be sure they follow a number of the Ten
Commandments of Emergency Medicine.

Specifically (1) Assume the Worst, (2) "Trust No One, Believe Nothing, Not Even Yourself" and (3) When in Doubt, Always Err on the Side
of the Patient.

Assume the Worst

The best thing the patient might be is just drunk, but the worst thing might
be something far more serious. Thus whenever you are faced with a patient
who appears drunk, even if they smell of alcohol, be sure to assess the
patient for the other causes of AMS.

Although there are many ways to classify AMS, subdividing AMS into
five basic causes seems optimal. Since the first thing we do in EMS and
Emergency Medicine is Secure the ABCs, the first, potential cause of AMS
is *Vital Sign Abnormalities*. Patients should be assessed for relatively normal
blood pressure, pulse rate, respiratory rate, oxygen saturation, and whether
they feel very febrile or extremely cold. Shocky patients with profound
hypotension, bradycardiac patients with third-degree heart block and a
pulse of 30, hypercarbic patients with lung disease and hypoventilation,
hypoxic patients with fever and delirium can all appear to be intoxicated
with alcohol, some might have even been drinking too. Thus "a drunk" with
grossly abnormal vital signs needs all abnormalities addressed before care
is withheld due to erroneously attributing these alterations to alcohol.

After the ABCs are secured, we should always think about narcan and
glucose for AMS. This brings us to the second major category of AMS
causes: *Toxic-Metabolic*. Although alcohol is one toxic-metabolic cause,
there are more important diseases to think about first. A fingerstick glucose estimate must be done on every "drunk", every time, every patient.
Hypoglycemia may look initially exactly like alcohol intoxication, but can
cause irreversible brain damage and even death if not recognized and

treated. Diabetic ketoacidosis (DKA) and severe hyperglycemia and dehydration can also make a severely ill patient appear intoxicated. DKA can even be caused by alcohol binging and not using enough, or any, insulin. Other toxic-metabolic causes include cocaine, amphetamines, PCP, thyrotoxicosis, and withdrawal syndromes. All of us have to remember that chronic intoxication and alcohol dependence can make the alcoholic at risk for Wernicke's encephalopathy. This syndrome may cause a staggering gait, eye findings and also AMS that may make the patient appear intoxicated.

The third category of AMS is *Structural*. This includes anything within the brain and central nervous system. Head trauma causing a subdural hematoma, epidural bleed, cerebral contusion or any intracranial bleeding can make a patient appear intoxicated. Even worse, drunks fall and hit their heads making them both drunk and having an expanding mass lesion intracranially!

The fourth category for causing AMS that may mimic being drunk is *Infectious Causes*. This includes enchephalitis, sepsis syndrome, early meningitis, and any infection that can cause fever, dehydration, and confusion.

The final category of AMS is *Psychiatric*. Although not usually life threatening, it is important to remember that psychiatric illness may make a patient appear intoxicated. These patients like all others, should be treated with respect and patience so that they do not become agitated or defensively violent.

Trust No One. Believe No One. Not even Yourself

Please be careful. If you decide someone is just drunk, observe them carefully during transport. If anything changes abruptly—don't blame it on the effects of alcohol—restart your evaluation for the real cause of the deterioration.

When in Doubt, Err on the Side of the Patient

Our job is to help all patients and the public. If there is any chance at all that the patient might be more than just suffering from alcohol intoxication, do your best to help that patient even if it means doing more rather than less.

I believe five rules apply to evaluating and treating any patient who appears intoxicated and is likely "just drunk."

1) Always assess and treat any significant vital sign abnormality.
2) All patients with altered mental status must have their glucose checked and the use of narcan considered for lethargy or coma.

3) Alcohol intoxication does not cause focal neurologic findings or unequal pupils—think trauma or CNS disease.

4) Most alcoholics have multiple medical problems—evaluate every patient the same way with a full history and physical examination.

5) Always transport an intoxicated patient, or be sure they are going to get care, detox or observation by some other public or private entity.

SELECTED READINGS

Lacherade JC, Jacqueminet S, Preiser JC. An overview of hypoglycemia in the critically ill. *J Diabetes Sci Technol.* 2009;3(6):1242–1249.

Marx JA. The varied faces of Wernicke's encephalopathy. *J Emerg Med.* 1985;3:411–413.

Meador SR, Slovis CM, Wrenn KD. EMS Bill of Rights: What every patient deserves. *JEMS.* 2003;28(3):70–75.

O'Malley GF. Emergency department management of the salicylate-poisoned patient. *Emerg Med Clin North Am.* 2007;25:333–346.

Wrenn K, Slovis CM. The ten commandments of emergency medicine. *Ann Emerg Med.* 1991; 20:1146–1147.

118

CONSIDER NEUROLEPTIC MALIGNANT SYNDROME AND SEROTONIN SYNDROME IN PSYCHIATRIC PATIENTS

ELIZABETH M. LICALZI, MD

AMANDA G. WILSON, MD

The transport of patients with psychiatric disease is becoming more common as is the use of psychotropic medications. With that in mind, it is important for EMS personnel to be aware of potentially life-threatening side effects that some psychiatric medications possess. Two relatively uncommon, but potentially lethal adverse drug reactions include serotonin syndrome and neuroleptic malignant syndrome (NMS). Both of these syndromes involve mental status changes, autonomic hyperactivity, and neuromuscular abnormalities. Since early mild symptoms are commonly overlooked, it is essential that EMS providers be aware of the clinical features and treatment of these syndromes in order to initiate therapy and prevent further deterioration (see *Table 118.1*).

DIAGNOSIS AND CLINICAL FEATURES

Serotonin syndrome results from excess serotonin in the central nervous system causing a number of abnormal clinical findings. It may result from an increase in a serotonergic agent or a drug interaction. Serotonin syndrome occurs rapidly and may also occur from an overdose of a serotonergic agent. About 60% of patients with serotonin syndrome present within 6 hours after taking the medication. Common drugs associated with serotonin syndrome include monoamine oxidase inhibitors (MAOIs), tricyclic antidepressants (TCAs), selective serotonin uptake inhibitors (SSRIs), opiates, dextromethorphan, and drugs of abuse, that is, MDMA (ecstasy). The typical patient with serotonin syndrome is taking psychotropic medications for a psychiatric disorder. Mild cases of serotonin syndrome can be easily missed due to early nonspecific symptoms including tachycardia, diarrhea, and diaphoresis. If the offending medication is not removed, or the dose is increased, symptoms can rapidly worsen. On neurologic examination providers may note clonus and hyperreflexia, especially in the lower extremities, which are more specific clinical findings in serotonin syndrome. In addition, an unusual head-turning behavior described as repetitive rotation of the head with the neck in moderate extension has been described. Severe cases of serotonin syndrome can exhibit hypertension, tachycardia, agitated delirium, muscular rigidity, and hyperthermia.

TABLE 118.1 COMPARISON OF SEROTONIN SYNDROME AND NMS

	MEDICATION	TIME COURSE	VITALS	MUSCLE TONE	REFLEXES	MENTAL STATUS	LAB FINDINGS
SEROTONIN SYNDROME	SSRI, MAOI, TCA taken within 5 wks	Acute <12 hr	Fever Hypertension Tachycardia Tachypnea Mydriasis	Increased tone (>lower extremities)	Tremor Hyperreflexia Clonus Horizontal ocular clonus	Irritability Agitation Confusion	Rhabdomyolysis ↑Creatinine Metabolic acidosis DIC
NMS	Antipsychotic taken within 7 days (2–4 wks for depot)	Subacute 1–3 days	Hyperthermia Hypertension Tachycardia Tachypnea	"Lead pipe" rigidity in all muscle groups	Bradyreflexia	Stupor Mutism	Rhabdomyolysis ↑CPK Myoglobinuria ↑WBC Metabolic acidosis DIC

NMS results from a decrease of dopamine in the central nervous system due to medications that act as dopamine antagonists. It may occur in the context of a rapid increase in a neuroleptic medication. Common drugs associated with NMS include typical antipsychotics such as haloperidol (haldol) and chlorpromazine (thorazine) and atypical antipsychotics such as olanzapine (zyprexa), quetiapine (seroquel), and risperidone (risperdal). One should suspect NMS in a febrile patient after administration of a neuroleptic. Similar to serotonin syndrome, mild symptoms of NMS may be overlooked. Typical cases of NMS exhibit hyperthermia, altered mental status, mutism, autonomic symptoms, and muscle rigidity, which develop over a few days. As opposed to serotonin syndrome, individuals with NMS will exhibit rigidity that can become "lead pipe" in nature and will have bradyreflexia.

TREATMENT

Both serotonin syndrome and NMS are self-limiting illnesses. The most important aspect of treatment is removing the offending agent and providing supportive care such as intravenous fluids and correction of expected vital sign abnormalities. For serotonin syndrome, benzodiazepines should be used for agitation and myoclonus. Benzodiazepines, such as midazolam, lorazepam, or diazepam, may improve survival by decreasing autonomic tone (blood pressure and heart rate) and temperature. For NMS, specific drug therapies such as dantrolene, amantadine, and bromocriptine have an uncertain role in treatment and are not readily available in the prehospital setting. Aggressive cooling measures should be initiated if hyperthermia is present. It is important to avoid using restraints as much as possible in patients with serotonin syndrome or NMS, because they may cause lactic acidosis or an increase in temperature as the patient fights against them. In both conditions, rhabdomyolysis can lead to hyperkalemia and renal failure. It is important to have these patients on the monitor, so the ECG changes seen in hyperkalemia can be rapidly identified. These include peaked T waves, loss of the P wave, and a wide QRS complex. When severe, serotonin syndrome and NMS can lead to death from medical complications.

While serotonin syndrome and NMS are uncommon clinical entities it is important for EMS providers to consider the diagnosis in the right clinical setting. Rapid recognition will allow for prompt initiation of treatment that can be life saving. Psychiatric patients, who have abnormal vital signs, abnormal head or body movements, or who are stiff, should be carefully evaluated and discussed with medical control.

Pitfalls

- Not considering serotonin syndrome and NMS with psychiatric patients that present with any of the following: Altered mental status, vital sign changes, or neuromuscular abnormalities.

- Not recognizing that serotonin syndrome can result from an overdose of medications or illicit substances such as meperidine (demerol), dextromethorphan, and MDMA.

- Not documenting a good physical examination in patients suspected of having NMS or serotonin syndrome.

- Inappropriate use of physical restraints, which can worsen serotonin syndrome and NMS.

- Not promptly initiating supportive care, as both NMS and serotonin syndrome can be lethal.

Selected Readings

Boyer E, Shannon M. The serotonin syndrome. *N Engl J Med.* 2005;352:1112–1120.

Fricchione G, Huffman J, Bush G, et al. Catatonia, neuroleptic malignant syndrome, and serotonin syndrome. In Stern TA, Rosenbaum JF, et al., eds. *Massachusetts General Hospital Comprehensive Clinical Psychiatry.* New York: Mosby; 2008.

Nisijima K, Shioda K, Iwamura T, Neuroleptic malignant syndrome and serotonin syndrome. *Progr Brain Res.* 2007;162:81–103.

119

DON'T MISS THE DIAGNOSIS
OF EXCITED DELIRIUM

JOSEPH EUGENE HOLLEY, JR, MD, FACEP

Excited delirium is a temporary disturbance in consciousness and cognition, patients are disoriented, have very disorganized and inconsistent thought processes, are unable to distinguish reality from hallucinations, have disturbances in speech, and are combative or violent. The typical patient with excited delirium is often aggressive and agitated, confrontational, and misdiagnosed. They present tremendous challenges to law enforcement and EMS providers. The rapid changes in mental status seen in patients with excited delirium are frequently thought to be due to drug ingestion, alcohol, head injury, hypoglycemia, or psychiatric illness. In addition, these patients often seem to be impervious to pain, and are usually hyperthermic, and tachycardic. Due to their uncontrolled behavior, excited delirium patients are often the victims of law enforcement efforts to control their behavior with physical attempts to subdue them. The use of TASERs is common in this group of patients, and EMS providers must be cognizant of the consequences of an aggressive response by law enforcement.

The greatest pitfall pertaining to caring for the patient with excited delirium is failure to consider the diagnosis and rule out other underlying causes of delirium and agitation such as hypoxia, hypoglycemia, and trauma. Starting with behavior reported in 9-1-1 calls, an American College of Emergency Physicians (ACEP) task force said Prehospital Excited Delirium Syndrome should be presumed, if a patient is disoriented or not making sense, constantly physically active, impervious to pain, has superhuman strength, is sweating and breathing rapidly, has tactile hyperthermia, and fails to respond to a police presence. Attempts to gain insight into possible other causes, such as a history of hypoglycemia, can be obtained from callers, bystanders, or family members at the scene. Obvious signs of trauma or head injury may be visible from a safe distance, and EMS providers can also assess the scene for indications of alcohol or substance abuse, or other clues to alternate diagnoses.

Another pitfall in the care of patients with excited delirium is the lack of recognition of the serious, and potentially lethal, nature of the syndrome. Excited delirium is a medical entity, not solely a law enforcement issue, and providers must resist the temptation to just have these patients restrained and arrested. Potential complications of excited delirium include hyperthermia, hypovolemia, acidosis, rhabdomyolysis, and hyperkalemia. EMS agencies should have protocols for aggressively treating patients with excited delirium. The ACEP task force recommends immediate medical assessment and treatment once physical control is obtained. "Initial assessment should include . . . vital signs, cardiac monitoring, IV access, glucose measurement, pulse oximetry, supplement oxygen, and careful physical examination," the White Paper noted. Treatment should include rapid capture of the patient by law enforcement and administration of a sedative by EMS to calm the patient and allow for treatment. Many services use a benzodiazepine such as Versed via the needleless mucosal atomizer device, which allows for drug delivery with minimal risk of accidental needlestick to EMS and rapid drug delivery to the patient. Once the patient is calm and accessible, an IV of cooled normal saline is initiated and rapidly infused. Some services administer a prophylactic 1 amp of sodium bicarbonate for possible acidosis that results from prolonged struggle. If possible, cardiac monitoring is crucial so that ECG changes consistent with hyperkalemia, such as peaked T waves and a widening QRS, can be rapidly recognized and appropriately treated. It is also important to recognize that patients with excited delirium are at risk for sudden death so patients who unexpectedly become "quiet" need immediate attention.

In summary, patients with excited delirium must be quickly recognized and aggressively treated. Chemical sedation is important, as is aggressive rehydration, cooling, correction of metabolic disturbances, prevention of self-harm, careful monitoring, and rapid response in the event of a catastrophic deterioration in the patient's condition.

SELECTED READING

White Paper Report on Excited Delirium Syndrome, ACEP Excited Delirium Task Force, September 10, 2009.

120

KEEP YOURSELF SAFE ON THE SCENE

AMANDA G. WILSON, MD

Violence in the workplace is popularly discussed in the media today. But what if your workplace is someone's home, place of business, or a street corner? There is little discussion in the literature about violence in the pre-hospital setting. However, it has been found that violent situations occur in 5% of calls and that EMS personnel commonly under-document violence. The most common type of violence noted is verbal aggression. The EMS setting is unfortunately by its very nature a potential setup for violence against any responder as 14% of all EMS calls occur as a direct result of violence (*Table 120.1*). EMS providers have an occupational fatality rate that is higher than the general population and is similar to that of police officers and fire fighters (estimated at 12.7 fatalities per 100,000 EMS workers annually). This illustrates the need for EMS providers to be alert to scene and personal safety. **You must "size up the scene."** (*Table 120.2.*)

HOW TO HANDLE THE VIOLENT PATIENT

1) Tell the patient you are there to help. Avoid intense eye contact that may be perceived as threatening.
2) Acknowledge that they seem upset. Ask what is troubling them. Listen empathetically.
3) Don't be defensive or take statements personally.
4) Listen to your "gut." Those little hairs on the back of your neck are going up for a reason. If you sense this, back away and reassess the situation.
5) Don't play along with delusions, but don't try to challenge the delusion either.
6) Be honest. Don't lie.
7) Keep a comfortable distance (a leg length) while talking to the patient.
8) Don't make sudden moves. As you are talking and performing an assessment, explain calmly what you are doing along the way.
9) While performing an examination, don't forget to intermittently scan the scene and reassess for any potential danger.
10) Involve family/friends if they are comforting (remember they can be destabilizing as well).
11) Ask for police assistance if patient appears combative/violent.
12) If the patient does not respond to de-escalation techniques, restraints and/or medications may be necessary.

TABLE 120.1   TYPICAL VIOLENT CALL FEATURES

- Young patient
- Male sex
- ETOH/drugs involved
- Presence of police
- Apparent presence of gang members
- Perceived psychiatric disorder

- More likely to refuse transport
- Violence most likely to come from patient
- Violence may come from others on the scene

THE B-52 BOMBER AND BEYOND

- Remember that an emotionally disturbed patient may refuse treatment.
- If you perceive the patient to be at a reasonable risk to harm themselves, others, or are so impaired that they cannot care for themselves, you may provide needed care and/or transport even if they refuse.
- Benzodiazepines are the safest medications to use in the combative patient and have minimal side effects. They will treat agitated withdrawal states, combative psychiatric patients, and will not worsen NMS.
- A tried-and-true regimen in the hospital is the "cocktail regimen" of haloperidol 5 mg + lorazepam 2 mg + benztropine 1 mg PO or IM. Haloperidol works synergistically with lorazepam to produce a sedative effect. This combination produces a rapid tranquilization that is effective within 30 minutes and may be repeated in 30 minutes if needed. Patients may develop akathisia, dystonic reactions, and more rarely, NMS.
- You can start therapy in the field with lorazepam, or if you don't carry it then with either IV diazepam or with IV or IM midazolam. Diazepam cannot be given IM. Dosages vary, but 5 mg of diazepam IV is a common starting dose, as is 5 mg IM of midazolam or 2 mg IV.
- Avoid restraints if possible, as they are associated with increased morbidity and death.
- Have police present, if possible, when restraints are required.

TABLE 120.2   RED FLAGS FOR VIOLENCE WHEN SIZING UP THE SCENE

- Presence of weapons
- Yelling, cursing, loud voice
- Clenched fists, frequent movement, dilated pupils
- Hitting or throwing objects

- Posturing, moves from sitting to standing
- Staring, period of silence
- Invading personal space
- Verbally threatening
- Bystanders give history of violence

PITFALLS

- Not assessing the scene *before* care delivery.
- Failure to continually assess the environment as you are treating the patient.
- Not recognizing that you CAN (and should) defend yourself if an emotionally disturbed patient becomes assaultive.
- Failure to utilize chemical sedation if needed for provider and patient safety. Keep in mind that any of the benzodiazepines at the doses listed above work well for rapid tranquilization.

EMS providers often have to care for patients in less than ideal settings and it is important to remember that no matter how urgent the call, scene safety must prevail. Scene assessment must occur prior to patient assessment. Never forget that if you fail to keep yourself safe, you will not be able to provide care to your patients.

SELECTED READINGS

Allen MH, Currier GW, Hughes DH, et al. Treatment of behavioral emergencies: a summary of the expert consensus guidelines. *J Psychiatr Pract*. 2003;9(1):16–38.

First Responder National Standard Curriculum, www.nhtsa.gov/people/injury/ems/pub/frnsc.pdf.

Hughes D. Acute psychopharmacological management of the aggressive psychotic patient. *Psychiatr Serv*. 1999;50(9):1135–1137.

Hughes D, Kleespies P. Treating aggression in the psychiatric emergency service. *J Clin Psychiatry*. 2003;64(suppl 4):10–15.

Mock EF, Wrenn KD, Wright SW, et al. Prospective field study of violence in emergency medical services calls. *Ann Emerg Med*. 1998;32:33–36.

121

RECOGNIZE THE MALINGERER!

AMANDA G. WILSON, MD

Malingering is not considered a medical or psychiatric disorder, but rather the feigning of symptoms or disease to obtain something tangible. A common example is the person caught on video tape by an insurance company lifting heavy objects while on worker's compensation.

DIAGNOSIS AND CLINICAL FEATURES

The DSM-IV TR, which is the official disease defining document used by psychiatrists and psychologists, defines malingering as:

"... the intentional production of false or grossly exaggerated physical or psychological symptoms, motivated by external incentives such as avoiding military duty, avoiding work, obtaining financial compensation, evading criminal prosecution, or obtaining drugs."

By far, the most commonly malingered symptom is vague pain. Pain is by nature a subjective complaint and therefore difficult to confirm. Typical examples of pain complaints include: Lower back pain, chest pain, whiplash injury/neck pain, abdominal pain, tooth pain, headache, and post-concussive syndrome. Although the precise prevalence of malingering is unknown and is thought to be underdiagnosed, it is thought to be more common in men than women and more common in settings such as prisons, the military, and worker's compensation review boards. Malingering is most suspected by clinicians when they see a patient with a chronic pain complaint. EMS providers should know the "red flags" for malingering listed in *Table 121.1*.

CLINICAL APPROACH

The biggest potential pitfall when dealing with this group of patients in the prehospital setting is to assume that they are just malingering. A nonjudgmental and neutral approach should be utilized, and the EMS provider must be vigilant not to miss a true diagnosis in this challenging population. It is not uncommon for EMS providers to transport these patients on a recurrent basis (the "frequent flyer") and it is easy to become complacent and assume nothing is wrong again. However, it is critical that these patients be treated like everyone else and have an appropriate workup initiated on the basis of presenting complaint. For example, the patient whose chest pain is only relieved with "IV dilaudid" (hydromorphone) may still really be having an acute myocardial infarction (MI). EMS

TABLE 121.1 "RED FLAGS"

- Antisocial personality disorder
- Uncooperativeness during evaluation
- Involvement of worker's compensation, disability, or other litigation
- Objective findings that are not consistent with the patient's disability
- Presenting during "off hours" such as nights, weekends, holidays when it is harder for the ER to obtain medical records
- Dramatic or atypical presentation
- Requests for a specific drug—"the only medicine that has worked for me is IV dilaudid…"
- History of substance misuse
- Angry, yelling, hostile, or demanding
- Eagerly endorses the presence of all symptoms asked by the EMS provider
- Anger at a "clean bill of health"
- Lack of adherence to a treatment regimen

providers must recognize that angry feelings toward the patient can lead to faulty and potentially dangerous medical decisions. Objective tests are necessary when malingering is suspected, but one also must avoid iatrogenesis in the process.

During examination, make note of:

- Exaggerated facial expressions of pain
- Superficial or nonanatomic pain with palpation
- Lack of symptoms of distress when the affected area is examined while the patient is distracted
- Overreaction
- Symptoms produced with axonal loading or rotation

TREATMENT

The patient has no investment in "being well." The symptoms do not typically resolve until the patient has attained his or her desired goal, that is, the patient gets pain medications. Try to avoid confronting the patient in the prehospital setting because it will often compromise rapid care and transport and cause unnecessary conflict. The EMS provider must be aware of the potential for manipulation and avoid acting as an accomplice in the patient's deception such as administering pain medications when not indicated. Instead, transport the patient and let them know they can be better evaluated once they reach the emergency department.

PEARLS

- Malingering is the feigning of symptoms or disease for secondary gain such as disability, narcotics, worker's compensation, or food and shelter at the hospital.
- The most common EMS presentations are a vague pain complaints including "Chest Pain."
- Confrontation is not advised.
- Objective testing in line with the patient's complaints.
- Do not let anger towards a patient influence your decision making.
- "Frequent Flyers" should be transported for evaluation. Do not assume that they are always malingering.

SELECTED READINGS

Ford CV. Factitious disorders and malingering. In: Ebert MH, Loosen PT, Nurcombe B, Leckman JF, eds. *Current Diagnosis and Treatment: Psychiatry*. 2nd ed. New York: McGraw-Hill; 2008.

McDermott BE, Feldman MD. Malingering in the medical setting. *Psychiatr Clin North Am.* 2007;30:645–662.

Mendelson G, Mendelson D. Malingering pain in the medicolegal context. *Clin J Pain.* 2004;20:423–432.

Smith F. Factitious disorders and malingering In: Stern TA, Rosenbaum JF, et al., eds *Massachusetts General Hospital Comprehensive Clinical Psychiatry*. Philadelphia, PA: Mosby; 2008.

122

Be wary of the suicidal patient!

Amanda G. Wilson, MD

Suicide is intentional harm to oneself with the intent of death and suicidal patients are considered a medical emergency. EMS providers must have a good understanding of this entity in order to deal with patient's threatening suicide and those who attempt it. Suicide is the 11th leading cause of death in the United States. Suicide attempts account for more than 500,000 emergency department visits per year and completed suicides account for more than 30,000 deaths per year. It is estimated that as many as two–thirds of suicide completers visit a physician within one month of suicide. Women *attempt* suicide more frequently; however, men *complete* suicide more often than women. Almost 20% of suicide completers are intoxicated at the time of death. The most common means of suicide completion is by firearms, suffocation is the second most common cause, and poisoning is the third. Drug ingestion is the most common cause of an unsuccessful attempt at suicide. All EMS providers should know the "Red Flags" for suicide (*Table 122.1*).

Clinical Approach

During initial evaluation, the EMS provider's goal is to *develop a good working relationship* and rapport. Try to *gather information* from available family and friends as possible. *Ask specifically about suicidal thoughts* or plan to commit suicide in any patient you suspect is at risk. If possible get the details of the suicide plan, and ask questions like "where were you going to do it, do you have a gun, have you written a suicide note" etc. Remember that asking about suicide does not put the idea in a patient's mind. Evaluate how much preparation has been put into the suicide plan. Ask about recent stressors or acute events in the patient's life. Look for hopelessness or anhedonia (lack of interest). Please note that if you deem the situation to be life or death, obtaining formal consent before speaking to a patient's loved ones may not be necessary to assure or investigate safety.

In the prehospital setting, always note the following:

- Presence of weapons, pill bottles, or poisons on the scene
- A suicide note (bring with the patient)
- Presence of illicit substances
- Conditions at the scene, comment on the scene if the living environment was in disrepair, pill bottles were scattered across the floor, etc.

TABLE 122.1 "RED FLAGS" RISK FACTORS FOR SUICIDE

- Male gender
- Older than 65 years of age
- White or Native American
- History of suicide attempts
- Widowed or divorced
- Firearms in the household
- Co-morbid medical disease
- Substance abuse
- Clinical depression or schizophrenia
- Recent adverse event, such as job loss or death of a loved one
- Recent hospital discharge
- Family history of suicide

Examples of questions to ask about suicide:

- Have you had thoughts of giving up or wished you could go to sleep and never wake up?
- Have you had any thoughts of killing yourself? How often? When was the last time?
- Have you thought of a plan? What steps have you taken for it?
- Do you have a gun or other weapons?
- How close have you come to going forward with it? Have you held the gun or knife in your hands? Have you held the pill bottle in your hands?
- Do you use any alcohol or other substances?
- Has anything changed in your life recently?
- Have you ever attempted suicide before? Has anyone in your family committed suicide?
- Have you been diagnosed with depression, anxiety, or another mental disorder?
- Are you hearing any voices? Are they commanding you in any way?

TREATMENT

First assure a safe environment, then address any acute medical issues and stabilize the patient medically. The patient may need to be searched and detained as needed for safety reasons. A patient at risk for suicide who threatens to leave before a suicide assessment is made may be detained involuntarily in accordance with the state statutes that deal with those at imminent risk to themselves or others. This allows the patient to be transported to a facility where a thorough psychiatric evaluation can commence. Pitfalls in the prehospital setting:

- Leaving the patient alone
- Not assuring a safe environment
- Once the patient is secured, not searching the patient for any objects of self-harm, pills, etc.

- Inappropriate use or lack of thorough documentation of physical or chemical restraints
- Allowing a patient who you deem at risk for suicide to refuse care
- Not communicating important patient or family comments about suicide to Emergency Department staff

PEARLS

- Suicidal patients should be evaluated emergently.
- Use a nonjudgmental, empathetic approach to the suicidal patient.
- Specific questions about whether someone has suicidal thoughts, plan, and intent must be asked.
- A suicidal patient may require involuntary detainment for further assessment and management.
- For 24-hour nationwide hotline access, call 1–800–SUICIDE (1–800–784–2433) or 1–800–273–TALK (1–800–273–8255) or visit the website (http://www.suicidehotlines.com/).

SELECTED READINGS

Brendel RW, Lagomasino IT, Perlis RH, et al. The suicidal patient. In: Stern TA, Rosenbaum JF, Fava M, et al., eds. *Massachusetts General Hospital Comprehensive Clinical Psychiatry.* 1st ed. Philadelphia, PA: Mosby; 2008.

Hirschfeld R., Russell J. Assessment and treatment of suicidal patients. *N Engl J Med.* 1997; 337:910–915.

Shader RI. Assessment and treatment of suicide risk. In: Shader RI, ed. *Manual of Psychiatric Therapeutics.* 3rd ed. Philadelphia, PA: Lippincott Williams & Wilkins; 2002.

123

DON'T MISS PULMONARY EMBOLISM IN THE PREGNANT PATIENT!

ANDERS APGAR, MD, FACOG

Shortness of breath is a pregnancy complaint so ubiquitous that it is possible for the caregiver to become complacent when assessing the acuity of the patient's clinical situation. While commonly a nonthreatening symptom, shortness of breath may overshadow a variety of other potentially lethal problems because physiologic adaptations in pregnancy occur in every major organ system of the body. In the pulmonary system, normal physiologic changes occur and offset each other to maintain the inspiratory capacity. Although it is intuitive that the growing uterus would impede the diaphragm during inspiration, changes that occur in the ribcage negate the inhibitory effects of the gravid uterus on the diaphragm. Specific etiologies for shortness of breath in pregnancy, real or perceived, are not known. The pulmonary system compensations play a significant role in maintaining lung capacity and oxygenation in the pregnant patient.

COMPENSATORY CHANGES

Changes in the cardiac and hematologic systems cannot be discounted when considering shortness of breath in the pregnant patient. Necessary increases in cardiac output are created by increases in both heart rate and stroke volume. Blood volumes increase throughout most of the pregnancy, beginning in the first trimester. To accommodate this volume, the capacitance of the circulatory system increases, including the left ventricle of the heart. Edema caused by this increase in blood volume may potentiate venous stasis. The activity of certain clotting factors in the coagulation cascade is increased in pregnancy while others are unchanged or decreased. Overall, there is no change in clotting or bleeding times in the normal pregnant patient. Decreases in exercise tolerance caused by shortness of breath during activities of daily living and the resultant sedentary behavior can potentiate deep venous thrombosis and therefore pulmonary embolus. Furthermore, lower extremity swelling, caused by deep venous thrombosis, may be incorrectly interpreted as normal physiologic changes. Virchow's triad of risk factors for thromboembolism applies as aptly in pregnancy as in other pathophysiologic conditions. Venous stasis, vascular injury, and hypercoagulability: These common factors mandate that EMS providers consider pulmonary embolus early in the evaluation of the pregnant patient complaining of shortness of breath.

Signs and Symptoms

The pregnant patient suffering from a pulmonary embolus will commonly present with chest pain and shortness of breath. The patient may appear anxious, diaphoretic, and may verbalize an impending sense of doom. Alternatively, respiratory symptoms such as cough or tachycardia may be quite subtle and underwhelming. Lung sounds are usually normal though rales may be found on physical examination. The most common, but nonspecific, ECG finding in the setting of pulmonary embolism is sinus tachycardia. A large, hemodynamically significant pulmonary embolism may result in tachycardia and right heart strain (right axis deviation) on the ECG. Finally, the presence of a large S wave in lead 1, a Q wave in lead 3, and T wave inversions in lead 3 (the "S1Q3T3" pattern) may enhance provider suspicion of pulmonary embolism. Definitive diagnosis of a blot clot is usually made in the hospital setting. Although the patient suffering from shortness of breath may not be able to give an extensive past medical history, it is important to elicit as much information as possible from anybody on the scene, and pay particular attention to events preceding the symptoms. A thorough medical history might include questions about pulmonary disease, a prior deep venous thrombosis, or an autoimmune disorder such as lupus or rheumatoid arthritis. These factors may increase a clinician's suspicion for pulmonary embolism.

Treatment

Presumptive treatment in the field is appropriate and without significant sequelae if the diagnosis should be inaccurate. Mortality from pulmonary embolus is significant (approximately 10%) and medications for treatment present comparatively little threat to the mother or fetus. Initial prehospital intervention should focus upon maintaining maternal oxygenation, intravenous access, hydration, and pain relief. Protocols may exist for anticoagulant therapy in the prehospital setting, but this should only be considered after communication with the receiving hospital. In the hospital setting, patients will frequently require treatment with heparin. Critically ill patients may receive systemic thrombolytics or surgical embolectomy (clot removal).

Summary

Although shortness of breath is a frequent complaint in normal pregnant and postpartum patients, it is important to consider pulmonary embolism early in the evaluation of a patient with any pulmonary or cardiac complaints. There exists a multitude of common non–cardiac, non–circulatory etiologies of shortness of breath in pregnancy, including asthma, upper respiratory infections, and anxiety. Shortness of breath, however, should not be evaluated without first considering pulmonary embolism in the differential diagnosis.

SELECTED READINGS

American College of Obstetricians and Gynecologists. *Practice Bulletin #19: Thromboembolism in Pregnancy*. Washington, DC: American College of Obstetricians and Gynecologists; 2000.

Clark SL, Phelan JP, Hankins G, et al. *Handbook of Critical Care Obstetrics*. Boston, MA: Blackwell Scientific Publications; 1994:79–88.

Cunningham FG, Gant NF, Leveno KJ, et al. *Williams Obstetrics*. 21st ed. New York, NY: McGraw-Hill; 2001:1234–1240.

Gabbe SG, Niebyl JR, Simpson JL. *Obstetrics: Normal and Problem Pregnancies*. 3rd ed. New York, NY: Churchill Livingstone; 1996:1019–1021.

Leveno KJ, Cunningham FG, Gant NF, et al. *Williams Manual of Obstetrics*. 21st ed. New York, NY: McGraw-Hill; 2003:506–512.

124

DON'T GET TANGLED UP IN A CORD EMERGENCY!

MORGAN M. WALKER, BA, RN, BSN

Many cord complications are difficult to recognize in the prehospital setting without the use of fetal monitoring. However, some cord emergencies can occur during delivery, especially precipitous deliveries outside of a labor and delivery department. Understanding how to manage these conditions will help avert maternal and fetal complications. The two most significant abnormal cord presentations encountered in prehospital settings are cord prolapse (vasa previa) and the nuchal cord.

Cord prolapse, or vasa previa, is a rare but serious situation in which the umbilical cord precedes (overt) or is present alongside (occult) the presenting part during attempted vaginal delivery of the fetus. This is an emergency because cord compression compromises blood–gas exchange and increases risk of vessel rupture leading to fetal exsanguination. Cord prolapse, if severe and untreated, can lead to fetal demise. Vasa previa can occur at any cervical dilation. Only overt prolapse is diagnosed during pre-hospital care, either through visualization of the protruding cord or palpation of the cord during examination. A thorough patient assessment should include maternal vital signs, evaluation of fetal heart rate (FHR) when possible (reminder: Normal FHR 110–160), and examination for vaginal bleeding and labor status. Internal vaginal exams are discouraged in the prehospital setting. Contractions that occur less than two minutes apart and crowning of the fetal head may herald imminent delivery. Delivery of the fetus is imperative. The priority of prehospital care therefore remains transport to a facility capable of performing an emergent cesarean section. Cesarean delivery is considered mandatory especially in the presence of severe vaginal bleeding. In general, the faster this is accomplished the better, but there are some conflicting data showing presence of acidemia in neonates even when delivered within this suggested time frame. Prehospital providers should initiate large-bore intravenous access in anticipation of maternal complications and the need for immediate operative intervention. Acidosis, or a low blood pH, is associated with fetal distress and poor oxygenation. Neonates with persistently low pH levels are at risk for cardiologic, neurologic, and pulmonary complications. In the time before the infant can be safely delivered, there are two primary recommendations for management to improve fetal outcome:

- Funic decompression—The most common method of indirectly restoring flow through a compressed umbilical cord. The examiner's hand is maintained in the vagina to elevate the presenting part off of the cord. Steep Trendelenburg or knee–chest positions can also help alleviate pressure. Manipulation of the cord is not recommended due to the risk of vessel rupture.

- Bladder filling—Through a Foley catheter, 500 to 700 mL of NS is infused into the bladder to elevate the presenting part. The patient is maintained in the Trendelenburg position. One study showed that this technique, when combined with a tocolytic, was 100% effective in 51 cases with a mean interval from diagnosis to delivery of 35 minutes.

Risk factors that can be determined outside of the hospital through interview with the client or physical assessment include multiparity, multiple gestation, prematurity, fetal malpresentation, polyhydramnios, placenta previa, pregnancies conceived following use of assistive reproductive technologies, and rupture of membranes. Lack of prenatal care could mean that this information is deficient. According to one case series, neonatal survival was reported in 59/61 cases (97%) when vasa previa was suspected antenatally. When vasa previa was not considered, survival was reported in only 41/94 (44%) cases. Efficient diagnosis, management, and cesarean delivery are key interventions in the management of vasa previa. Asking about risk factors and obtaining a thorough gynecologic history can help you prepare for the possibility of a cord emergency.

A nuchal cord is defined as a loop of the umbilical cord 360 degrees around the fetal neck. This is a more common finding during delivery, with a prevalence of 15% to 34% as compared to cord prolapse (<1%), and can lead to similar negative fetal outcomes. A single nuchal cord is most common but the umbilical cord may be wrapped several times. There are two types, "A" (able to undo itself) and "B" (cannot undo itself). The nuchal cord may be mild to severely constricting, greater severity evidenced by disruption of the smooth contour of the fetal neck referred to as the "divot sign."

Again, it is impossible to diagnose this condition in a prehospital environment prior to active delivery, but may have been shown on ultrasound if the patient has had sufficient prenatal care. Interview questions should include frequency of fetal movement, and as always management should include rapid transport to a C-section capable facility. If vaginal delivery is necessary prior to hospital arrival, management should not differ from traditional delivery protocols. The nuchal cord should be gently unwrapped as soon as there is sufficient room to do so in order to prevent possible rupture or the adverse effects of cord compression. If you are unable to unwrap the cord gently, do not forcefully attempt to untangle the cord because rupture, avulsion, and serious fetal/neonatal hemorrhage can occur. Regional protocols and medical direction may authorize you to clamp and cut a cord that is severely constricting. There are many potential obstetric complications during pregnancy and delivery which can lead to negative outcomes for the mother and fetus. Being mindful of these possibilities, providers should perform a thorough history and physical examination in order to fully evaluate any present situation. Knowledge of effective interventions and care in their execution will improve the outcome for mother and fetus alike. Don't get all tangled up in an umbilical cord emergency!

PREHOSPITAL PEARLS

- Ask about maternal history: This may clue you in to problems during labor.
- Cord prolapse is an emergency! Elevate the presenting fetal part off of the cord and transport to a facility with emergency obstetric capabilities.
- Gently attempt to unwrap the nuchal cord. If unsuccessful, clamp and cut the cord according to local protocol and medical direction.

SELECTED READINGS

Barss V. Precipitous birth not occurring on a labor and delivery unit. UpToDate website. http://www.uptodate.com/contents/precipitous-birth-not-occurring-on-a-labor-and-delivery-unit?source=search_result&selectedTitle=1%7E17. Updated October 2009. Accessed June 2011.

Belogolovkin V, Bush M, Eddleman K, et al. Umbilical cord prolapse. UpToDate website. http://www.uptodate.com/contents/umbilical-cord-prolapse?source=search_result&selectedTitle=1%7E15. Updated January 2009. Accessed June 2011.

Lockwood CJ, Russo-Steiglitz K. Vasa previa and velamentous umbilical cord. UpToDate website. http://www.uptodate.com/contents/vasa-previa-and-velamentous-umbilical-cord?source=search_result&selectedTitle=1%7E14. Updated November 2010. Accessed June 2011.

Schaffer L, Zimmerman R. Nuchal cords. UpToDate website. http://www.uptodate.com/contents/velamentous-umbilical-cord-insertion-and-vasa-previa?source=search_result&search=VASA+PREVIA+AND+VELAMENTOUS&selectedTitle=1%7E16. Updated August 2010. Accessed June 2011.

125

DON'T THROW YOUR HANDS UP JUST YET: WHAT YOU NEED TO KNOW ABOUT HYPEREMESIS

MORGAN M. WALKER, BA, RN, BSN

BENJAMIN J. LAWNER, DO, EMT-P, FAAEM

INTRODUCTION

It is anticipated that expectant mothers may experience nausea and vomiting during their pregnancy. "Morning sickness" is a well-known term to most all pregnant women, and many people consider vomiting to be an unavoidable part of the first trimester. However, there are situations in which vomiting indicates a more serious underlying disorder. This chapter will help you understand when nausea and vomiting in pregnancy can represent a true medical emergency.

Approximately 70% to 85% of women in their first trimester may experience nausea and vomiting. Usually, these symptoms are self-limiting and pose little or no threat to mother and child. Intractable vomiting, however, places the patient at risk for serious complications, including dehydration and acidosis, and also poses serious risk for the fetus. Prematurity, low birth weight, and reduced APGAR scores have all been reported in fetuses of mothers affected by hyperemesis. The condition of hyperemesis gravidarum occurs most commonly at 8 to 12 weeks gestation. Rarely does it persist beyond 20 weeks. Patients report weight loss, poor appetite, weakness, and uncontrolled vomiting. Pain is unusual in the presentation of hyperemesis. Patients reporting abdominal pain or who present with these symptoms in their late second or early third trimesters should be assessed for other conditions. For example, an ectopic pregnancy should be considered in pregnant patients who report pain and bleeding during their first trimester.

HOW IS IT DIAGNOSED?

Hyperemesis gravidarum is usually diagnosed during the initial history and physical examination. Pregnant women report an inability to tolerate oral intake. Weakness, tachycardia, and poor skin turgor may indicate mild to moderate dehydration. The physical examination may also reveal dry oral mucosa. In a patient who has not progressed to a state of clinical dehydration, the vital signs and physical examination may show no abnormalities. Therefore, it remains important to consider the diagnosis of hyperemesis when the patent reports episodes of protracted vomiting. It is possible that symptoms developing over the course of 24 to 48 hours may result in hyperemesis.

HOW DO I TREAT HYPEREMESIS?

Depending upon local protocols, prehospital providers may have several options available for the treatment of hyperemesis. Obtain vital signs and permit the patient to remain in a position of comfort. Advanced life support providers should consider starting an intravenous line and administering normal saline or lactated ringers. Dehydrated patients may benefit from an infusion of 1 to 2 L of isotonic crystalloid. Symptomatic relief in the form of antiemetics will help break the vicious cycle of nausea, vomiting, and dehydration. Follow your local protocols with respect to the administration of antinausea medications. Uncontrolled emesis stimulates the breakdown of fatty acids which in turn activate the brain's vomiting center. *Table 125.1* shows the commonly utilized medications that have proven their effectiveness and safety in the setting of hyperemesis.

LABORATORY FINDINGS

Occasionally, hyperemesis may be a sign of a more severe underlying disorder. The emergency department may order additional tests to confirm the

TABLE 125.1	MEDICATIONS FOR THE TREATMENT OF SUSPECTED HYPEREMESIS	
MEDICATION	**DOSE**	**MECHANISM**
Ondansetron (Zofran)	4–8 mg IV, may be repeated in 30 min	This medicine acts directly on the brain's vomiting center. It may also have peripheral action on the small bowel and vagus nerve to further decrease vomiting.
Promethazine (Phenergan)	12–25 mg IV, repeat every 4–6 h	Promethazine is a dopamine receptor antagonist. It acts on the brain's "chemoreceptor trigger zone" to reduce the vomiting stimulus. This medicine also has direct action on dopamine receptors in the gastrointestinal tract.
Metoclopramide (Reglan)	10 mg IV	Metoclopramide is a pro–motility agent that has a well–established safety record. A small percentage of patients may experience tremors or involuntary movements following dose administration. Diphenhydramine may be co–administered with this medicine to minimize side effects.
Corticosteroids	IV	There are some data to suggest that steroids may help reduce symptoms associated with hyperemesis. These drugs are not as well studied in acute hyperemesis and are generally used for patients with protracted and severe symptoms. The mechanism of action is unclear.

diagnosis of hyperemesis. Blood testing evaluates for electrolyte imbalance and urine tests can detect ketones, which are metabolic byproducts of fatty acid breakdown. Ketones may indicate a state of dehydration and starvation.

SUMMARY

Nausea and vomiting are common complaints occurring during the first trimester of pregnancy. Though usually self-limiting, persistent vomiting defines the abnormal condition of hyperemesis gravidarum. Prehospital providers should recognize historical factors and physical signs associated with hyperemesis and have a low threshold for the treatment and transport of pregnant patients. Vomiting, if unchecked, may cause electrolyte abnormalities, acidosis, and could pose a threat to the well-being of the unborn fetus. Treat patients with boluses of intravenous fluid and antiemetics. Medications that have a demonstrated safety record in pregnancy include metoclopramide and ondansetron. Promethazine and prochlorperazine are other agents used for the treatment of hyperemesis, and steroid injections may be administered in severe or refractory cases.

SELECTED READINGS

Lee NM, Saha S. Nausea and vomiting of pregnancy. *Gastroenterol Clin North Am.* 2011; 40(2):309–334.

Sonkusare S. The clinical management of hyperemesis gravidarum. *Arch Gynecol Obstet.* 2011;283(6):1183–1192.

Wilcox SR. Pregnancy, hyperemesis gravidarum. Emedicine website. http://emedicine.medscape.com/article/796564-overview. Updated January 2010. Accessed June 2, 2011.

126

DON'T DISMISS HEADACHES IN THE POSTPARTUM PATIENT

ANDERS APGAR, MD, FACOG

Preeclampsia is a disease of high blood pressure in pregnancy. It can occur in almost any pregnant patient but is most common in primiparous patients at the extremes of age. Teenage patients and those patients 35 and older are considered higher risk for preeclampsia in pregnancy. At its worst, preeclampsia affects the liver, kidneys, and hematopoietic system of the expectant mother and ultimately the fetus, which, for simplicity, is considered an end-organ in the pregnant patient. Hallmarks of preeclampsia include edema, proteinuria, and high blood pressure. Additional information that supports the diagnosis of eclampsia includes elevation in liver enzymes, elevation in serum uric acid, high normal hematocrit, and low platelets. Ultimately, if left unchecked, preeclampsia can develop into eclampsia. The latter simply involves a grand mal type of seizure.

While surveillance for preeclampsia during pregnancy requires vigilance, making the diagnosis of postpartum preeclampsia requires an alert clinician. Many of the common complaints in the unaffected postpartum patient can also be found in the same patient who is developing postpartum preeclampsia or nearing the seizure threshold. Postpartum preeclampsia can affect the patient up to 6 weeks after delivery but is most common within the first 2 weeks. In patients who have been successfully discharged from the hospital, an eclamptic seizure may be the first indicator that the postpartum mother ever had preeclampsia because her symptoms, when explained over the phone, are often too nonspecific to effectively make the diagnosis. Generally, patients who call their doctors are advised to monitor their symptoms. Uncommonly, their condition deteriorates and the EMS system is called to attend to a rather sick or seizing new mother.

Patients with postpartum preeclampsia commonly complain of a severe, frontal, unrelenting, band-like headache. There may be flashes of light and photophobia associated with the headache. Many postpartum mothers experience headaches due to exhaustion, dehydration, and side effects of epidural or spinal anesthesia used during delivery. The preeclamptic headache, in contrast to the headache associated with regional anesthesia, has no relationship to patient position. Anesthesia-related headaches will worsen when the patient sits up and improve when the patient is in the dorsal supine position. Headaches may respond to analgesics, and the patient may have access to narcotics prescribed appropriately in the postpartum mother, but any headache in the postpartum patient should be evaluated in the context of preeclampsia.

FACTORS ASSOCIATED WITH PREECLAMPTIC HEADACHE

- Unremitting despite analgesics, bed rest, and position change
- Band-like nature around the head, at the level of the eyes
- Photophobia
- Persistent nausea and vomiting
- Emotional sense of impending doom

Another common complaint associated with normal postpartum course is swelling. Due to the collection of fluid throughout the pregnancy and the resultant third spacing that occurs in the third trimester, patients can develop significant lower extremity edema. This edema may actually worsen after delivery due to the mobilization of third space fluid. Patients may complain of numbness or tingling in the lower extremities and feet, walking may be uncomfortable in the first 72 hours after delivery. However, swelling that occurs in the upper extremities, especially in the eyes, should be considered a symptom of preeclampsia.

The preeclamptic patient, by definition, has elevated blood pressure. Blood pressures approaching, or in excess of 140/90 meet criteria for preeclampsia. Blood pressures higher than 160/110 indicate severe preeclampsia and should prompt immediate intervention with intravenous fluids, hydralazine for blood pressure control, and intravenous magnesium sulfate for seizure prevention. In the hospital setting, elevated blood pressure is aggressively managed in order to avoid eclampsia. Magnesium sulfate is commonly administered intravenously at a loading dose of 4 to 6 g. The bolus is typically followed by a maintenance dose of magnesium at 2 g of magnesium sulfate per hour.

TABLE 126.1	FEATURES OF ECLAMPSIA
SIGN OR SYMPTOM	**DESCRIPTION**
Seizure	Seizures or post ictal presentation most common
Headache	Usually frontal in location
Generalized edema	Non dependent swelling in hands, feet
Visual disturbances	Blurred vision, light sensitivity
Abdominal pain	Usually in the right upper quadrant, associated with nausea
Hypertension	Usually sustained >160/110 mm Hg
Rales	
Abnormal reflexes	

Eclampsia, by definition, presents with a single clinical sign: Seizure. Should the patient develop a seizure, or be seizing upon arrival of EMS, the goals of therapy are to prevent injury to the patient, protect the airway, ensure oxygenation of the patient, and minimize the occurrence of subsequent seizures. Some prehospital protocols may authorize the administration of benzodiazepines such as diazepam. The use of anti-convulsants to break the initial seizure can have deleterious cardiac or pulmonary side effects in the newly postpartum patient and should only be used as intervention after IV access is obtained and the patient's airway is adequately protected. As an alternative to anti-convulsants in the hospital setting, subsequent seizure risk can be reduced by intravenously administering 6 g of magnesium sulfate over 15 minutes.

Postpartum preeclampsia can be a confusing presentation due to the similarity of the pathologic symptoms of disease to the common maladies associated with a normal postpartum course. Headache and swelling in the postpartum mother in the first 6 weeks after delivery should be considered a symptom of preeclampsia until proven otherwise. Have a low threshold to transport pregnant patients to the hospital! Carefully monitor their blood pressure, consider starting an intravenous line, and be prepared for the occurrence of seizures.

SELECTED READINGS

American College of Obstetricians and Gynecologists. Practice Bulletin #33. Diagnosis and management of preeclampsia and eclampsia. Washington, DC: American College of Obstetricians and Gynecologists; 2002: 99(1):159–167.
Clark SL, Cotton DB, Hankins GD, et al. *Handbook of Critical Care Obstetrics*. Boston, MA: Blackwell Scientific Publications. 1994:123–138.
Gabbe SG, Niebyl JR, Simpson JL. *Obstetrics: Normal and Problem Pregnancies*. 3rd ed. New York, NY: Churchill Livingstone Inc.; 1996.

127

IT CAN STILL BE A SURPRISE, EVEN AFTER NINE MONTHS! DO NOT FAIL TO PREPARE FOR THE EMERGENT DELIVERY

THERESA GALLO, NREMT-P
KEVIN G. SEAMAN, MD, FACEP

Don't be surprised by an unanticipated delivery! Learn from other providers' experiences. Think about pregnancy and its complications during the initial evaluation of any female of childbearing age. Labor should be considered as a potential cause of any episodic or recurring pain from the pubic bone to the xiphoid process. The patient may or may not know she is pregnant, or may attempt to conceal a pregnancy in the presence of others. The prehospital provider should attempt to obtain possible pregnancy history in private and explain the importance of truthful and honest historical interview. Of particular importance are factors such as the patient's menstrual history, the presence or absence of positive home pregnancy tests, and any prenatal care the patient may have received. A pregnant patient should be questioned about the stage of her pregnancy and estimated due date, but the provider should consider the possibility of labor regardless of the due date's proximity. Also key is whether this pregnancy is the patient's first, as second and subsequent pregnancies can progress from cervical dilation to active delivery *very* quickly. Other pertinent historical information includes pregnancy-related complications or the possibility of a twin or multiple gestation. Questions related to an imminent delivery might include:

- Has your water broken?
- Have you passed a mucous plug or any meconium?
- Do you feel the need to push or have a bowel movement?

To Peek or Not to Peek

As a prehospital provider facing a potentially emergent delivery, the first issue to consider is: *To peek or not to peek*. You do not know how close your patient is to delivering without taking a look. Certainly, if she says she feels like pushing you will know where you stand. Sometimes, the intensity of labor pain may foretell of an impending delivery. The best course of action is simply to ask for permission when you suspect an emergent delivery: "I would like to take a look and see how close you are to delivery" is a good start.

SHOULD I STAY OR SHOULD I GO?

The ambulance is a suboptimal setting for delivery, but so is the bathroom, an elevator, or the lobby of a movie theater. Nevertheless, if your patient is crowning you have an imminent delivery and you should stay put. If your patient is not crowning then drive on, in the hope that you reach the optimal setting for delivery, an obstetrical delivery suite. Certain factors dictate the decision in favor of immediate transport such as an abnormal presenting part (any presenting part of the baby other than the head), a prolapsed umbilical cord, meconium staining of the amniotic fluid, or rupture of the patient's membranes more than 24 hours previously. A prolapsed umbilical cord should prompt not only immediate transport, but also patient transport in the head down, buttocks up position. *If the infant is crowning with a prolapsed cord present you must keep pressure off the umbilical cord by placing two fingers in the mother's vagina, one on either side of the cord.*

PREPARE FOR THE WORST, HOPE FOR THE BEST

Laboring women who present to EMS are far more likely to have serious complications than women who deliver in the obstetrical unit of a hospital. Studies have shown that these women have higher rates of complex presentations, maternal, and perinatal morbidity. The prehospital provider should strongly consider these facts when deliberating on the adequacy of available resources. Even delivery of a single infant will generate two patients: mother and baby. Emergency medical service personnel operate with a "*prepare for the worst, hope for the best*" mentality, and this is not a time to stray from those guidelines. Have extra hands available and consider the need for additional ambulances or fire department personnel. Remember that extra resources can always be returned to service in the event of an uncomplicated delivery.

Are you familiar with what is included in your OB kit? You should be. Take it out. Look through it. Know what is there, and what is not. If you are preparing for immediate delivery, dress appropriately. Deliveries are messy and place you at risk for exposure to blood and body fluids. Absolutely, positively wear a mask and eye protection. Put on an infection control gown. If time permits, drape both the delivery area and the patient's legs with a disposable cover from your OB kit. Control the delivery of the baby's head by applying gentle pressure. Remember that babies are very slippery, and be prepared. If the amniotic sac is still intact you must tear it to permit the baby to breathe. Slide your finger around the head and neck and palpate for the umbilical cord. If it is wrapped around the baby's neck do your best to slip it over the head and shoulder. If it is wrapped so tightly that you are unable to do this you must clamp the cord in two places about 2 in. apart and cut the cord to allow delivery to proceed. Suction the infant's mouth and nose with a bulb syringe.

As the baby's body begins to deliver gently guide the head downward to facilitate delivery of the upper shoulder. As that shoulder passes you may lift the infant upward to allow the upper shoulder to deliver. After that, the rest of the body should deliver without incident. Clamp the umbilical cord approximately 7 and 10 in. from the baby and cut in between, if you have not done so already. Re-suction as necessary. Dry the baby *completely*, paying particular attention to the baby's head and face. Place the infant skin-to-skin with the mother and cover them both.

The usual maternal blood loss from delivery is about 1 pint. Monitor both mother and infant, and wait for the placenta to deliver. If it does deliver prior to your arrival at the hospital place it in a container and bring it with you to the obstetrical unit for evaluation.

PEARLS

- Do not fail to consider pregnancy as a cause for other symptoms.
- Do not fail to recognize the signs of imminent delivery.
- Know the conditions that should prompt immediate transport.
- Do not fail to prepare for imminent delivery, including securing adequate manpower and resources.

SELECTED READINGS

Bernhard M. Prehospital obstetrical emergencies in a physician-staffed ground-based emergency service. A retrospective analysis over a 5-year period. *Anaesthesist.* 2009;58(4):353–361.

Bledsoe BE, Porter RS, Cherry RA. *Paramedic Care, Principles and Practice.* 3rd ed. Upper Saddle River, NJ: Pearson Education, Inc.; 2009:749–757.

DeCock MF. Early arrivals. Premature infant delivery in the prehospital setting. *JEMS.* 2007; 32(2):72–83.

Moscovitz HC, Magriples U, Kessling M, et al. Care and outcome of out-of-hospital deliveries. *Acad Emerg Med.* 2000;7(7):757–761.

Stallard TC, Burns B. Emergency delivery and perimortem C-section. *Emerg Med Clin North Am.* 2003;21:679–693.

NEUROLOGIC EMERGENCIES

129

Pediatric altered mental status: Did you think about the possibility of child abuse?

Gilberto Salazar, MD

The child with acute neurological dysfunction may present a number of challenges that are often not encountered in adults. The ill child may cause an EMS provider anxiety, uncertainty, and at times, insecurity as regards clinical skills in caring for pediatric patients. This is due in part to the relative rarity of encounters with ill children, or the thought that the stakes are higher for kids who have a long future ahead of them. Furthermore, history taking and physical examination of the ill child is more difficult for many providers.

Pitfalls for providers include differences in vital signs for various pediatric age groups, the small size of the patients as regards procedures such as airway control and venous access, and dosing issues as regards medications rarely given in children by most EMS providers. It is critical that the EMS provider gain a good foothold on the assessment of the neurological status of various pediatric age groups. A pitfall to be avoided is failing to recognize "inconsolability" in a pediatric patient, especially in a baby or toddler. The child is telling the provider that something is wrong and that a close look needs to be taken at this situation.

Altered mental status in a child most often represents an organic process, meaning that a psychiatric process is probably not the working differential diagnosis for the patient. For example, the child who seizes for the very first time may well have a primary neuronal firing abnormality secondary to a congenital problem including primary epilepsy. Certain the syndrome of the child who experiences a convulsion in the presence of fever—the suspected "febrile convulsion"—is familiar to the EMS providers. Other causes of new onset convulsions in the pediatric age group include metabolic, infectious, vascular (e.g., intracranial hemorrhage), or toxin related. The EMS provider caring for the child must be highly trained in the pathophysiology of neurologic dysfunction in this age group, the potential causes, physical assessment of the pediatric patient, and modes of treatment.

Once a child has been assessed, initial treatment has been implemented, and an appropriate transport decision has been made, the EMS provider must be vigilant of another problem which may result in further injury or death in that child. Child abuse is a silent killer that affects those most vulnerable. The potential psychological causes are numerous, and maintaining a healthy sense of awareness is vital for the prehospital provider taking care of children. For example, a child with an altered level of consciousness—suspected of having intracranial hemorrhage due to external physical forces as well as focal findings on the neurological examination—should prompt the EMS provider to consider trauma as part of the list of causes.

Focal findings on neurologic examination should prompt the EMS provider to consider trauma as part of the list of causes. If trauma is indeed suspected, the EMS provider must instinctively think of possible mechanisms and document what the caretaker states. An inconsistent story and a mechanism that does not match clinical findings are often clues that should make the provider suspicious. These suspicions should be communicated in private to the accepting physician or nurse.

Trauma is only one example of child abuse. Examples of other causes of potential abuse would include suspected toxic ingestion of adult medications, noncompliance with anti-convulsant medications, unexplained weight loss, or obvious dietary indiscretions in the setting of a chronically ill child whose diet must be carefully controlled. The provider should remember that negligence goes hand-in-hand with child abuse.

As the providers size up the situation that prompted the EMS call, it is vital to observe the family interactions to see if elements of control and anger appear to be present. A parent seemingly unwilling to relate a medical history or whose story is inconsistent with that of another family member gives one pause to reflect and wonder what the real truth to the story is.

Medical providers of all levels have a duty to report suspected child abuse if they are acting in good faith concern for the welfare of the child. That reporting can be initiated through the emergency department receiving staff, but it is important that providers who suspect potential abuse follow through with a report through the chain of command of the EMS agency. It is so much better to be safe than to be sorry in these situations.

Failing to consider and report suspicion of child abuse in the child with acute neurological deficit is a major pitfall. The EMS provider is legally liable to report reasonable suspicions. It would be a tragedy for that child about whom the provider is concerned to later be injured or killed at the hands of family or other perpetrators when there existed clear signs of abuse in the past. Excellent EMS care of the ill child should always involve consideration of the child's psychosocial condition and overall safety.

Selected Readings

American College of Emergency Physicians. Clinical policy for the initial approach to patients presenting with altered mental status. *Ann Emerg Med* 1999;33(2):251–281.

Rubenstein JS. Initial management of coma and altered consciousness in the pediatric patient. *Pediatr Rev* 1994;15(5):204–207.

130

Remember that drugs, toxins, and meds can cause AMS

Gilberto Salazar, MD

The patient with acute neurological dysfunction (AND) presents particular challenges. A critical reason for this challenge is that the patient may not be able to interact appropriately with the EMS provider. Potential manifestations of AND include altered level of consciousness, confusion, seizure activity, dysarthria (difficulty in articulating words), and a constellation of other signs and symptoms that may all prevent the patient from communicating. The provider is thus forced to assess, treat, and transport the patient, based only on the information obtained from physical assessments, family members, and the scene itself. The EMS provider will commit an error and possibly harm the patient (and potentially get injured in the process) if all of the possible reasons for AND are not considered.

An aging population, with increasing numbers of medical problems, has prompted tremendous advances in pharmacology. Medications and interventions to combat disease, however, do not come without side effects. Increased availability of illicit drugs and improper or even illegal use of prescription drugs truly bring a potential cache of agents that may negatively affect normal brain function. Indeed, the prescribing of an additional medication to an elderly person is a set-up for potential side effects that may cause altered mental status in the patient. The addition of a new antihypertensive medication to a frail old patient might be forgotten in the setting of a patient now acutely delirious due to diminished blood flow to the brain. Or in another case, a patient and family might naturally resist sharing the medical history of the patient's chronic use of benzodiazepines that have recently run out, resulting in a withdrawal delirium. It may certainly be said that the EMS provider must carefully examine the history of present illness, the past medical history, and perform careful physical assessments to attempt to get a handle on the patient's condition and how to safely treat it.

Toxic environmental agents such as carbon monoxide, lead, and arsenic are somewhat less common, presenting a challenge to the EMS provider to make the assessment, especially in time to be able to help the patient. A relatively common syndrome is the setting of a family in which headaches and vomiting have begun over the last few hours. They naturally think that the problem is a "virus" or food poisoning, not remembering that the weather has gotten cooler and they have turned the gas heater on in the house for the first time in months. The EMS provider, indeed, can become "at risk" in this scenario, and so it is critical that syndromes such as these are fresh in the memory of field personnel.

The EMS provider responding to patients with neurological dysfunction must have a standing knowledge of the common etiologies, but must also take into account medications, drugs, and toxins. The EMS provider may be the sole witness to a potential cause of neurological dysfunction. For example, as mentioned above, a newly lit furnace as a source of heat during the winter may lead to accumulation of carbon monoxide in the home of an unresponsive patient. A collection of hydrocarbon sources such as toluene used for sniffing may be found at the side of a patient with weakness or delirium. A child with decreased level of consciousness may be found with scattered hypoglycemic agents belonging to an adult caretaker.

One of the dreaded consequences of public service is injury or death in the line of service. Firemen who enter burning buildings are placed in great hazard due to potential smoke inhalation. Smoke is composed of innumerable chemicals, many of them toxic. A fireman who is pulled from a burning building who experiences acute confusion followed by coma and shock could be suspected of having had a severe carbon monoxide inhalation. The EMS provider should remember, though, that this presentation is also consistent with cyanide inhalation, which can be one of the products carried in smoke from a burning building. A current challenge in the management of this syndrome is whether "cyanide kits" are made available in the field. The patient in cardiovascular collapse from smoke inhalation may benefit from cyanide kit administration in the field. The victim of smoke inhalation whose initial symptoms are clearing and the patient who appears to be recovering likely will not benefit from a cyanide kit administration. Carbon monoxide toxicity, however, should always be suspected, and the recently emerged ability to use new monitors with carbon monoxide detection capability may prove a benefit to field analysis of these scenarios over time.

The EMS provider should be aware of the pitfall of failure to recognize, document, and transmit information regarding the role of medications, drugs, and environmental toxins in patients with neurological dysfunction. Hospital clinicians rely heavily on information provided by EMS providers, especially when the patient is unable to provide an accurate history and the clinical picture is obscure. A potentially treatable condition may prove fatal unless vital scene information is relayed to hospital personnel. Diligence in the art of observation can prevent unnecessary patient morbidity.

Selected Readings

Barillo D. Diagnosis and treatment of cyanide toxicity. *J Burn Care Res.* 2009;30(1):148–152.

Chapleau W, Burba AC, Pons PT, et al. *The Paramedic,* Update Edition, McGraw-Hill Publishers, 2011.

Sanders MJ. *Mosby's Paramedic Textbook.* 3rd ed. Chapter 31 – Neurology, 2007.

131

DID YOU THINK ABOUT EXCITED DELIRIUM AS THE CAUSE OF THAT PATIENT'S AGITATION?

GILBERTO SALAZAR, MD

Excited delirium is a syndrome now recognized as a dangerous medical condition with an associated high morbidity and mortality. The hallmark of excited delirium is altered mental status, but there are numerous other clinical findings associated with this condition. Excited delirium should be considered an acute neurological dysfunction, one which often takes the shape of combativeness and aggressiveness in the setting of a patient who may be seriously ill from drug intoxication, alcohol withdrawal, or serious forms of illness such as encephalitis.

The patient with excited delirium presents one of the greatest challenges to prehospital providers. These patients are often wildly agitated and delirious, indeed dangerous to both the providers as well as to other citizens and to public safety officers who assist in attempting to control these individuals. One of the great challenges in dealing with these patients is in being able to control their agitation so that measures can be taken to calm them and control the scene, while initiating a medical workup to attempt to reveal the source of the problem.

One critical pitfall that must be mentioned early is that the prehospital provider must avoid personal injury when dealing with these patients. These patients are capable of extreme violence, and it is a pitfall in the management of these patients for the provider to be placed in harm's way. Thus, avoiding the pitfall includes getting enough help to control the patient so that sedation can be initiated.

CONSIDERATIONS

The causes of excited delirium are numerous, and are best understood using a systems approach. One useful categorization is:

1) metabolic—such as hypoglycemia and hyponatremia;
2) infectious—such as sepsis and meningitis;
3) toxins—such as illicit drug use and alcohol intoxication; and
4) primary CNS—such as stroke and intracranial hemorrhage.

The EMS provider must have a basic understanding of the pathophysiology of conditions within each category, and understand their roles in excited delirium.

Most EMS providers recall patient encounters involving a high level of patient excitation, with their safety compromised as a result. Unfortunately, it is during these types of anxious moments that a pitfall is encountered. Many patients with an organic cause for excited delirium are found to be agitated, and are immediately believed to have a primary psychiatric problem such as acute psychosis. The patient might then be transported to a facility responsible for managing patients with psychiatric complaints, and the true etiology goes unrecognized.

Patients suffering from excited delirium are often quite ill due to whatever caused the agitation. Sympathomimetic drugs such as cocaine and methamphetamine can cause profound excited delirium. These patients are often difficult and dangerous to manage. The interaction with them is often near violent, with multiple public safety officers holding the patient down in handcuffs for control. The positioning of these patients is important, and a pitfall for the provider to avoid is to have the patient in a prone position for any prolonged periods. The prone position—especially with a number of individuals holding the patient in place—can in fact cause respiratory embarrassment for the patient and has been associated with cardiac arrest.

Patients in excited delirium due to substance abuse often have some or all of these features:

1) Extreme agitation
2) Hyperthermic (at temperatures approaching heat stroke)
3) Hyperkalemia (due to muscle cell breakdown, known as rhabdomyolysis)
4) Hypoglycemia
5) Extreme sympathetic outflow, with hypertension and tachycardia
6) Dehydration
7) Commonly have coronary artery disease (CAD, either diagnosed or occult)
8) Have likely been smokers and may have COPD
9) Often have a history of an infectious disease such as Hepatitis C, putting all responders at risk

Thus, when the providers finally manage to gain control of this individual, it is critical to remember that this patient is hot, tachycardic, hypertensive, likely with elevated potassium, and low blood sugar. Each of these conditions—especially in the setting of a patient with known or occult CAD—is at a greater risk of sudden death due to cardiac arrest. The patient must be sedated until controlled, allowed to cool off, have a blood sugar checked, and hooked to a monitor to evaluation for signs of hyperkalemia (peaked T waves, prolonged QRS complex, or AV dissociation).

EMS providers must be vigilant when encountering patients who exhibit a high level of agitation. Agitation and other forms of abnormal behavior must be considered an acute neurological condition with an organic etiology until proven otherwise. It is a major pitfall for the EMS provider to fail to recognize excited delirium, consider its many causes, and treat the patient appropriately. As difficult as these patients are to manage, they are still the patients of the EMS system and deserve to be treated humanely and in a manner consistent with acceptable clinical standards.

SELECTED READINGS

Otahbachi M, Cevik C, Bagdure S, et al. Excited delirium, restraints, and unexpected death: A review of pathogenesis. *Am J Forensic Med Pathol.* 2010;31(2):107–112.

Takeuchi A, Ahern TL, Henderson SO. Excited delirium. *West J Emerg Med.* 2011;12(1):77–83.

White Paper Report on Excited Delirium Syndrome, ACEP Excited Delirium Task Force, September 10, 2009.

132

Always remember to consider hypoglycemia!

Gilberto Salazar, MD

Hypoglycemia is a condition in which serum glucose levels are below normal, resulting in diminished metabolic nutrient supply to vital organs, most notably the brain. The cellular make-up of the brain relies heavily on a constant supply of nutrients and oxygen to carry out its intricate and complex activities. The brain is highly sensitive to changes in this supply of nutrients. When serum glucose levels drop significantly below normal, a wide spectrum of signs and symptoms may develop.

Hypoglycemia is a common cause of acute neurologic dysfunction including altered mental status. It is very useful to think of hypoglycemia as a "great imitator." Signs of hypoglycemia may take various forms, but the most significant signs may include acute paresthesias, cranial nerve dysfunction, severe confusion, behavioral changes, obtundation, and even coma. Clearly, it is evident that acute hypoglycemia can present a clinical condition that can be virtually identical to many other conditions, including acute stroke, meningitis, encephalitis, acute drug and/or alcohol intoxication, thermal emergencies, malingering, delirium of other causes, and many more.

The EMS provider should be well versed in the neurologic presentation and treatment of hypoglycemia. Generally, it is reasonable to say that the patient presenting with acute hypoglycemia is diabetic, and the EMS providers will generally find that piece of information out as they go along. One important pitfall then is if the EMS provider does not take an adequate enough medical history to find this out. Complicating this factor, of course, is that the patient may not have a significant other available to give this history. The inability to recognize hypoglycemia and treat it appropriately may result in erroneous decisions in transport, triage, and even therapy. Imagine the devastating effects of hypoglycemia that may incur if the patient, who exhibited odd behavior and paranoid ideations, was transported to a psychiatric care facility without having blood sugar being checked. Consider the consequences of initiating a stroke treatment pathway on a patient with hypoglycemia who presented with facial droop, altered mental status, and hemiparesis, who might have been spared this workup, treatment, and expense had a blood sugar merely been taken.

Patients may be acutely hypoglycemic for many reasons, and it is a pitfall for EMS providers not to consider many of the causes. The severe alcoholic who has been drinking for a long period and then goes off of alcohol may be quite hypoglycemic and may even become altered, this in the absence of a history of diabetes. A nondiabetic patient may have taken someone else's medication that turned out to be a diabetic medication, either accidentally or in a self-harm attempt, including self-injecting with insulin in a suicide attempt. Insulin-secreting tumors may rarely occur, causing profound hypoglycemia. Thus, it is a pitfall for the provider not to take a careful history, perform a proper physical assessment, identify the low blood sugar and treat it, and then look for causes of the problem.

It is common for diabetic patients on medication to develop low blood sugar. EMS is frequently activated for these patients, responding to the scene, finding the low blood sugar, and treating the problem with oral or intravenous glucose and possibly glucagon. When these patients come to full awareness after treatment, it is very common that they will refuse transport to a hospital facility, will sign a patient refusal form, and the EMS crew will depart the scene and complete their medical record.

The very critical pitfall for the EMS provider to remember in this scenario is this: Why did this diabetic patient become hypoglycemic? For a diabetic on medication to have been doing well and then to suddenly develop hypoglycemia to the point of activating EMS means that something has happened:

- The patient took the diabetic medication without eating a meal. This is an especially important consideration in the insulin–dependent diabetic (IDDM). This is an information problem for the patient who requires remediation so that this won't occur again. Some IDDM patients really try to keep their glucose levels under tight control, often balancing their dose of insulin against the timing of their next meal. Sometimes they don't get it quite right, and they end up dropping their glucose very low. This requires re-education on the patient's part.
- Occasionally, a patient will have had a medications change, which then caused the hypoglycemia. Just giving a dose of glucose to this patient to bring the blood sugar up is not going to solve the fact that there is something about the medications that has brought about this problem. It is a pitfall for the EMS provider not to ask about this issue and possibly contact the physician. Certain of the diabetic medications can cause blood glucose levels to remain low for a long time, long after the dose of glucose you gave goes away!
- Sometimes when diabetic patients become ill with another problem— such as pneumonia or a urinary tract infection—they will drop their

blood sugars. The pitfall here is if the EMS provider doesn't take a more thorough "history of present illness" to find that the patient may have been having problems before dropping the blood sugar. Such patients should be transported for hospital evaluation.

The standard of care in EMS for the patient exhibiting acute neurologic dysfunction is to assess, resuscitate, and among other things, check the blood glucose level to assess for hypoglycemia. Transport decisions should be based on local agency protocols. Failure to recognize hypoglycemia in these patients is indeed a significant pitfall.

SELECTED READINGS

Augustine JJ. Thanks, I'll stay here. A hypoglycemic episode is quickly resolved – but what about transport? *EMS Mag.* 2008;37(9):36, 39–40.

Murphy P, Colwell C. Prehospital management of diabetes. *Emerg Med Serv.* 2000;29(10): 78–85.

Socransky SJ, Pirrallo RG, Rubin JM. Out-of-hospital treatment of hypoglycemia: refusal of transport and patient outcome. *Acad Emerg Med.* 1998;5(11):1080–1085.

133

REMEMBER THAT HYPOXIA MAY BE CAUSING THAT ALTERED MENTAL STATUS!

GILBERTO SALAZAR, MD

The brain relies on a large and continuous supply of oxygen and nutrients to perform optimally, actually consuming, in the resting state, some 25% of the total energy produced by the body. The brain is exquisitely sensitive to changes in oxygen supply to its tissues. Hypoxia is a highly dangerous state that deprives end organs of a healthy supply of oxygen, and the cause of hypoxia (such as a shock state, chronic lung disease exacerbation, or pulmonary embolism) not uncommonly decreases removal of carbon dioxide from the tissues as well. Since the brain tissue is so oxygen dependent, hypoxia has significant negative effects on the brain, decreasing its metabolism and often leading to the patient demonstrating an altered level of consciousness.

The main causes of hypoxia can be divided into two broad categories: (1) barriers to oxygen delivery, and (2) ventilatory insufficiency. Barriers to oxygen delivery include the disruption of the mechanism by which oxygen enters the airway, then the lungs, crossing the alveolar–capillary membrane, and is transported to the periphery on hemoglobin. The disruption may be due to a number of factors including lung damage or fluid and vascular system dysfunction such as shock. "Oxygen deficit" refers to a condition in which decreased oxygen exchange occurs in the lungs, leading to a decrease of oxygen in the blood and thus hypoxia.

Ventilatory insufficiency means that the movement of air through the tracheobronchial tree is inadequate to provide for a sufficient supply of oxygen and removal of carbon dioxide (CO_2). Generally, a given amount of air must be moved per minute to optimize oxygen supply and CO_2 removal. This is called "minute ventilation," which is computed by multiplying the respiratory rate times the size of the breaths being taken (known as "tidal volume"). A pitfall for EMS providers is in not assessing "adequacy" of ventilation. Said another way, the provider must ask "is the patient moving sufficient air each minute to maintain oxygen delivery and CO_2 removal?" This is a skill requiring appropriate training as well as the willingness of the provider to employ this assessment, especially in critically ill patients.

When oxygenation and ventilation are diminished, the patient may decompensate rapidly. This may take the form of abnormal behavior, combativeness, sensorimotor disturbances, obtundation, and apnea. The EMS provider's main responsibility when assessing such a patient is to consider organic causes, treat them appropriately, and transport while maintaining treatment and ongoing assessment. Hypoxia may be highly responsive to simple maneuvers, such as ensuring the airway is patent, providing supplemental oxygen, or assisting ventilations through applying positive airway pressure. As the oxygen supply to the brain improves, improvement in an altered level of consciousness may occur.

The EMS provider must be aware of situations in which hypoxia is present, but not typically suspected. Examples include unfavorable methods of restraining patients (hog-tie position or kneeling on a patient's thorax in the setting of the management of a violently agitated patient suffering from excited delirium), decreased respiratory drive (such as may occur under the influence of drugs, due to a brain injury, or from shock of any cause), and abnormal oxygen exchange states (such as carbon monoxide poisoning, chemical pneumonitis, pulmonary edema, severe pneumonia, COPD exacerbation, or pulmonary embolism). Each of these conditions may result in hypoxia, leading to brain ischemia.

A major pitfall in the care of the patient with altered level of consciousness is the failure to consider hypoxia as a cause, followed by the failure to attempt to reverse hypoxia. The EMS provider—after ensuring the safety of the response team—must then perform standard physical assessments. If a patient with AMS is identified, hypoxia is one of the many causes that must be considered for this physical sign. Every precaution must then be taken to ensure that hypoxia is not iatrogenic (i.e., caused by the healthcare provider or other members of the team, such as public safety officers restraining a patient). The next step is to ensure the adequacy of ventilation, applying supplemental oxygen, searching for any other obvious causes of hypoxia, and continuously re-evaluating the patient while preparing for transport.

Increased morbidity and increased incidence of mortality—not to mention increased medicolegal liability—may be significant should the provider fail to address the presence of hypoxia in the patient with an altered level of consciousness.

Finally, the critical pitfall for the EMS provider is the failure to link the patient with AMS with other findings present on physical assessment, including pulse oximetry, while failing to assess for adequacy of ventilation. Through applying all of these findings into a comprehensive assessment, the provider may often be able to determine the cause of the altered mental status, or at least develop a working differential diagnosis that can guide further assessment and treatment.

SELECTED READINGS

Bota GW, Rowe BH. Continuous monitoring of oxygen saturation in prehospital patients with severe illness: the problem of unrecognized hypoxemia. *J Emerg Med*. 1995;13(3):305–311.

New A. Oxygen: kill or cure? Prehospital hyperoxia in the COPD patient. *Emerg Med J*. 2006;23(2):144–146.

Stahel PF, Smith WR, Moore EE. Hypoxia and hypotension, the "lethal duo" in traumatic brain injury: implications for prehospital care. *Intensive Care Med*. 2008;34(3):402–404.

134

THOSE MAY BE STROKE SYMPTOMS AND THE PATIENT SHOULD GO TO A STROKE CENTER!

GILBERTO SALAZAR, MD

Acute stroke is a diagnosis that is time sensitive. It has two forms, ischemic and hemorrhagic, both of which warrant immediate assessment, appropriate diagnostic modalities, and definitive therapy. Signs and symptoms of acute stroke are variable, and include paresthesias (tingling sensations), weakness or paralysis, sensory changes, visual changes, cranial nerve abnormalities, and altered mental status. It is absolutely critical that the prehospital provider have a standardized approach to examining patients so that the primary survey and the secondary surveys quickly reveal neurologic findings that may be consistent with a medical crisis such as stroke.

EMS providers have become reliable and knowledgeable clinicians in the field of stroke, utilizing clinical tools—such as the NIH stroke scale in some systems or more abbreviated scales such as the Cincinnati or the FAST scales—to determine the clinical probability of acute stroke, its timing, and its acuity. Furthermore, major metropolitan EMS systems have made the treatment of patients with stroke an organized, highly effective process. This process relies on a network of hospitals and providers that meet accepted criteria demonstrating their capacity to treat stroke. The designation of a facility as a stroke center certifies it as a place with advanced diagnostic and therapeutic techniques.

Most EMS systems, especially urban ones, have protocols delineating the assessment and transport of patients with signs and symptoms that may be consistent with stroke. The EMS provider has the responsibility to ensure that such patients be transported to the closest appropriate facility, which in the setting of acute stroke should be a certified Stroke Center.

A principal issue in the setting of the patient with acute neurologic changes is to determine if, in fact, the primary etiology of the problem is neurologic. It is common that patients will develop altered mental status, for example, in conditions that appear to be stroke-like in nature but, in fact, are being caused by a condition that mimics acute stroke but in fact is not. A good example is the acute altered mental status that is associated with severe hypoglycemia, usually in a diabetic patient. The provider must always be thorough in the assessment of patients with altered mental status and be sure to perform a blood glucose check. Failure to do so could keep the patient in a profound hypoglycemic state during a "lights and sirens" run to the nearest Stroke Center, only to find at the hospital that an ampule of 50% dextrose given intravenously caused the resolution of what had appeared to be a potential stroke state.

Being thorough in the workup of the patient with acutely altered mental status includes the performing of a 12-lead ECG. It is not uncommon for elderly patients who develop altered mental status to do so because of suffering from acute myocardial ischemia or infarction in the absence of chest pain. In that setting it would be critical for the prehospital provider to try to ascertain which organ system was the culprit for causing the changes in mental status. It would not be in the best interest of a patient having a STEMI to be transported to a Stroke Center that did not also have available emergency cardiac catheterization capabilities, especially given the modern emphasis on the concept of "time is muscle." On the other hand, if the patient has acutely altered mental status—and especially in the setting of a nondiagnostic 12-lead ECG and perhaps the presence of a neurologic finding such as limb weakness—then transport to a Stroke Center would be appropriate.

Failure to transport a patient with signs and symptoms of stroke to a designated Stroke Center is a major pitfall. Accredited Stroke Centers rely on protocols that dictate prompt emergency department assessment, rapid imaging with computed tomography and possibly magnetic resonance imaging, immediate access to a neurology team, and in the setting of "comprehensive Stroke Centers," state-of-the-art catheterization laboratories where advanced therapeutic techniques can take place quickly. The latter therapies include intra-arterial clot retrieval or thrombolysis. These centers also have dedicated Stroke Units, allowing close monitoring of these patients, providing followup imaging techniques where indicated, carefully monitoring swallowing studies, and ensuring that the patient's discharge planning is appropriate and adequate to the level of the patient's deficits, if any. These facilities also have extensive rehabilitation programs to attempt to optimize the patient's final outcome as regards motor deficits, speech deficits, swallowing difficulties, and assistance where indicated for the activities of daily living.

Many hospitals do not meet these robust requirements. Therefore, EMS providers must be well versed in their Medical Director's protocols, be familiar with the location of the local Stroke Centers, and avoid when at all possible the transport of these patients to a facility incapable of providing comprehensive and appropriate stroke care.

SELECTED READINGS

Durant E, Sporer KA. Characteristics of patients with an abnormal glasgow coma scale score in the prehospital setting. *West J Emerg Med.* 2011;12(1):30–36.

Millin MG, Gullett T, Daya MR. EMS management of acute stroke—out-of-hospital treatment and stroke system development. *Prehosp Emerg Care.* 2007;11(3):318–325.

Patel MD, Rose KM, O'Brien EC, et al. Prehospital notification by emergency medical services reduces delays in stroke evaluation: findings from the North Carolina stroke care collaborative. *Stroke.* 2011;42(8):2263–2268.

135

THE PATIENT WITH HEADACHE: WHAT MIGHT BE THE CAUSE?

GILBERTO SALAZAR, MD

The differential diagnosis of headache is broad and encompasses a range of medical conditions from benign to life-threatening. One of the main challenges with dealing with a patient with headache is that the physical examination may be completely normal in a patient who actually is seriously ill. Therefore, headache should be considered a neurologic emergency, and a potentially critical condition must be presumed until proven otherwise.

Many factors must be considered in the assessment of headache, including the fact that many patients both perceive and tolerate pain differently from other patients. Another important challenge is in the level to which a patient volunteers useful clinical information. It is well know that many patients are not great historians when it comes to the EMS provider trying to get a reliable history of present illness (HPI). Thus, the EMS provider must rely on clinical suspicion to gauge the severity of the problem, to allow the provider to make an informed decision regarding possible treatments and what transport modalities should be utilized.

One of the most frightening clinical conditions that occurs in EMS is in the patient who has suffered an acute intracranial hemorrhage (ICH). This dangerous problem is one cause of headache that is exceptionally time sensitive. Patients with ICHs due to such conditions as subarachnoid hemorrhage, epidural hematoma (typically due to trauma), subdural hematoma (which may occur spontaneously), arteriovenous malformation rupture, and aneurysm rupture may experience headache ranging from a dull ache to the worst headache of their lives.

The EMS provider must be very careful in gaining the HPI on victims of potential ICH. The provider must not forget to ask some specific questions that may elicit important information:

- Did the headache begin suddenly, or was it gradual in onset?
- Does the patient have a history of headaches, and, if so, is this one similar to previous headaches? (Remember, though, that a previous similar headache might have been a "sentinel bleed" associated with a previous bleeding intracranial aneurysm.
- Has there been trauma that preceded the onset of the headache?
- Have there been other associated symptoms, such as nausea, vomiting, fever, or rash?

- Has the patient noted any signs of neurologic deficits such as weakness of the face or of an extremity, alterations in speech, or altered mental status?

Ischemic stroke (due to an obstructed artery in the brain) may also be associated with headache, so the provider should be vigilant about getting the appropriate history while at the same time preparing the patient for transport in an expeditious manner. The headache may be accompanied by a neurologic finding or deficit found on physical examination. These findings include altered mental status, paresthesias, paralysis, or cranial nerve abnormalities. Patients with ICH commonly have vomiting associated with the headache, a condition that can make initial assessment difficult. The provider should especially remember that the syndrome of the abrupt onset of headache in a patient who appears to be in a lot of pain, associated with vomiting, in the setting of no prior history of such headaches, has an ICH until proven otherwise.

Patients believed to have serious etiologies underlying their headache must be assessed promptly, resuscitated appropriately, and transported to a facility with the capacity to treat the patient. The EMS provider must document a physical examination that details the neurologic function at the time of encounter, which will help hospital clinicians determine the progression of disease process. In the setting of both ischemic stroke as well as ICH, the patient's airway may become compromised. The provider should have suction available and standing by. Aspiration can occur during the setting of stroke, being a source of increased likelihood of death or disability in the stroke victim.

The patient with severe headache associated with fever—especially if a purplish dot-like rash or bruises are found on the skin—may have an infectious etiology causing the headache. In addition to the usual modes of assessment, treatment, and preparation for transport, the provider must not forget to use appropriate personal protective equipment in such cases, as serious (and potentially deadly) infectious organisms may be causing this condition, including bacterial meningitis.

It is a pitfall to assume that the patient with headache is unlikely to have severe intracranial pathology. The EMS provider must remember that headache may be the only symptom present. The patient with ICH has a high propensity to deteriorate rapidly. Again, a pressing concern is the airway, so vigilance as regards airway protection is essential for the prehospital provider to remember. In addition, the intracranial lesion may cause a significant increase in intracranial pressure, which may lead to apnea or decreased ventilatory effort. If the provider fails to consider this etiology, the results may be disastrous. Finally, prompt mobilization of patients with headache to the appropriate medical facility is critical. Strong consideration should be given to transporting these patients to certified Stroke Centers, especially if neurologic deficits accompany the headache.

SELECTED READINGS

Rinaldi S, Bulmer K. The splitting headache. Prehospital assessment and treatment of acute head pain. *JEMS.* 2006;31(3):102–118.

Wiemokly G. Just a headache? What EMS providers need to know about the signs and symptoms of headaches. *EMS Mag.* 2009;38(6):56–59.

136

THE PATIENT WITH CNS INJURIES: DID YOU REMEMBER TO IMMOBILIZE?

GILBERTO SALAZAR, MD

The central nervous system (CNS) is a delicate, complex network of communication pathways. The brain and the spinal cord are largely responsible for the appropriate relay of information throughout the body. When the CNS is compromised by acute traumatic events, then the results can be devastating, frightening, long lasting, and even fatal.

The EMS provider is regularly asked to assess and treat the patient with CNS compromise due to trauma. CNS trauma may be caused either by blunt trauma, penetrating trauma, or combinations of both. These conditions encompass the majority of acute CNS injury, though other causes exist, such as hypoxic brain damage that can occur during drowning, for example. These events commonly occur quickly, and rapid assessment and management techniques are required for even the most sophisticated EMS technician. Standardized assessment techniques and a vital command of specific skills are necessary to optimize the care of these head-injured patients.

The EMS provider must exercise sound clinical judgment based on excellent training and extensive field experience when assessing patients with suspected CNS injury due to trauma. Signs and symptoms are variable, but the presence of concerning findings warrants treatment modalities that optimize neurologic outcome. The finding of an acute neurologic deficit in a patient with suspected CNS injury may take the form of a patient complaint (back pain, headache, or tingling or weakness in an extremity) or a physical examination finding (paresthesia, paralysis, priapism, etc.).

It is important for the EMS provider to always complete the assessment surveys, to avoid examination short cuts, and to take full note of findings that may be present, unless some clinical emergency with the patient is preventing further assessment until it is managed. It is frequent, for example, to find a victim of a motor vehicle accident in which substantial energy was transmitted to the vehicle and on to the occupant through the mechanism of the crash. The acute back pain, for example, of which a patient in such a crash complains due to an acute vertebral fracture, might mask the fact that the patient has weakness in one or both of the lower extremities acutely since the accident. This finding may indicate spinal cord trauma and/or compression, a potential surgical emergency and one that would suggest that this victim might be mobilized to a higher level of care on the first transport rather than opting for interfacility transport from the primary receiving facility. So, when it is possible to complete the full assessment of the victim, the provider must not fail to notice acute neurologic findings, bearing in mind always that the patient's primary complaint—in this example acute posttraumatic back pain—may be a distracting injury to the much more subtle finding in the lower extremity.

Immobilization is a mandatory and proven initial intervention which should be applied in the field when CNS injury is suspected. Failure to immobilize a patient may result in outside forces acting on the CNS system, particularly the spinal cord. These unnecessary forces have the potential to worsen a bony or spinal cord deformity, and eliminate any residual neurologic function. Significant debate is ongoing in the EMS world now about how immobilization should be performed. Work out of Ben Taub Hospital in Houston, TX has found that typical cervical immobilization devices may in fact cause "distraction" of vertebra when soft-tissue injuries are present in the neck, meaning that the vertebra are stretched apart by the force of the collar. One new paradigm is emerging: "Cervical splinting." This is a method of "holding the head still" without stretching the neck and possibly, though unintentionally, causing spinal cord injury.

The Cochrane Collaboration has stated that it is unclear at this time which spinal immobilization techniques provide optimal immobilization with the least risk of causing additional harm to an already badly injured victim. The pitfall to be avoided here is, of course, that if the patient's pain seems to worsen while immobilization is in process or after it has taken place, then it would be wise to consider repositioning the victim. Certainly, if a neurologic finding—weakness in an extremity, for example—seems to worsen during or following immobilization, then it would be wise to alter the immobilization approach to attempt to prevent the patient's condition from worsening.

The astute EMS provider must take into account that a neurologic deficit suspected to be the result of brain injury does not exclude the possibility of spinal cord injury. It is a pitfall not to immobilize the patient with altered mental status after traumatic head injury, with the considerations mentioned above about not putting traction onto the cervical spine. CNS injury is a dynamic process necessitating a high level of vigilance, sharp clinical skills, and prompt treatment.

SELECTED READINGS

Domeier RM. Indications for prehospital spinal immobilization. *Prehosp Emerg Care.* 1999; 3(3):251–253.

Kwan I, Bunn F, et al. Spinal Immobilisation for Trauma Patients. In *The Cochrane Library,* published online January 2009.

Streger MR. Spinal immobilization. *Emerg Med Serv.* 2001;30(3):34.

137

Remember! That back pain may be due to a spinal cord problem!

Gilberto Salazar, MD

Back pain is a common cause of EMS calls and visits to the emergency department. It is also a common acute complaint after motor vehicle collisions and other forms of blunt trauma. Perhaps due to how common it is, back pain isn't typically considered a presenting physical sign and symptom of acute neurologic dysfunction. Despite the severity of the pain, and even despite back tenderness on examination, many clinicians and EMS providers dismiss the possibility of spinal cord injury in favor of a diagnosis of musculoskeletal origin.

Back pain, particularly after trauma, should be considered neurologic in nature until proven otherwise. The types of spinal cord injury are numerous, but back pain is one of the most common symptoms reported when cord injury is present. Complaints of other types of neurologic dysfunction, ranging from numbness and tingling to neurogenic shock (also known as spinal shock), lend support to the diagnosis of cord injury. However, the absence of additional symptoms should not decrease the level of suspicion of the EMS provider. Patients with back pain and suspected cord injury, even those with mild symptoms, should be immobilized, resuscitated appropriately, and transported to a facility with the capacity to care for such patients. As mentioned elsewhere in this text, the EMS provider should take care during immobilization. Should the nature of the pain worsen or if neurologic symptoms that may be related to the back injury worsen during immobilization, it would be prudent of the EMS provider to reposition the patient, padding the long spine board or cot appropriately in an attempt to decrease both pain as well as worsening neurologic deficits.

Another important pitfall for EMS providers is forming a belief during the examination that a patient's pain may not be associated with a spinal injury. It is often difficult for providers to change their impressions as more information becomes available. Hanging onto earlier impressions as other evidence become available that refutes the original impression is called "anchoring." It is especially common for the provider to "anchor" regarding a patient impression when the provider may have run on a patient previously, including for the same or a related complaint. It is a pitfall for an EMS provider to anchor on a clinical impression.

The determination that a patient's back pain isn't associated with a spinal cord injury should only be made after considering the patient's risk factors and comorbidities, the mechanism of injury, and conducting a thorough primary and secondary survey on the patient. Note should be made of any alterations in the level of consciousness, possibly making the physical examination less reliable. The patient may have been medicated for pain, possibly heavily, and the provider must weigh the possibility of the patient having a narcotic analgesic in their system. Specific questions should be asked about any numbness or weakness of any of the extremities. It would be helpful to know if the patient had had prior back surgeries, especially any associated with compression of the spinal cord, herniated discs, or previous vertebral fracture.

Providers should be aware that compression of the lower spinal cord—after it separates into filaments at the level of the second lumbar vertebra (where the spinal cord is then named the "cauda equina")—can produce a clinical condition called the "cauda equina syndrome" (CES), a condition that may present with very subtle yet serious features. CES is commonly, though not exclusively, associated with low back pain, and the patient may or may not have had a history of trauma. Indeed, back pain may be absent. The patient with CES may experience urinary retention or urinary incontinence. The provider should ask if the patient has experienced any difficulty in urination or dribbling of urine. Numbness in the perineal area (between the genitalia and the anus) can be reported. Weakness and loss of reflexes in the lower extremities may result. Thus the pitfall in this syndrome would be in the failure to ask about urinary problems, numbness in the perineal area, or leg weakness in a patient with back pain. Conversely, should the patient volunteer these symptoms in the absence of back pain, the provider should not fail to take note of these complaints. Agency protocols and Medical Director guidance must also be utilized during the decision-making process. The provider should carefully document his or her reasoning and advise the patient of the plan of care.

Failure to treat back pain as a symptom of potential cord injury may have long-standing catastrophic consequences for a patient. It is important that the EMS provider recognize that cord injury may present exactly like benign causes of back pain and use sound clinical knowledge when evaluating such patients. The EMS provider should also pay attention to other clinical clues that may point to spinal cord injury, such as deteriorating vital signs, increasing motor or sensory losses, extremes of age, and mechanism of injury.

SELECTED READINGS

Domeier RM, Evans RW, Swor RA, et al. Prehospital clinical findings associated with spinal injury. *Prehosp Emerg Care.* 1997;1(1):11–15.

Mattera CJ. Spinal trauma: New guidelines for assessment and management in the out-of-hospital environment. *J Emerg Nurs.* 1998;24(6):523–534.

138

ALWAYS REMEMBER TO THINK ABOUT INCREASED ICP AND MANAGE THE AIRWAY APPROPRIATELY!

GILBERTO SALAZAR, MD

The EMS provider will be presented from time to time with a patient who exhibits potential or even confirmed increased intracranial pressure (ICP). The prehospital personnel must treat this condition with the utmost respect when it is present. Increased ICP may arise from many causes including intracranial hemorrhage, mass effect (from tumors, etc.), abnormal drainage of cerebrospinal fluid into the spinal canal, and other conditions. EMS providers are often asked to participate in the care of patients with increased ICP once the patient has received care in a hospital, especially in the setting of a patient for whom interfacility transport is anticipated or ordered. Most often in this setting, the plan is to transfer such a patient to a facility with neurosurgery services, and the transport is planned to send the patient to a higher level of care.

Not uncommonly, a patient with increased ICP may be asymptomatic. On the other hand the patient may present with numerous overt signs and symptoms of increased ICP. Such signs include headache, visual changes, various neurological symptoms, vomiting, and altered mental status. Thus, should any of these signs be present in a patient for whom the prehospital provider is caring—such as headache and visual changes—it is reasonable to anticipate that this patient might be having increased ICP as the cause of these findings. Occasionally, the provider will get the history that a patient has had a previous cause of increased ICP, such as a previous condition like hydrocephalus which has been treated with a "ventriculoperitoneal shunt." This shunt leads from the brain into the abdominal cavity, and occasionally these shunts malfunction, sometimes even becoming completely obstructed. Another relatively common cause of increased ICP is a patient with "pseudotumor cerebri," a condition called "idiopathic intracranial hypertension" in which pressure increases inside the cranial cavity, commonly treated by performing a spinal tap to remove an amount of spinal fluid that will allow the patient's ICP to decrease. These patients typically do NOT develop altered mental status but rather severe headache, and visual changes may result due to pressure on the optic nerves.

This unpredictability is one of the aspects that makes an increase in ICP especially dangerous. A patient who appears initially well may suddenly exhibit acute neurological dysfunction, ranging from paresthesias and cranial nerve dysfunction to more concerning signs such as seizure and obtundation. This speaks to the need for careful initial assessments being aware of conditions such as these that may occur, and performing frequent reassessments, especially on the patient whose condition appears to be rapidly changing. Consultation with online medical control (OLMC) if available may be helpful.

Rapid neurological deterioration may be accompanied by the patient's loss of airway control and the subsequent inability to oxygenate and ventilate adequately. If this occurs en route to a hospital destination, the EMS provider may suddenly be faced with the possibility of having to treat several conditions, often under difficult circumstances and possibly alone in the back of a moving ambulance. The patient who experiences a convulsion, for example, will need treatment for the seizure activity but also for the airway compromise that may be present. The EMS provider might then have to instrument a trachea against clenched teeth, an obstructed airway, and possibly vomitus. This setting is perhaps one of the most challenging for the prehospital provider.

One of the key pitfalls in the setting of the patient who is experiencing a changing mental status in the failure to recognize the change. It is natural to "anchor" on an initial impression, and it takes a very skilled and experienced provider to note gradual mental status deterioration and to anticipate the procedures and treatments that may be necessary, for example, to prevent the patient's airway status from suddenly deteriorating. It has been shown that in the setting of head-injured victims, advanced airway placement may be associated with decreased survival. One of the likely reasons for this decrease in survival is in the excessive manipulation often required to place an advanced airway in the setting of a patient with altered mental status. The pitfall to be avoided here is not having BVM ventilation and suction readily available for the patient with worsening mental status.

Failure to protect the airway of a patient with suspected increased ICP prior to or during transport (especially long transports) may lead to potentially devastating consequences. Hypoxia during a state of increased ICP is harmful to the patient, leading to decreased chance for neurologic recovery, permanent loss of function, and even death. Therefore, a timely decision to place an advanced airway in a patient with suspected increased ICP may need to be made by the EMS provider in conjunction with the guidance of the Medical Director and agency protocols.

SELECTED READINGS

Duncan T, Krost WS, Mistovich JJ, et al. Beyond the basics: Brain injuries. *EMS Mag.* 2007;36(7):65–69.

Stiver SI, Manley GT. Prehospital management of traumatic brain injury. *Neurosurg Focus.* 2008;25(4):E5.

Note: Page numbers followed by "t" indicate table; those with "f" indicate figure.